IVERMECTIN Testimonials by Clinicians Worldwide

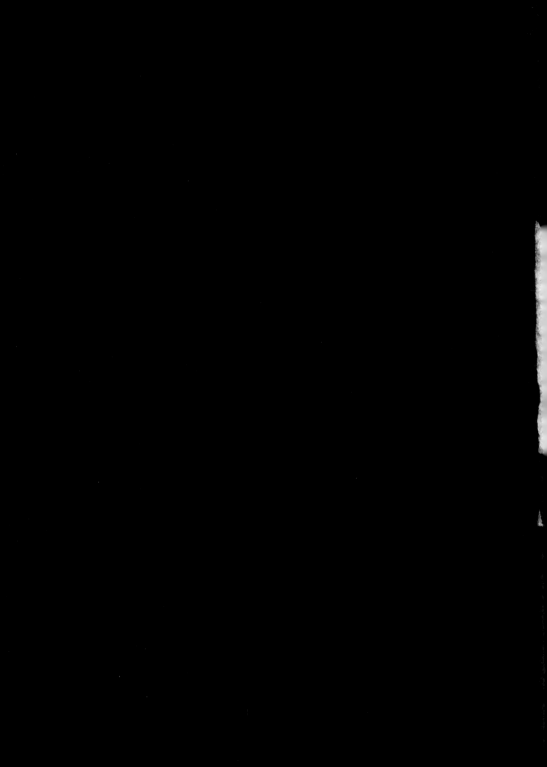

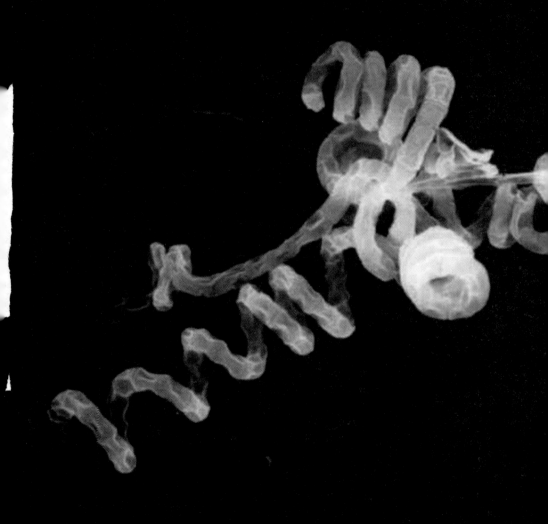

Streptomyces avermectinius (S. avermitilis)

IVERMECTIN Testimonials by Clinicians Worldwide

Edited by Dr. Paul E. Marik

IVERMECTIN — Testimonials by Clinicians Worldwide

©2024 by Paul E. Marik, Alan F. Bain, Jennifer Hibberd, M. Gilberta St. Rose, Flávio A. Cadegiani, Héctor E. Carvallo, Roberto R. Hirsch, Kazuhiro NAGAO, Katsuhiko FUKUDA, Allan A. Landrito, Julian Fidge, Kavery Nambisan, Rob Elens, Philip Chidi Njemanze, Jackie Stone, Colleen Aldous, E.V. Rapiti

All rights reserved. No portion of this book may be reproduced, stored in a retrieval system, or transmitted in any form or by any means—electronic, mechanical, photocopy, recording, scanning, or other—except for brief quotations in critical reviews or articles.

Published in Tokyo, Japan by Nantosha Co., Ltd.

E-mail ishimic0511@gmail.com

Phone +81-80-6260-0853

Printed by SANEI PRINTERY CO., LTD.

Book Design: Yukimasa MATSUDA

Produced by Kenji TORII

Edited by Paul E. Marik, and Eiichiro ISHIYAMA

Any Internet addresses, phone number, or company or producer information printed in this book is offered as a resource and are not intended in any way to be or to imply an endorsement by Nantosha, nor does Nantosha vouch for the existence, content, or services of these sites, phone numbers, companies, or products beyond the life of this book.

Publication Data

Name: Paul E. Marik, Representative Author

Title: IVERMECTIN — Testimonials by Clinicians Worldwide

Description: Clinical records and testimonials from physicians worldwide who prescribed Ivermectin to patients during the COVID-19 pandemic.

Identifier: ISBN978-4-8068-0776-6

Subject: LCSH Paul E. Marik, Medical doctors testimonials

First Edition

— *Dedicated to those who lost their lives in COVID-19.* —

We try to remember that medicine is for the patient. We try never to forget that medicine is for the people. It is not for the profits. The profits follow, and if we have remembered that, they have never failed to appear. The better we have remembered it, the larger they have been.

Nor is medicine for the politicians, except insofar as they are statesmen.

I could add that medicine also is not for the professions, unless it is for the patient — first and last. How can we bring the best of medicine to each and every person?

It won't be solved by wrangling with words and it won't be settled by slogans and by calling names. We will fall into gross error with fatal consequence unless we find the answer — how to get the best of all medicine to all the people.

It is up to us in research work, in industries and in colleges and other institutions, to help keep the problem in this focus. We cannot step aside and say that we have achieved our goal by inventing a new drug or a new way to help those who suffer from malnutrition, or the creation of ideal balanced diets on a worldwide scale. We cannot rest till the way has been found, with our help, to bring our finest achievement to everyone.

— George W. Merck, December 1, 1950

All I want to do is help people and save lives. But politics, driven by fear, is keeping me from doing my job and fulfilling my oath. Thousands of doctors across the country face the same perils every day. We must take these life and death decisions out of the hands of politicized administrators and place them where they belong, with the patients who bravely face the worst and the physicians who care for them.

— Dr. Paul E. Marik, November 22, 2021

A message for the publication

Ivermectin has taken a different path from other anti-infective drugs, from the time of its discovery to the recent consideration of its indication of extension to new respiratory infections (COVID-19).

Ivermectin is generally known as the drug that successfully controlled nematode-induced tropical diseases such as onchocerciasis (river blindness) and lymphatic filariasis (elephantiasis), which are common in Africa and South America. It has been used for about 20 years as the specific drug for treating particular types of infections — human strongyloidiasis and scabies.

In the veterinary field, Ivermectin has also been widely used as an anthelmintic for companion animals such as dogs and cats, as well as livestock such as cattle and sheep. It is therefore often thought of as a "parasiticide" or "veterinary" drug, but it is effective in both human beings and animals.

Ivermectin is already known to have antiviral activity against many types of viruses, and its therapeutic effect against COVID-19 has now been investigated. Furthermore, it is now being confirmed that the therapeutic and prophylactic effects of Ivermectin against COVID-19 are not only due to its antiviral activity, but also to its ability to suppress the abnormal increase in the patient's immune response, known as the cytokine storm, which causes COVID-19 to become more severe.

This is due to the fact that the chemical structure of Ivermectin is what is known as a macrolide skeleton. The reason I have made research on macrolide compounds my life's work, since returning from my study in the United States in April of 1973 to head a new laboratory at the Kitasato Institute, is because I have experienced that macrolide compounds have an unexpectedly wide range of biological activities.

Since the first case report in Wuhan, China at the end of December 2019 to date, numerous clinical trial results and statistical analyses of these results have been published demonstrating the efficacy of Ivermectin against COVID-19, which is raging around the world.

We have decided to document the results of global research on Ivermectin during the emergency situation of a pandemic; in March of 2021 and March of 2023, we published review articles entitled "Global Trends in Clinical Trials of Ivermectin for COVID-19," in The Japanese Journal of Antibiotics, a peer-reviewed journal.

One story illustrates the nature of Ivermectin in a nutshell: When Dr. Paul Marik, the co-founder of The Frontline COVID-19 Critical Care (FLCCC) Alliance and editor of this book, was in dialogue with The New York Times bestselling author Michael Capuzzo, Dr. Marik was asked what the perfect properties of a drug should be for COVID-19 should be, and Dr. Marik replied:

"I think it could be something that's safe, that's cheap, that's readily available, and that has anti-viral and anti-inflammatory properties. People would say, 'That's ridiculous. There could not possibly be a drug that has all of those characteristics. That's just unreasonable.' But we do have such a drug. The drug is called Ivermectin."

In time, actual science will clarify the role of Ivermectin in the prevention and treatment of COVID-19. This book is truly a record of valuable testimony that only a physician who has treated COVID-19 patients and prescribed Ivermectin in clinical practice could know. The voices of these physicians cannot be ignored.

I want those who have doubts about the efficacy of Ivermectin to know the truth.

I have been fortunate to be involved in the discovery of Avermectin and the development of Ivermectin — it has become my life's work.

In conclusion, I would like to contribute this statement as a message to this book, expressing my respect and deep gratitude to the physicians and other healthcare professionals worldwide who are sincerely confronting COVID-19.

Early Spring, 2024

— *Satoshi ŌMURA*

Satoshi ŌMURA, Ph.D.

Born July 12, 1935, Yamanashi Prefecture, Japan.
Nobel Laureate in Physiology or Medicine 2015; Member of the Japan Academy: Distinguished Emeritus Professor, Kitasato University: Honorary President, Joshibi University of Art and Design; Max Tischler Professor Emeritus, Wesleyan University, USA. ; the President of the Japan Essayists Club; the Honorary Director of the Robert Koch Institute; the Honorary Member of the Royal Society of Chemistry of the United Kingdom; the Emeritus Editor-in-Chief of the Journal of Antibiotics; the Foreign Members of the U.S. National Academy of Sciences, French Academy of Sciences, and the Chinese Academy of Engineering; the Members of the German National Academy of Sciences Leopoldina, the European Academy of Sciences, and the Russian Academy of Sciences.

During a career spanning more than 50 years, he has discovered exceeding 520 new natural organic compounds from microorganisms. 26 of those compounds, including avermectin and staurosporine are widely used worldwide as pharmaceuticals, veterinary drugs, agrochemicals and reagents in biochemical research.

Other major research achievements include the elucidation of the structures of macrolide antibiotics including leucomycin, spiramycin, tylosin etc., the creation of a new substance, mederrhodin, by the world's first producing bacteria gene manipulation, and the elucidation of the mechanism of action of the fatty acid biosynthesis inhibitor, cerulenin.

He also has a deep knowledge of art and built the Nirasaki Ōmura Art Museum in 2007 based on his longtime collection. In 2008, he donated the museum building and 4,000 works from his collection to his hometown, Nirasaki City, Yamanashi Prefecture, Japan to help promote culture and art.

CONTENTS

Chapter 1

My Journey to Discovering Ivermectin
Nature's Gift to Humanity
Dr. Paul E. Marik / US ⋯⋯⋯⋯⋯⋯⋯⋯⋯⋯⋯⋯⋯⋯⋯⋯⋯⋯ 001

Chapter 2

Straight From the Horse's Mouth and the Unvaccinated Doctor
Dr. Alan F. Bain / US ⋯⋯⋯⋯⋯⋯⋯⋯⋯⋯⋯⋯⋯⋯⋯⋯⋯⋯ 019

Chapter 3

Canada: 'The Land of the Free'? You Decide
Dr. Jennifer Hibberd / Canada ⋯⋯⋯⋯⋯⋯⋯⋯⋯⋯⋯⋯⋯⋯ 039

Chapter 4

Ivermectin Endangered and Recovering
Dr. M. Gilberta St. Rose / Saint Lucia ⋯⋯⋯⋯⋯⋯⋯⋯⋯⋯ 085

Chapter 5

Ivermectin and Brazil
A Love-hate Story in COVID-19
Dr. Flávio A. Cadegiani / Brazil ⋯⋯⋯⋯⋯⋯⋯⋯⋯⋯⋯⋯⋯⋯ 119

Chapter 6

Ivermectin on COVID-19 in Argentina
Dr. Héctor E. Carvallo and Dr. Roberto R. Hirsch / Argentina ···· 171

Chapter 7

Encounter and Experience with Ivermectin
Dr. Kazuhiro NAGAO / Japan ··· 189

Chapter 8

Flash in Japan
Survival Wisdom from a Vaccidemic Superpower
Dr. Katsuhiko FUKUDA / Japan ·································· 203

Chapter 9

The Philippine Experience on Ivermectin During and After the Pandemic
Dr. Allan A. Landrito / Philippines ······················· 245

Chapter 10

Ivermectin in Australia
Dr. Julian Fidge / Australia ······································· 267

Chapter 11

The Pandemic and the Rural Doctor
Dr. Kavery Nambisan / India ····································· 285

Chapter 12

My Experience with Ivermectin
Dr. Rob Elens / Netherlands ⋯⋯⋯⋯⋯⋯⋯⋯⋯⋯⋯ 305

Chapter 13

A Tale of Ivermectin, Prayer, and Resilience in a Monastery During the COVID-19 Pandemic
Dr. Philip Chidi Njemanze / Nigeria ⋯⋯⋯⋯⋯⋯⋯ 321

Chapter 14

An Ethical, Clinical, and Regulatory Analysis
Ivermectin in COVID-19 Treatment in Zimbabwe
Dr. Jackie Stone and Professor Colleen Aldous /
Zimbabwe & South Africa ⋯⋯⋯⋯⋯⋯⋯⋯⋯⋯⋯ 329

Chapter 15

Ivermectin Saved My Patients with Severe COVID and the Vaccine Injured
Dr. E.V. Rapiti / South Africa ⋯⋯⋯⋯⋯⋯⋯⋯⋯ 355

Producer's Note

And Yet it Works
Kenji TORII / Japan ⋯⋯⋯⋯⋯⋯⋯⋯⋯⋯⋯⋯⋯ 449

North America

Chapter

1

US

Dr. Paul E. Marik

My Journey to Discovering Ivermectin
Nature's Gift to Humanity

Ivermectin was a gift from nature handed to us to solve many of the devastating diseases of this planet. It is a multi-functional drug having numerous biological properties. Furthermore, it is an exceedingly safe pharmaceutical product. Ivermectin is truly a "Wonder drug". It is on the World Health Organization's (WHO) list of essential medicines and together with penicillin and aspirin, Ivermectin is amongst the most important medicines ever used on human beings. In this paper, I outline the journey that led to the discovery of Ivermectin.

Ivermectin was not developed in a pharmaceutical/drug development laboratory; rather it is a product of nature. Streptomyces avermectinius (S. Avermectinius) the microorganism that produces the avermectins was discovered in 1973 by Satoshi Omura in the soil of a golf course just outside of Tokyo Japan.[1-4] Satoshi Omura sent the soil specimen to William Campbell, at Merck Pharmaceuticals™ in the USA, to identify and characterize the compound he found in the soil.[5, 6] A safer and more effective derivative of Avermectin, named Ivermectin, was subsequently commercialized, entering the veterinary, agricultural and aquaculture markets in 1981.

When the avermectins were discovered, they represented a completely new class of compounds called 'endectocides', so designated because they killed a diverse range of disease-causing organisms, as well as pathogen vectors, both inside as well as outside the body.[1] Avermectins bind selectively to glutamate-gated chloride ion channels in invertebrate nerve and muscle cells thus paralyzing the cells. The first publication on avermectin appeared in 1979, describing it as a complex mixture of 16-membered macrocyclic lactones produced by fermentation of the actinomycete Streptomyces avermectinius.[7] Ivermectin is a safer, more potent semisynthetic mixture of two chemically modified avermectins, comprised of 80% of 22,23-dihydroavermectin-B1a and 20% 22,23-dihydroavermectin-B1b.[1]

The drug's life-saving potential was confirmed in 1987 when it was approved by the US Food and Drug Administration (FDA) and immediately provided free of charge by Merck Company (branded as Mectizan) to help control Onchocerciasis (River Blindness) and lymphatic filariasis around the globe. For most of this century, some 250 million people have been taking Ivermectin annually to combat these two disfiguring and debilitating parasitic diseases.[1] Over the past three decades, approximately 3.7 billion doses of Ivermectin have been distributed worldwide.[1-4]

There are but a few drugs that can seriously lay claim to the title of 'Wonder drug'. Penicillin and Aspirin are two pharmaceuticals that have perhaps had the greatest beneficial impact on the health and wellbeing of mankind because of its effectiveness in fighting a wide range of life-threatening diseases. Ivermectin can also be considered alongside these 'germ fighters'. Ivermectin continues to help hundreds of millions of the world's poorest people. (see Figure 1).[4] Because of Ivermectin's contributions to pharmacology, scientists William Campbell and Satoshi Omura were awarded a Nobel Prize in 2015 for their 1975 discovery of Ivermectin.

Ivermectin is a multi-function, multi-purpose drug with truly remarkable pharmacologic properties.[5, 8-16] Ivermectin is unique amongst the thousands of pharmaceutical products available in that it has a diverse range of pharmacodynamic properties which include, anti-parasitic activity against a wide variety of parasite, antiviral properties against a spectrum of RNA viruses, potent anti-inflammatory properties, ant-cancer activity, activation of autophagy and it positively influences the microbiome.[5, 8-16] What makes this drug even more unique is its remarkable safety profile.

The safety of Ivermectin is unparalleled.[17-20] Ivermectin ranks as one of the safest medicines on the planet. It is well tolerated in humans up to 2.0 mg/kg.[17] Minor side effects include pruritis, fever, rash and arthralgia.[18] The safety of Ivermectin as compared to penicillin, Aspirin (ASA) and a number of other interventions is listed in Figure 1 (data obtained from the WHO pharmaco-vigilance database, https://www.vigiaccess.org/, updated June 10, 2023). While Vigiacess™ lists 25 deaths associated with the use of Ivermectin, a detailed and comprehensive analysis of these cases indicates that these patients likely died from overwhelming parasitic infection rather than from Ivermectin itself (communication with Jacques Descotes MD, PharmD, PhD Professor Emeritus, Claude Bernard University of Lyon, Fellow, US Academy of Toxicological Sciences).[18]

My interest in Ivermectin began with the outbreak of COVID-19 in January 2020. As an intensive care unit (ICU) physician and Chief of the Division of Critical Care Medicine at my University (Eastern Virginia Medical School) my responsibility was to develop a treatment approach for the management of critically ill patients hospitalized with SARS-CoV-2. At that time the recommendations of the World Health Organization (WHO), National Institutes of Health (NIH), Center for Disease Control and Prevention (CDC) as well as almost every health care agency across the globe were supportive care alone. This therapeutic nihilism was surprising, considering the fact that ventilated patients with COVID-19 pneumonia had a reported mortality of close to 80%.[21] Furthermore, there is no disease than an intensivist cannot attempt to treat. As COVID-19 was characterized by uncontrolled inflammation (cytokine storm) and macro- and micro-vascular clotting our original protocol included Methylprednisolone, Ascorbic Acid, Thiamine and

Heparin, also called the MATH+ protocol.[22, 23] The MATH+ protocol was an adaptation of our Hydrocortisone-Ascorbic acid-Thiamine-Melatonin (HAT-m) protocol for the treatment of patients with septic shock.[24-27] Following the development of the MATH+ protocol our attention turned to the early outpatient treatments of COVID-19. It became clear to us that the key to controlling (and ending) the pandemic involved early outpatient treatment. At this time, we began developing an outpatient protocol for COVID-19 (originally called I-MASK then renamed I-CARE, see www.flccc.net).

In April of 2020, the publication by Caly and colleagues attracted our interest with regards to the use of Ivermectin for the treatment of COVID-19. These authors published a preprint entitled *"The FDA-approved drug Ivermectin inhibits the replication of SARS-CoV-2 in vitro"* which demonstrated that Ivermectin potently inhibited the replication of SARS-CoV-2.[28] In a VERO monkey kidney cell model, after 2 hours post infection with SARS-CoV-2, Ivermectin resulted in a 5,000-fold reduction in viral RNA at 48 hour. It was previously known that Ivermectin inhibited the replication of a wide spectrum of RNA viruses including, Yellow Fever virus, West Nile virus, Dengue virus, Respiratory Syncytial Virus, Hendra virus, Newcastle virus, Venezuelan Equine encephalitis virus, Chikungunya virus, Semliki Forest virus, Sindbis virus, Influenza virus including influenza A virus (H5N1), Human Immunodeficiency Type 1 virus, Pseudorabies virus and BK Polyomavirus. This study sparked my curiosity and interest in Ivermectin. The lack of clinical data at that time was a major limiting factor. However, I was interested in the mechanisms of the drug's antiviral activity. Viruses must enter the nucleus of a cell to use the nucleus's machinery to replicate or multiply. To enter the nucleus, however, viruses need to hitch a ride on transport proteins. In the case of SARS-CoV-2, it needs to bind with importin (IMP) α and importin β.[29-31] The SARS-CoV-2-IMP α/β complex then passes through the nuclear wall's nuclear pore complex (NPC) to enter the nucleus. Once inside the nucleus, the SARS-CoV-2 replicates in the millions or billions, and succeeding generations entering other host cells to continue replicating. In the study by Caly et al., Ivermectin binds to the transport protein, importin α to prevent the SARS-CoV-2-IMPα/β from forming.[29, 30] This action prevents the entry of viral proteins into the nucleus, so that the immune system can continue to fend off the virus. As discussed below, We will soon find out that Ivermectin has multiple antiviral mechanisms.

In July 2020, Khan et al published the preprint of their paper entitled *"Ivermectin treatment may improve the prognosis of patients with COVID-19"* (paper subsequently published in December 2020).[32] This retrospective study enrolled 248 consecutive patients hospitalized with SARS-CoV-2 infection in a hospital in Bangladesh between April to June 2020. In this study 115 patients received Ivermectin plus standard care while 133 received standard care alone. Hospital mortality was significantly lower in the Ivermectin group (0.9% vs, 6.8%; $p < 0.05$). In addition, patients in the Ivermectin group became SARS-CoV-2 negative more rapidly (4 vs 15 days; $p < 0.001$) and had a significantly shorter length of hospital stay (9 vs 15 days, $p < 0.001$).

Similarly in July 2020, in a preprint publication, Gorial et al published an observational clinical trial conducted in hospitalized adult patients with mild to moderate COVID-19.[33] In this study, 16 patients received a single dose of Ivermectin (0.2 mg/kg) on admission day and as add on therapy to the standard of care at that time. These patients were compared with 71 control patients matched in age, gender, clinical features, and comorbidities. The primary outcome was the percentage of cured patients, defined as symptoms free to be discharged from the hospital and two consecutive negative PCR tests. All the patients of IVM group were cured compared to 97% in the control group (NS). The mean hospital length of stay was significantly lower in the Ivermectin group compared with the control group (7.6 ± 2.7 versus 13.2 ±5.9 days, p< 0.001). This ground breaking paper remains as a preprint which is typical of "positive" studies using repurposed drugs, it is interesting to note that le negative studies get rapidly published in highly ranked peer-reviewed journals,[34-38] although most of them are methodologically flawed.[39]

In August of 2020, Shouman et al published the results on ClinicalTrials.gov (NCT04422561) of a study which investigated the role of Ivermectin in preventing COVID-19 infection in asymptomatic close contacts of patients with COVID-19.[40] This randomized open label-controlled study was conducted in Egypt between during June and July 2020. The intervention group received two doses of Ivermectin, spaced 72 hours apart. The dose of Ivermectin was adjusted according to body weight as follows: 15 mg/day for subjects of 40-60 kg; 18 mg/day for 60-80 kg; and 24 mg/day for those >80 kg. The Ivermectin group included 203 contacts while the control group included 101 contacts. In the treatment group 7.4% of contacts developed COVID-19 as compared to 58.4% in the control group (p<0.001).[41]

In September of 2020 Maurya posted a preprint entitled "*A Combination of Ivermectin and Doxycycline Possibly Blocks the Viral Entry and Modulates the Innate Immune Response in COVID-19 Patients*" (once again, this paper has yet to be published in a peer reviewed Journal).[42] This study used molecular docking studies to determine the binding affinity of both drugs. The author demonstrated that both Ivermectin and doxycycline had significant binding capacity with SARS-CoV-2, with Ivermectin having better binding than doxycycline. Furthermore, Ivermectin showed perfect binding to the spike-RBD and ACE2 interacting region. Ivermectin also exhibited significant binding affinity with several SARS-CoV-2 structural and non-structural proteins (NSPs). In addition, Ivermectin demonstrated significant binding with the RNA-dependent-RNA- polymerase (RdRp) indicative of its role in the inhibition of the viral replication. Additional studies have demonstrated that Ivermectin has significant binding affinity for the main viral protease (SARS-CoV-2 M[pro]), thus further limiting viral replication.[31] It should be noted that Ivermectin is a more potent inhibitor of M[pro] than Paxlovid (nirmatrelvir/ritonavir).[43-45]

Also in September 2020, Lehrer and Rheinstein published an experimental study which demonstrated that Ivermectin docks to the SARS-CoV-2 spike receptor binding domain attached to ACE2.[46] The authors suggested that the docking of Ivermectin to the spike-ACE2 complex may interfere with the attachment of the spike to the human cell membrane.

In October of 2020, Mahmud et al published the results of their study entitled *"Clinical trial of Ivermectin plus doxycycline for the treatment of conformed COVID-19 infection"* on ClinicalTrials.gov (NCT04523831).[47] This was a randomized, blinded, placebo-controlled trial in non-hospitalized patients with mild-to moderate COVID-19 symptoms who were randomly assigned to treatment (n=200) and placebo (n=200) groups. The treatment group received a single dose of Ivermectin 12 mg and doxycycline 100 mg, twice daily for 5 days, in addition to standard care. The primary outcome was duration from treatment to clinical recovery. The median recovery time was 7 days in the treatment group and 9 days in the placebo group (hazard ratio, 0.73; 95% CI 0.60–0.90). The number of patients with a < 7-day recovery was 61% in the treatment group and 44% in the placebo group (hazard ratio, 0.06; CI 0.04–0.09). The study was subsequently published in a peer reviewed journal.[48]

Chapter 1   My Journey to Discovering Ivermectin

Also In October of 2020, Jean-Jacques Rajter and colleagues published a preprint of an observational study which reported the outcome of Ivermectin in critically ill patients with COVID-19 infection (subsequently published in the Journal CHEST in January of 2021).[49]

Between March and May 2020 these authors treated 280 consecutive patients hospitalized at four Broward Health hospitals in Florida with confirmed COVID-19 infection. In this study 173 patients were treated with Ivermectin while 107 similar patients served as the control group. Most patients in both groups also received hydroxychloroquine, azithromycin, or both. Univariate analysis showed lower mortality in the Ivermectin group (15.0% vs 25.2%; OR, 0.52; 95% CI, 0.29-0.96; P =0.04). After multivariate adjustment for confounders and mortality risks, the mortality difference remained significant (OR, 0.27; 95% CI, 0.09-0.80; P=0 .03). The authors then performed a propensity-matched cohort (n=196). In the propensity matched analysis mortality was significantly lower in the Ivermectin group as compared to the control group (13.3% vs 24.5%; OR, 0.47; 95% CI, 0.22-0.99; P < .05).

This study by Rajter et al convinced me Ivermectin had a role in the management of COVID-19. The published data led me to believe that the inclusion of Ivermectin in an early treatment protocol would reduce the spread of SARS-CoV-2 and reduce hospitalizations and deaths from COVID-19, essentially ending the pandemic. In discussions with Dr. Pierre Kory, Ivermectin shot to the top of the FLCCC (www.flccc.net) list of repurposed drugs for the early treatment of COVID-19. It was at this time that I did a webinar with an international audience entitled *"COVID-19: Saving the Planet with Ivermectin"*. In this talk I presented a table outlining the efficacy of various pharmaceutical agents in the various phases of COVID-19 disease (see Figure 2). This talk had over 1 million YouTube views; however, shortly thereafter it was removed under the pretense of "misinformation". On December 8, 2020, Dr. Kory testified in US Senate hearings (under the Chairmanship of Senator Johnson) in which he proclaimed that "Ivermectin could end the pandemic". His testimony went "viral" with millions of views. Essentially, at this time the FLCCC put Ivermectin onto the map for the treatment of COVID-19. The retail sales of Ivermectin in the USA in temporal relationship to these FLCCC events is illustrated in Figure 3.[50]

In early 2021 FLCCC published a meta-analyses of 18 randomized controlled treatment trials of Ivermectin in COVID-19 in which we found a large, statistically significant reductions in mortality time to clinical recovery, and time to viral clearance.[51] At the same time Bryant et al published a similar meta-analysis of 15 trials reporting that Ivermectin reduced risk of death compared with no Ivermectin (average risk ratio 0.38, 95% confidence interval 0.19–0.73).[52]

The COVID-19 Early Treatment Group has performed a real-time analysis of 2,902 interventional studies for the treatment of COVID-19 (to date, June 2023).[53] Ninety-eight of these studies evaluated the role of Ivermectin in the treatment and prophylaxis of COVID-19. These 98 studies enrolled over 135,000 patients from 27 countries; 46 of these studies were randomized controlled trials. A meta-analysis of these studies demonstrated an overall benefit of 62% with a 50% reduction in mortality and a 34% reduction in hospitalization. The analysis remained robust and unchanged after excluding lower quality studies. Of all the drugs studied Ivermectin is the most clinically effective. The cost per life saved was $24 for Ivermectin while it is reported to be $39,035 for Paxlovid. This meta-analysis included the "Big Five" RCT's,[34-38] all of which were designed to "fail". Despite the scientific shenanigans in the design, conduct and interpretation of these studies, many were positive when evaluating the initial primary end-point (prior to post hoc data manipulation).[34, 38, 39]

Big Pharma and their collaborators have waged a war against repurposed drugs, and Ivermectin in particular.[54] Despite the millions of dollars spent in waging this war, Ivermectin has emerged triumphant. Ivermectin is simply the most effective, safest and cheapest drug to treat COVID-19.

VigiAccess™ Uppsala Monitoring Centre		WHO Collaborating Centre for International Drug Monitoring	
Medicine	Year stated reporting	Deaths	Adverse event
Ivermectin	1992	26	7097
Penicillin	1968	118	56003
Aspirin(ASA)	1968	1512	202423
COVID-19 vaccines	2021	25341*	5082447
Tetanus vaccine	1968	32	15647

* Underreporting by a fact of a least 30%

Figure1. Safety profile of Ivermectin, Penicillin and ASA as well as other compounds (data from WHO's Pharmacovigilance data base, VigiAccess @ https://www.vigiaccess.org/, updated June 10 2023)

	Pre-exposure/ Post-Exposure/ Incubation	Symptomatic Phase	Pulmonary/ inflammatory phase
Hydroxychloroquine	Unclear benefit	No benefit	?Trend to harm
Remdesivir	n/a	?? Reduced time to recovery No mortality benefit	No benefit
Lopivinar-Ritonavir	n/a	No benefit	No benefit
Interferon a/β	Inhaled? Benefit	No benefit	? Trend harm
Tocilizumab	n/a	n/a	?Trend to harm
Convalescent Serum	n/a	Unlikely	No Benefit
Corticosteroids	n/a	Trend to harm	BENEFIT
Ivermectin	BENEFIT	BENEFIT	BENEFIT

Figure 2. Failed and Successful Rx for COVID-19 by Phase of Illness (October 2020).

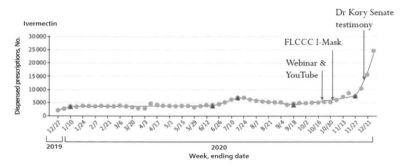

Figure 3. Retail Pharmacy Sales of Ivermectin in the USA according to FLCCC activity Adapted with permission from JAMA; from Geller AI, et al JAMA Intern Med 2021; 181: 869. (50)

Chapter 1　My Journey to Discovering Ivermectin

References

1. Crump A. Ivermectin: enigmatic multifaceted 'wonder' drug continues to surprise and exceed expectations. Journal of Antibiotics. 2021;70:495-505.
2. Omura S. Ivermectin: 25 years and still going strong. Int J Antimicrob Agents. 2008;31(2):91-8.
3. Omura S, Crump A. The life and times of ivermectin - a success story. Nat Rev Microbiol. 2004;2(12):984-9.
4. Crump A, Omura S. Ivermectin, "Wonder drug" from Japan: the human use perspective. Proc. Jpn. Acad. Ser. B. 87. 2011;13:13-28.
5. Campbell WC. Ivermectin as an antiparasitic agent for use in humans. Annu Rev Microbiol. 1991;45:445-74.
6. Campbell WC. History of avermectin and ivermectin, with notes on the history of other macrocyclic lactone antiparasitic agents. Curr Pharm Biotechnol. 2012;13(6):853-65.
7. Burg RW, Miller BM, Baker EE, Birnbaum J, Currie SA, Hartman R, et al. Avermectins, new family of potent anthelmintic agents: producing organism and fermentation. Antimicrob Agents Chemother. 1979;15(3):361-7.
8. Chhaiya SB, Mehta DS, Kataria BC. Ivermectin: pharmacology and therapeutic applications. Int. J. Basic Clin. Pharmacol. 2012;1:132-9.
9. Dominguez-Gomez G, Chavez-Blanco A, Medina-Franco JL, Saldivar-Gonzalez F, Flores-Torrontegui Y, Juarez M, et al. Ivermectin as an inhibitor of cancer stem-like cells. Mol. Med Rep. 2018;17(2):3397-403.
10. Dou Q, Chen HN, Wang K, Yuan K, Lei Y, Li K, et al. Ivermectin Induces Cytostatic Autophagy by Blocking the PAK1/Akt Axis in Breast Cancer. Cancer Res. 2016;76(15):4457-69.
11. Elkholy KO, Hegazy O, Erdinc B, Abowali H. Ivermectin: a closer look at a potential remedy. Cureus. 2020;12:e10378.
12. Jans DA, Wagstaff KM. Ivermectin as a broad-spectrum host directed anti-viral: The real deal. Cells. 2020;9:2100.
13. Yang SN, Atkinson SC, Wang C, Lee A. The broad spectrum antiviral ivermectin targets the host nuclear transport importin alpha/beta1 heterodimer. Antiviral Res. 2020;177:104760.
14. Zhang P, Li Xu W, Cheng J, Zhang C, Gao J. Immunotoxicity induced by ivermectin is associated with NF-kB signaling pathway on macrophages. Chemosphere. 2022;289:133087.
15. Zhang X, Song Y, Ci X, An N, Ju Y. Ivermectin inhibits LPS-induced production of inflammatory cytokines and improves LPS-induced survival in mice. Inflamm. Res. 2008;57:524-9.
16. Hazan S. Microbiome-based hypotheses on Ivermectin's mechanism in COVID-19: Ivermecting feeds Bifidobacteria to boost immunity. Front. Microbiol. 2022;13:952321.
17. Guzzo CA, Furtek CI, Porras AG, Chen C, Tipping R, Clineschmidt CM. Safety, tolerability, and pharmacokinetics of escalating high doses of ivermectin in healthy adult subjects. J. Clin. Pharmacol. 2002;42:1122-33.
18. Kircik LH, Del Rosso JQ, Layton AM, schauber J. Over 25 years of clinical experience with Ivermectin: An overview of safety for an increasing number of indications. J. Drugs

Dermatol. 2016;15:325-32.

19. Munoz J, Ballester MR, Antonijoan RM, Gich I, Coili E. Safety and pharmacokinetic profile of fixed-dose ivermectin with an innovative 18 mg tablet in healthy adult volunteers. PLoS Neglected Tropical Diseases. 2018;12:e0006020.

20. Navarro M, Camprubi D, Requena-Mendez A, Buonfrate D, Giorli G. Safety of high-dose ivermectin: a systematic review and meta-analysis. J. Antimicrob. Chemother. 2020;75:827-34.

21. Marik PE, Iglesias J, Varon J, Kory P. COVID-19 in-hospital mortality: a Concise Worldwide review. J. Community Medicine and Public Health Reports. 2021.

22. Kory P, Meduri GU, Iglesias J, Varon J, Cadegiani FA, Marik PE. "MATH+" multi-modal hospital treatment protocol for COVID-19 infection: Clinical and Scientific. Journal of Clinical Medicine Research. 2022;14:53-79.

23. Marik PE, Kory P, Varon J, Iglesias J, Meduri GU. MATH+ protocol for the treatment of SARS-CoV-2 infection: the scientific rationale. Exp. Rev. Anti. Infect. Ther. 2020.

24. Marik PE. "Vitamin S' (steroids) and Vitaminc C for the treatment of severe sepsis and septic shock! Crit. Care Med. 2016;44:1228-9.

25. Marik PE. Hydrocortisone, Ascorbic Acid and Thiamine (HAT therapy) for the treatment of sepsis. Focus on ascorbic acid. Nutrients. 2018;10:1762.

26. Marik PE. Vitamin C: An essential "stress hormone" during sepsis. J. Thorac. Dis. 2020;12 (suppl 1):S84-S8.

27. Marik PE, Khangoora V, Rivera R, Hooper MH, Catravas J. Hydrocortisone, Vitamin C and Thiamine for the treatment of severe sepsis and septic shock: A retrospective before-after study. Chest. 2017;151:1229-38.

28. Caly L, Druce JD, Catton MG, Jans DA, Wagstaff KM. The FDA-approved drug Ivermectin inhibits the replication of SARS-CoV-2 in vitro. Antiviral Res. 2020.

29. Caly L, Druce JD, Catton MG, Jans DA, Wagstaff KM. Ivermectin and COVID-19: A report in Antiviral Research, widespread interest, an FDA warning, two letters to the editor and the authors' response. Antiviral Research. 2020;178:104805.

30. Caly L, Wagstaff KM, Jans DA. Nuclear trafficking of proteins from RNA viruses: Potential target for antivirals? Antiviral Res. 2012;95:202-6.

31. Bello M. Elucidation of the inhibitory activity of ivermectin with host nuclear importin α and several SARS-CoV-2 targets. J Biomol Struct Dyn. 2022;40(18):8375-83.

32. Khan MS, Khan MS, Debnath Cr, Nath PN, Mahtab MA. Ivermectin treatment may improve the prognosis of patients with COVID-19. Archivos de Bronconeumologia. 2020;12:828-30.

33. Gorial FI, Mashhadani S, Sayaly HM, Dakhil BD, AlMashhadani MM. Effectiveness of Ivermectin as add-on therapy in COVID-19 management (Pilot Trial). medRxiv. 2020.

34. Naggie S, Boulware DR, Lindsell C, Stewart TG, Gentile N, Collins S, et al. Effect of ivermectin vs placebo on time to sustained recovery in outpatients with mild to moderate COVID-19. A randomized Clinical Trial. JAMA. 2022;328:1595-603.

35. Lim SC, Hor CP, Tay KH, Jelani AM, Tan WH. Efficacy of Ivermectin treatment on disease progression among adults with mild to moderate COVID-19 and comorbidities. The I-TECH randomized clinical trial. JAMA Intern. Med. 2022.

36. Lopez-Medina E, Lopez P, Hurtado IC, Davalos DM, Ramirez O. Effect of ivermectin

on time to resolution of symptoms among adults with mild COVID-19. A randomized clinical trial. JAMA. 2021.

37. Bramante CT, Huling JD, Tiganelli CJ, Buse JB, Liebovitz DM, Cohen K, et al. Randomized trial of metformin, Ivermectin and Fluvoxamine for COVID-19. N. Engl. J. Med. 2022;287:599-610.

38. Reis G, Silva EA, Silva DC, Thabane L, Milagres AC, Mills EJ. Effect of early treatment with ivermectin among patients with Covid-19. N. Engl. J. Med. 2022.

39. Scheim DE, Aldous C, Osimani B, Fordham EJ, Hoy WE. When characteristics of clinical trials require per-protocol as well as intention-to-treat outcomes to draw reliable conclusions: Three examples. J. Clin. Med. 2023;12:3625.

40. Shouman W. https://clinicaltrials.gov/ct2/show/NCT04422561. 2020.

41. Shouman WM, Hegazy AA, Nafae RM, Ragab ME, Samra SR, Anas D. Use of ivermectin as a potential chemoprophylaxis for COVID-19 in Egypt: A randomised clinical trial. Journal of Clinical and Diagnostic Research. 2020;15:OC27-OC32.

42. Maurya DK. A combination of Ivermectin and Doxycycline possibly blocks the viral entry and modulate the innate immune response in COVID-19 patients. ChemRxiv. 2020.

43. Alvarado YJ, Olivarez Y, Lossada C, Vera-Villalobos J, Paz JL, Vera E, et al. Interaction of the new inhibitor paxlovid (PF-07321332) and ivermectin with the monomer of the main protease SARS-CoV-2: A volumetric study based on molecular dynamics, elastic networks, classical thermodynamics and SPT. Comput Biol Chem. 2022;99:107692.

44. Arouche TDS, Martins AY, Ramalho TC, Júnior RNC, Costa FLP, Filho TSA, et al. Molecular Docking of Azithromycin, Ritonavir, Lopinavir, Oseltamivir, Ivermectin and Heparin Interacting with Coronavirus Disease 2019 Main and Severe Acute Respiratory Syndrome Coronavirus-2 3C-Like Proteases. J Nanosci Nanotechnol. 2021;21(4):2075-89.

45. Mody V, Ho J, Wills S, Mawri A, Lawson L, Ebert M, et al. Identification of 3-chymotrypsin like protease (3CLPro) inhibitors as potential anti-SARS-CoV-2 agents. Commun Biol. 2021;4(1):93.

46. Lehrer S, Rheinstein PH. Ivermectin docks to the SARS-CoV-2 spike receptor-binding domain attached to ACE2. In Vivo. 2020;34:3023-6.

47. Mahmud R. https://clinicaltrials.gov/ct2/show/NCT04523831. 2020.

48. Mahmud R, Rahman M, Alam I, Ahmed KG, Kabir H, Sayeed SK, et al. Ivermectin in combination with doxycycline for treating COVID-19 symptoms: a randomized trial. J. Int. Med. Res. 2021;49:1-14.

49. Rajter JC, Sherman MS, Fatteh N, Vogel F, Sacks J, Rajter JJ. Use of ivermectin is associated with lower mortality in hospitalized patients with Coronavirus Disease 2019. The Ivermectin in COVID Nineteen study. Chest. 2021;159:85-92.

50. Geller AI, Lovegrove MC, Lind JN, Datta SD. Assessment of outpatient dispensing of products proposed for treatment or prevention of COVID-19 by US retail pharmacies during the pandemic. JAMA Intern. Med. 2021;181:869-72.

51. Kory P, Meduri GU, Iglesias J, Varon J, Berkowitz K, Kornfeld H, et al. Review of the emerging evidence demonstrating the efficacy of ivermectin in the prophylaxis and treatment of COVID-19. Am. J. Ther. 2020;28:e299-e318.

52. Bryant A, Lawrie TA, Dowswell T, Fordham EJ, Mitchell S, Hill SR. Ivermectin for prevention and treatment of COVID-19 infection: a systematic review, meta-analysis, and trial sequential analysis to inform clinical guidelines. Am. J. Ther. 2021.
53. C-19 Early Treatment Group 2023;Pageshttps://c19early.org/.
54. Kory P, Mccarthy J. The War on Ivermectin. The Medicine that Saved Millions and Could Have ended the Pandemic. New York, NY: Skyhorse Publishing; 2023.

Paul E. Marik, MD, FCCP, FCCM

Dr. Marik received his medical degree from the University of the Witwatersrand, Johannesburg, South Africa. He was an ICU attending at Baragwanath Hospital, in Soweto, South Africa. During this time, he obtained a Master of Medicine Degree, Bachelor of Science Degree in Pharmacology, Diploma in Anesthesia as well as a Diploma in Tropical Medicine and Hygiene. Dr. Marik did a Critical Care Fellowship in London, Ontario, Canada, during which time he was admitted as a Fellow to the Royal College of Physicians and Surgeons of Canada. Dr. Marik has worked in various teaching hospitals in the US since 1992. He is board certified in Internal Medicine, Critical Care Medicine, Neurocritical Care and Nutrition Science. Until recently, Dr. Marik was a tenured Professor of Medicine and Chief of Pulmonary and Critical Care Medicine at Eastern Virginia Medical School. Dr. Marik has written over 700 peer-reviewed journal articles, 80 book chapters and authored four critical care books. He has been cited over 53,000 times in peer-reviewed publications and has an H-index of 111. He has delivered over 350 lectures at international conferences and visiting professorships. He has received numerous teaching awards, including the National Teacher of the Year award by the American College of Physicians in 2017. Dr. Marik is the co-founder of the Front-Line COVID-19 Critical Care (FLCCC) Alliance.

Chapter

2

US

Dr. Alan F. Bain

Straight From the Horse's Mouth and the Unvaccinated Doctor

As an internist for the last 30 years, I never envisioned that I would be a part of an important movement to support a drug, whose effectiveness is indisputable. This remarkable medicine was being added to treatment regimens that have saved people from the brink of death. My story began when I heard about trailblazing attorney Ralph Lorigo in New York who, with his associates Beth Parlato and Jon Minear, chose to fight for somebody's life over failing hospital protocols. I was reading about two or three cases in New York that Mr. Lorigo was working on. He fought for these patients to receive the drug Ivermectin. The cases were published in the news, and they reported that patients were able to get off a ventilator within 3-5 days by adding Ivermectin in the treatment. Curious, I decided to call the law office to confirm what really was going on.

Serendipitously, I would be asked to get involved with cases in Chicago where families were fighting for their loved one's lives to get hospitals to administer Ivermectin.

In May of 2021, I was asked by Dr. Pierre Kory to get involved with a patient who had been on a ventilator for at least 6 days. In September, I was asked to be an expert witness and the physician administrator of this well studied drug, Ivermectin, that had been given through the years over 3 billion times. In October, I was again an expert witness and the main administrator of this life-saving addition to a patient's regimen. In all three cases, the court ordered me to administer Ivermectin on ventilated patients who were at the brink of death. Thanks to Ivermectin, they were all able to go home to their families and back to their normal lives.

I was involved in a total of six court cases. But the real clinical heroes are those who testified in the U.S. Senate like Peter McCullough, the late Ramin Oskoui, George Fareed, Dr. Pierre Kory, Dr. Paul Marik, Dr. Harvey Risch, Dr. Ryan Cole, Nurse Nicole Sirotek, and even more physicians, clinicians, and researchers. Dr. Joseph Varon of Texas and Dr. Paul Marik of Virginia probably saved hundreds of ventilators dependent, acute COVID-19 cases from death with the addition of Ivermectin to their protocol.

Yet even after having shown how hundreds of lives were saved in this heroic fashion, the narrative is still considered unfounded and not worthy of further investigation.

Shame on public policy for the skewing the reports of this natural drug that has helped in saving countless lives. So-called "experts" continue to say that this is anecdotal and that many people have still died on ventilators after having tried Ivermectin. The success of Ivermectin treatments cannot be dismissed, especially when it happens repeatedly under optimal circumstances.

We doctors seek life for our patients at all costs and see life as a sacred bond between human and their creator. This oath we pledged should not be altered by any bias or ignorance from the government, or any corporate entity. This is not a matter of statistics but rather a discussion of clinical circumstances that determines whether a person will stay alive. This is therefore a story of simply trying to exhaust all possible options to save a life.

I was involved in court cases where, as an expert witness, I had to influence judges with bonafide research to allow a patient to receive Ivermectin. I had to quote a young surgeon's research article on the 20 different ways that Ivermectin was valuable in helping the body regain its healing capacity. I can tell you that of the cases, that I know of, that were publicly known and fought for, there are 6 more cases total where the patients were able to get off ventilators with adding this drug. And yet, in still unpublished reports, the number of lives saved are much more. Mine was just a small contribution to the stories about this amazing drug.

Dr. Joseph Varon of Texas and Dr. Paul Marik's success rate at getting many more people off ventilators with the addition of Ivermectin aptly places the drug in the category of observational and statistical legitimacy and relevance.

This is a story about "letting doctors be doctors," as Dr. Paul Marik would say. This is a story about heeding a physician's observational skills, over statistical "geniuses" who, apart from only observing from a cold, objective distance, think they can provide clinical care by just looking at numbers.

Researchers only must account for one variable in the human body when conducting a study but in reality, the human body does not work that way. One cannot give credit to one drug and say it was the total answer. But what I can say for sure is that the addition of Ivermectin with the other carefully prescribed medications was useful and profoundly lifesaving.

Ivermectin could not do what it was able to do for the patients if the ventilator, the steroids, and the blood thinning agents were not there. If the drug is not given at the right dosage for a long enough period, it also will not be as effective. Research must account for all the interrelated parts of the story of each patient at that specific point in time. When a publication comes out and decides that a drug does not work, it fails to account for all of the other factors, like the clinical adjustments that had to be made to save a life. Most of all, these studies do not honor the sacrosanct Human Condition that we call life.

Dr. McCullough, one of our heroes, has constantly urged us to treat COVID-19 as a multi-variant, multi-drug interventional journey. For the naysayers who believe that Ivermectin does not work, I say that nothing works alone. There are key ingredients for a system to work properly.

There are a multitude of biochemical processes that are going on at the same time to keep a person healthy and strong.

Making Ivermectin part of this medical symphony in my hospital cases allowed me to save my 3 patients' lives.

DESI AND HER MOTHER

Each one of my three hospital stories had its own unique learning opportunity. I came to understand human nature when I witnessed how each of the family members and their heroic allies stepped up to the plate to sacrifice what they could, to ascertain that their loved one would survive. Inserted in this chapter will be actual accounts of some of the family members' journey, shared in their own words.

The first story demonstrates the deep love of a daughter who fought the odds to save her mother's life. She pushed me to stay longer in the hospital so that her mother could win this battle.

This is the story of Desareta (Desi), our amazingly brave heroine. Bring it forward Desi.

On April 7, 2021, my mom was hospitalized because her oxygen saturation went down to 86 and severe coughing and shortness of breath. She was only on 3 liters of oxygen and maintained a stable 97 percent saturation O2 in the hospital. Twenty four hours later, she was given the first dose of Remdesivir and fresh plasma. This was the start of her downfall.

Mom was admitted to the ICU as her oxygen level dropped drastically. Suddenly, doctors were telling me that she might need to be intubated. They warned me that if she was not intubated, her heart could stop and that they might not be able to bring her back. They wanted to discuss every option with me, so I rushed to the hospital. I begged them to let me stay with her overnight in the hospital because they were unable to communicate with my mom who did not speak any English at all. Even though this was the worst nightmare of our life, the best thing about it all was that I got to stay with Mom for twenty four hours straight.

I was told that her lungs were damaged, so the intubation had to be postponed. My mom was on high flow (55 liters of oxygen per minute) and on an oxygen mask till April 28. I started my request to administer Ivermectin on her on April 20. But every doctor ignored my request. They argued that Ivermectin was only a political drug and was used only for outpatient purposes. I was told that it was not approved for the COVID-19 protocols at the hospital.

Frustrated, I thought about getting in touch with Mr. Ralph Lorigo who fought in court in New York for patients to receive Ivermectin. I was eventually able to contact him and hire him to help my mom and me. Not only did he win all those cases for other patients but also all made it out alive after using Ivermectin.

Mom was intubated on April 28. She had a cardiac arrest, but by the grace of God, the doctors revived her.

Our case got to court, and even after winning the court case with the Judge's order, the hospital still denied giving Ivermectin to Mom. I had no option but to take the story out to the media, hoping for a solution. We went to court a second time. Because of this, the hospital was forced to finally allow Ivermectin to be administered, but they could not find a doctor to do it.

The hospital claimed that 20 doctors were asked to administer the Ivermectin and all of them refused. But Dr. Bain, an outside doctor, agreed to help to administer it for her. Dr. Bain was our Angel who made all this possible. My mom is now home, and we could not be happier with the results, all because of Ivermectin. Mom started showing *improvement after the 3rd day of receiving Ivermectin. Although still on a ventilator, her oxygen intake was lowered. The results would have been better if Ivermectin had been administered earlier to her.*

Before the Ivermectin doctors gave her a zero chance of surviving, especially after her cardiac arrest. But God had other plans for my mom.

Ivermectin (the miracle pill), Dr. Bain, Mr. Lorigo and his team, and the love and prayers of everyone, gave us hope again. Thank God, my mom made it!

Desi's loyalty and tenacity to this day inspires me to keep on fighting for my patients and their family. Being at this hospital was a disappointing experience for me as I witnessed the lack of collegial atmosphere between myself as the outside doctor and the regular staff who had to follow protocol and didn't really look at the quality of life of the patient as much as they should. It seemed they just wanted to stymy an outside doctor from attending to the well-being of his patient. I was an outsider trying to be collegial but was being blocked by a hospital administrator whose ego surpassed the compassion that they should have had for Nurije Fype, Desi's mom. It was a blessing that the patient could not speak English, so that the daughter could stay with her mother all during this time.

This is also a story and celebration of the daughter, Desi. With a steadfast manner, she pushed back at the hospital's Infectious Disease specialist who called her out for her 'arrogance.'

Desi had the courage to accuse the doctor of playing God with her mother, as the latter offered shortsighted prognosis on Nurije if Desi did not follow orders.

It was in this hospital that I spent 20 days (about 3 weeks) giving Ivermectin every night after work. Since I did not want to get my family sick from COVID-19, I spent 24 days in a hotel.

LESLIE AND HER SIX DAUGHTERS

Leslie Pai and her six remarkable daughters represent what is profoundly good about humanity. They exude joy and give hope to all of those around them in their persistent joy for life.

Fighting for this family with Ivermectin's special gift, and being able to bestow it upon a family was my best reward.

Leslie Pai was on the ventilator and her higher level of consciousness pushed me to save her life. Her strong spirit was evident as it guided her family to do the right thing for her.

Her daughter Tiffany used her power of attorney in her fierce fight for her mother's survival. She made tough decisions to get her mother away from a hospital that was cold, calculating, and conniving in its processes to put a patient on a ventilator. Almost at the brink of death, Leslie Pai fought for her life. With frightfully low oxygen levels, she had the energy to push away the insensitive bullying of the doctors and verbally declare that she wanted to leave the hospital, no matter what.

Below is Tiffany and her family's account of what transpired, in their own words:

"Evidence-based medicine only." *These were the words the doctors kept repeating, on top of my pleas to them. My mom was admitted to the hospital for low blood oxygen levels due to COVID-19. Things were looking bleak. She whispered in fear to us over the phone that they were being rough with her, and they were not giving her anything that was helpful. They just gave her lots of morphine.*

We (her six daughters) were not allowed to see her except for a short 30-minute visit from one of us once a week. We were only allowed one update call with a nurse a day. If we exceeded the limit we would lose the privilege. They were not feeding my mom and refused to bring in any food that we delivered to her. We begged them to give her water on a sponge

Chapter 2   Straight From the Horse's Mouth and the Unvaccinated Doctor

because she was so thirsty. The annoyed nurses told us: "Only one swab we gave her one three hours ago." Then, they told us that they would need to intubate her, or she would die. They also agreed that her chances of survival after intubation were next to none due to her age (69). They scared her and told her she was surely dying. They blithely informed us that "Two of her six daughters could come in to say goodbye... and that was a very generous offer". Never have we experienced such a level of cold-hearted care.

My mother overheard them say sarcastically, "What a shame...the entire family is not vaccinated. This is what they get." Not one to lose hope, I pleaded with the doctor. "Please, can we do something? Imagine if this was your mother." The doctor rolled her eyes and sardonically replied, "Your mother is now under palliative care. If you do not want to intubate her, there is nothing more we could do."

My mother had already heard wonderful things about Ivermectin, and when she tested positive for COVID-19, a telehealth officer prescribed it. Unfortunately, the telehealth doctor had prescribed her a very low dose. The dose was lower than the prophylactic dose, so mom did not recover. She could not keep down any pills. She begged us to get Ivermectin for her. But when we brought it in for her, the doctors confiscated it and put it in a biohazard bag. They also refused her vitamin C tablets and vitamin D drops that we had packed for her. I begged them to try giving her a few doses of Ivermectin. I came prepared with articles and studies on how it was helping people with COVID-19 all over the world.

"My mom is dying and all you are giving her is morphine?" I asked. They brought another doctor in who told me that there was no evidence that Ivermectin worked for COVID-19 so that they would not administer it to her. Because of hospital rules, they would not administer it to her. They also would not read the articles or studies I brought. Their decision *was final.*

*"Then I will take her out of this hospital and administer it myself!"
I declared. But the hospital administrator said that my mom would be
a threat to the public by just being wheeled out of the hospital. When
I asked about a transfer, they said I would have a hard time finding a
hospital that would give her Ivermectin.*

*After several harrowing days, my mom was literally on death's
doorstep. We decided that she couldn't die in the hands of these cold-
hearted people so we got a lawyer who told us we could take her out of
the hospital as long as we paid for the very costly ambulance.*

*In a day, we got a crew of nurses to help us with the hospital breakout
to take my mom back home. Nevertheless, the nurses and doctors of the
hospital made it clear that they were not going to make us leave so easily.
They would not send her home with her IV lines, and they increased her
oxygen to a level we could not match in a home environment.*

*I was her person of authority for of health matters, but they kept
trying to get her to override the decisions which was already made. We
recorded their phone call where they told us she would most likely die
before she even reached the ambulance.*

*Luckily, we had a great ambulance company that took over
immediately when they ripped out her IV lines and oxygen. When we got
her home, she was getting cold in front of our eyes. Her mouth was dried
out like leather from dehydration. She was so weak and could not even
swallow any water. We decided to take her to another hospital to get the
oxygen that she needed and to buy more time. If the hospital wouldn't
give us the Ivermectin, then again we would fight the hospital with the
law to get it for her. That evening our mother almost died when her O2
level dropped to 46%!*

*We will never forget the blank look in her eyes. I ran alongside the
gurney as she was wheeled into the new hospital and promised her that*

Chapter 2   Straight From the Horse's Mouth and the Unvaccinated Doctor

if she agreed to be intubated once more, I would get her Ivermectin. She nodded weakly and whispered "I trust you" before she lost consciousness.

The hospital staff rushed in to revive her and then intubated her. I had no idea how I would keep my promise and I was afraid to appear contentious with the people that held my mom's life in their hands. I politely asked about administering Ivermectin, but the doctors refused. Undeterred, I tracked down the two sisters from New York who took their hospital to court and saved their mom by getting her Ivermectin. They referred me to their lawyers who were now swamped with similar cases all over the country. The lawyers told me that I needed to find a doctor that would vouch for the fact that this drug that could help my mother recover.

We called dozens of doctors but none would help as they were too afraid for their reputation. Finally, our lawyers told us about Dr. Alan Bain who was our first piece of good news in more than a month!

I begged Dr. Bain to take our case. Dr. Bain believed that Ivermectin could help our mom and so he agreed to take our case. We quickly prepared to take the hospital to court. The judge could not understand why the hospital would refuse to let a dying woman take a clinically proven safe medication, if the family wanted it. "What would be the harm?" he asked.

We won the case! And after the first dose of Ivermectin, we began seeing major improvement. But the hospital was not going to let this drug perform its healing powers. They told us it was causing my mom's blood pressure to drop to dangerous levels and took us back to court after our third dose. We feared that the hospital would go to any length to prove us wrong and make Ivermectin appear to be a dangerous drug. However, Dr. Bain was confident that with the 3 days' worth of medicine, would turn the tides and my mom would recover.

So, we didn't fight the hospital and agreed to stop administration of

Ivermectin.

On the other hand we did request for all the hospital records so we could confirm that my mom's blood pressure was dropping from or not from the Ivermectin. The court ordered that my mom's medical records be released to us. We were given 30 of 1,500 pages but they were not from the dates when Ivermectin was administered.

Our lawyers persisted and we got 900 more pages that we weeded through, only to find that they still did not include the Ivermectin treatments.

We realized that the hospital had locked her records. Thankfully, my mom's condition improved and we transferred her to a Long-Term Acute Hospital. Still, her new doctors were unable to access her previous medical records. My mom was a patient but was being treated like a prison inmate or a fugitive.

Finally, one day we marched into the hospital and talked to a girl who knew the HIPAA (Health Insurance Portability and Accountability) laws. She confided "I don't know who you pissed off, but I do know that the HIPAA laws say you can have your medical records" as she handed my mom's medical records to us.

We discovered from reading the medical records that Ivermectin did not cause my mom's blood pressure (BP) to drop. Rather, her BP rate was dropping because of the suppressors they gave her.

Our suspicions were right. They were using other medications to make my mom's blood pressure drop after her Ivermectin had been administered and putting the blame on Ivermectin.

Fast forward to today, after months of physical therapy, my mother enjoys a full and normal life with her 6 daughters, and now 19 grandchildren. She travels, hikes, and cooks for her family, like she used to. We owe her life to Ivermectin and the people who helped us fight to get it to her when she needed it.

Side note

I was always confused about why COVID-19 was so dangerous and how serious it really was. I know now from my experience why all of those millions of COVID-19 deaths took place in the hospitals. The hospital protocols were depriving the patient of human contact, nutrition, hydration, and the proper protocol, which included inhaled steroids and Ivermectin, which could have greatly eased their difficulty. Instead, patients were getting pain killers, intrusive ventilators, and coma-inducing medications that are very hard to recover from.

Desi and Tiffany described their similar experiences of courage to find an unconventional but effective treatment for their mothers.

When Leslie informed the hospital of her wish to be discharged, the hospital's refusal was appalling.

Leslie informed the hospital of her wish to be discharged. The hospital's refusal was appalling.

Leslie and Tiffany knew that the hospital staff were aware of studies the lifesaving benefits of adding Ivermectin to her mother's regimen.

It is an outright crime for hospitals to knowingly deny this powerful option.

Tiffany spoke of the freedom of choice which is guaranteed by law.

This argument was used in court cases I participated in. Depriving patients of fluids and helpful medicines are anti-life.

In the case of Leslie Pai, the opposing attorneys were trying to claim that Ivermectin was lowering Leslie's blood pressure and they tried to stop the administration after 3 days. The medical team even made up stories about the results of my Ivermectin dosing. We did not fight for more days as I thankfully had witnessed important signs of healing with my initial administration of Ivermectin in that short period of time.

After the first administration of Ivermectin, Leslie on the very next day, went from being on her stomach for 6 days to being strong enough to be placed on her back. I considered this a very positive sign. I administered 2 more dosages and watched the pulse oximetry improve right before my eyes. Slowly but surely, she was successfully weaned off the ventilator.

Consequently, she was transferred to a more compassionate Wisconsin nursing home care where her family was granted more time to visit. Leslie is now fully recovered back with her family, and happy and healthy.

Given our country's advanced medical system, turning our homes into hospitals is counter-intuitive. Never again should we ever witness such medical dereliction of duty as was described by Tiffany, our heroine in this true story.

UNVACCINATED ARE OFF-LIMITS

Like the earlier stories, the third case was been eloquently reported by Mary Beth Pfeiffer, an investigative journalist. It is about how I, an unvaccinated doctor, was thwarted from entering a hospital even after the judge ruled that I could administer Ivermectin on patient. For one seemingly long weekend, we waited to reconvene with the judge to allow me to get a PCR test. Hospital protocol states I needed to test negative on a PCR test.

I arrived at the hospital an hour before midnight, only to be turned away. I witnessed in shock and disappointment, the administrative bias and ignorance of a medical specialist who should know more than I about Ivermectin. This doctor was blaming Ivermectin for the fevers. It turned out that the doctor misread the case report and that the fevers were coming from the utilization of antibiotics.

I chose to remain unvaccinated because of my family history of cancer. Along with reasons I abstained from receiving this so-called vaccine, which I consider a hastily cobbled concoction, a product of poor research, and with a questionable safety record.

In my opinion, somebody should have put the brakes on the roll-out of the COVID-19 vaccines. Because it is reported to be causing rare cancers in many patients.

Despite claims that vaccines are 'safe and effective', we are discovering the opposite.

According to research coming out of the Cleveland clinic, the more vaccine shots given to health workers, the greater their chances of contracting COVID-19.

Specialization is not the only requirement for doctors to find a successful outcome to a medical problem. More than that, it is through keen and unbiased clinical observation that successful outcomes are achieved. The daughter of my patient, an accomplished academic, successfully fought for her sick father to be given Ivermectin. This allowed me to administer Ivermectin on the patient for 5 days.

The miraculous part came when, four minutes after receiving Ivermectin, the patient's pulse oximetry reading improved from 93% to 100%.

We must reconsider how so-called specialists are permitted to render opinions that can affect public policy when they do not have sufficient background information or context. Statisticians will not be able to view the totality of the body's response to multiples medications prescribed together.

This is a failure of the medical system. Evidence-based medical research only recognizes independent variables responding to controlled changes. What was equally daunting in my experience was trying to save the lives of patients who refused to go to the hospital. Many of them knew that Ivermectin was going to help them in some way. They wanted me to prescribe it. Their fear of being ventilated was sobering and chilling because of the other protocols that were being offered.

Now we know that Remdesivir was authorized prematurely and dangerously to the public. Dr. Paul Marik in his testimonies has described in detail how research was tampered to make Remdesivir look effective.

Moving the endpoint in midstream is totally unacceptable in research; this is what happened in the Remdesivir trial. I therefore believe it is grossly unfair and dangerous to use Remdesivir research to guide our decisions.

We could have used a simple natural medicine that comes from the ground to really help us.

Instead, the more affordable Ivermectin, got vilified because it was more effective than the laboratory produced drug that cost us $3,000.00 per dosage.

Is there not something terribly wrong with this equation?

I came to believe that since the hospital protocols centered on this dangerous drug called Remdesivir, along with reduced fluid resuscitation, it is now more dangerous for patients to undergo hospital treatment. So, I tried very hard to fight for people to stay out of hospitals as long as they knew the consequences of their decision.

Doctors are not prepared to create a hospital environment in the home. But the pandemic showed us that this could be a better option. I certainly had to do that on three to four occasions. Patients refused to go to the hospital; instead they wanted me to take care of them.

In 2021 Coleman McDonough was released from the hospital and given anticoagulation medicine. Records of his illness show that, for a short period of time, he began to feel better. But on the 8th to 9th day, the cytokine storm began, This overreaction of the immune cells could cause severe organ damage or death for the patient unless the right medications are given. Despite his dire condition, he was adamant about home care. Racing against time, I had to call oxygen and IV companies to deliver fluids and medications to him quickly. He was on 5 to 7 liters of oxygen with very low saturation at 88%. Methylprednisolone, the drug suggested in the Front Line COVID-19 Critical Care (FLCCC) Alliance protocol, was helping the patient.

And of course, Ivermectin and hydroxychloroquine were on the medical menu. Slowly but surely, Coleman needed a lower dosage of the steroids, and eventually, less oxygen support. I know of many many other cases like his all over the country.

A vital observation I would like to share is the fact that COVID-19 patients mainly need fluids in the beginning. For patients with heart disease, one has to be more careful. The ignorance of our medical community in not understanding that fluids would be 40 to 60% of the treatment protocol was a blind spot that needed to be investigated with strong research. We are learning now that COVID-19 was more a vascular attack around the lung tissues than an airway attack. Introducing more fluids would increase the blood flow to the lung tissue, which would in turn, help more oxygen into the lungs.

My diligent nurse Katherine Pagan Roman was there to administer the fluids and she recorded the wonderful changes in the pulse oximetry. As the patient was hydrated, the pulse oximetry reading moved up, decreasing the need for additional oxygen. We saw this over and over again: the hospital protocols were actually causing many patients to dehydrate and weaken. If fluids were introduced at the onset of treatment, thousands of lives could have been saved.

For example, the blood thinners, fluids, and oxygen contributed to one of my patient's survivals. And this was a case where Ivermectin was never used. So we understand that treating patients for acute COVID-19 is more of a coordinated menu, an ensemble of medications. Ivermectin may be part of the mixture.

There are many more quiet heroes all over the world who were able to help people get off the ventilators using different Ivermectin delivery systems. They used their innovativeness and knowledge to quietly fight for the lives of their patients. When health workers are restrained under threat of reprisal or ridicule, we have the beginnings of an autocratic environment that may be detrimental to the medical profession.

We are intelligent citizens of the world who should not be manipulated by those with vested interests. Sadly and horrifyingly, the actions of powerful show that they truly do not care about the greater good.

In conclusion, this pandemic has taught me that in very crucial times, we need to use our own God-given common sense. Real-world evidence has shown that Ivermectin has saved thousands of lives, yet its benefits have been ignored. Helpful drugs like Ivermectin and hydroxychloroquine have been tainted with political misinformation by organizations threatened by its potential.

We must remain steadfast in the truth and protect each other from forces that would disingenuously manipulate our right to fight vigorously for liberty, personal survival, and unobstructed self-determination. Vilifying an innocent drug like Ivermectin is a grave disservice to science and medicine. We must remember that doctors are committed to each and every one of their patients. Relying upon 'experts' who cling desperately to manipulated statistics and data is a travesty. Let us all join in this quest to reverse this dangerous practice. Amen.

Chapter 2 Straight From the Horse's Mouth and the Unvaccinated Doctor

Alan F. Bain, DO

Dr. Alan Bain, DO, is an internal medicine specialist in Chicago, IL and has 35 years' experience. He graduated from CHICAGO COLLEGE OF OSTEOPATHIC MEDICINE OF MIDWESTERN UNIVERSITY in 1988 and completed a residency at the University of Illinois Hospital. He currently runs his own practice at Chicago Health and Wellness Alliance and is affiliated with Ascension Saint Joseph - Chicago.

Chapter

3

Canada

Dr. Jennifer Hibberd

Canada:
'The Land of the Free'?
You Decide

IVERMECTIN TREATMENT FOR COVID-19?
MAINSTREAM MEDIA "EXPERTS" SAY NO!

That was the beginning of a mind-bending cover up of epic proportions. The fallout continues…

You will read about important aspects of the history of Ivermectin as it happened in Canada through the declared COVID-19 pandemic. I will share my experiences and those of colleagues in this 'Land of the Free'. My intention is to provide the public with a very different view of Ivermectin in relation to the world of healthcare, ethics, and the media, which is not being shared through mainstream channels such as legacy media and the medical 'industry'. We are experiencing a medical crisis like no other. Our whole world has been brought to its knees through the mishandling of a supposed 'health crisis' that has altered humanity.

I am a dental surgeon, a specialist in pediatrics, and a university educator with extensive clinical and academic experience. I am also a freelance editor and have written several papers with leading doctors and scientists, notably, during this pandemic period. Below is a selection of papers I co-authored, all based on very noteworthy studies focused on the pandemic, including impressive country-wide Ivermectin studies. I am highlighting these studies because they stand out as the largest studies done on Ivermectin to date. Notably, they were conducted prior to the initiation of the COVID-19 vaccine program.

1. **Regular Use of Ivermectin as Prophylaxis for COVID-19 Led Up to a 92% Reduction in COVID-19 Mortality Rate in a Dose-**

Response Manner: Results of a Prospective Observational Study of a Strictly Controlled Population of 88,012 Subjects

Lucy Kerr • Fernando Baldi • Raysildo Lobo • Washington Luiz Assagra • Fernando Carlos Proença • Juan J. Chamie • Jennifer A. Hibberd • Pierre Kory • Flavio A. Cadegiani

- https://www.cureus.com/articles/111851-regular-use-of-ivermectin-as-prophylaxis-for-covid-19-led-up-to-a-92-reduction-in-covid-19-mortality-rate-in-a-dose-response-manner-results-of-a-prospective-observational-study-of-a-strictly-controlled-population-of-88012-subjects?utm_medium=email&utm_source=transaction#!/

In this study, an evaluation was done with participants who used Ivermectin prophylactically for COVID-19, to determine if regular use, when compared to irregular use, impacted the degree of reduction in COVID-19 infection, hospitalization, and mortality rates. Regular and irregular Ivermectin users were also compared to non-users to evaluate evidence of a dose-response pattern of efficacy.

Non-use of Ivermectin was associated with a 12.5-fold increase in mortality rate and a seven-fold increased risk of dying from COVID-19 compared to the regular use of Ivermectin. This dose-response efficacy reinforces the prophylactic effects of Ivermectin against COVID-19.

2. **Ivermectin Prophylaxis Used for COVID-19: A Citywide, Prospective, Observational Study of 223,128 Subjects Using Propensity Score Matching**

Lucy Kerr • Flavio A. Cadegiani • Fernando Baldi • Raysildo B. Lobo • Washington Luiz O. Assagra • Fernando Carlos Proença • Pierre Kory • Jennifer A. Hibberd • Juan J. Chamie-Quintero

- https://www.cureus.com/articles/82162-ivermectin-prophylaxis-used-for-covid-19-a-citywide-prospective-observational-study-of-223128-%20subjects-using-propensity-score-matching?utm_medium=email&utm_source=transaction#!/

Based on the studies suggesting efficacy in prophylaxis, combined with the known safety profile of Ivermectin, a citywide prevention program using Ivermectin for COVID-19 was implemented in Itajaí, a southern city in Brazil, in the state of Santa Catarina. The objective of this study was to evaluate the impact of regular Ivermectin use on subsequent COVID-19 infection and mortality rates.

Conclusion

In this large Propensity Score Matching (PSM) study, regular use of Ivermectin as a prophylactic agent was associated with significantly reduced COVID-19 infection, hospitalization, and mortality rates.

3. **COVID-19 Excess Deaths in Peru's 25 States in 2020: Nationwide Trends, Confounding Factors, and Correlations with the Extent of Ivermectin Treatment by State**

Juan J. Chamie • Jennifer A. Hibberd • David E. Scheim

- https://www.cureus.com/articles/172991-covid-19-excess-deaths-in-perus-25-states-in-2020-nationwide-trends-confounding-factors-and-correlations-with-the-extent-of-ivermectin-treatment-by-state?utm_medium=email&utm_source=transaction#!/

In Peru, an opportunity to track the efficacy of Ivermectin (with a close consideration of confounding factors) was provided through data for excess deaths as correlated with Ivermectin use in 2020, under semi-autonomous policies in the country's 25 states.

The natural experiment that was put into motion with the authorization of Ivermectin use for COVID-19 in Peru in May 2020. An analysis of the data on excess deaths by locality and by state from Peruvian national health centers, shows strong evidence of the drug's effectiveness. Several potential confounding factors, including effects of a social isolation mandate imposed in May 2020, variations in the genetic makeup of the SARS-CoV-2 virus, and differences in seropositivity rates and population densities across the 25 states, were considered but did not appear to have significantly influenced these outcomes.

These studies gave such conclusive results, they appear to have inevitably triggered the publishing of the 'TOGETHER trials'. This happened shortly after each Ivermectin country study was published. The TOGETHER trials refuted the resounding conclusions that Ivermectin is effective against COVID-19.

Please note, the TOGETHER trials were initiated from McMaster University in Ontario, Canada, whose research facilities are known to be recipients of millions of dollars of funding by the Bill and Melinda Gates Foundation.

These TOGETHER platform trials were unfortunately published with errors in their methodology and overall study designs. See one of many critiques of the TOGETHER trials:

When Characteristics of Clinical Trials Require Per-Protocol as Well as Intention-to-Treat Outcomes to Draw Reliable Conclusions: Three Examples

Scheim DE, Aldous C, Osimani B, Fordham EJ, Hoy WE. When Characteristics of Clinical Trials Require Per-Protocol as Well as Intention-to-Treat Outcomes to Draw Reliable Conclusions: Three Examples. J. Clin. Med. 2023;12:3625.

- https://www.mdpi.com/2077-0383/12/11/3625.

And then read one of the TOGETHER platform trial papers featured in this next link:

- https://www.nejm.org › doi › full › 10.1056 › NEJMoa2115869

I have added another publication on the questionable nature of the COVID-19 vaccines, positioned for potentially serious neurological effects on the vaccinated.

4. **How Does Severe Acute Respiratory Syndrome-Coronavirus-2 Affect the Brain and Its Implications for the Vaccines Currently in Use**

Philip R. Oldfield 1, Jennifer Hibberd 2 and Byram W. Bridle

- PDF Version: https://www.mdpi.com/2076-393X/10/1/1/pdf

This mini-review focuses on the mechanisms of how SARS-CoV-2 affects the brain, with emphasis on the role of the spike protein in patients with neurological symptoms. Patients with a history of neurological complications may be at a higher risk of developing long-term neurological conditions associated with the α-synuclein prion, such as Parkinson's disease and Lewy body dementia. Compelling evidence has been published to indicate that the spike protein, which is derived from SARS-CoV-2, and generated from the vaccines currently being employed, is not only able to cross the blood–brain barrier but may cause inflammation and/or blood clots in the brain. Consequently, should vaccine-induced expression of spike proteins not be limited to the site of injection and draining lymph nodes, then there is the potential of long-term implications following inoculation that may be very similar to that of patients exhibiting neurological complications after being infected with SARS-CoV-2.

How could this not be mentioned here? The blocking of Ivermectin, along with other effective treatments, falsely positioned the vaccines as the primary available therapy, under the Emergency Use Authorization (EUA), fully disregarding important protocols normally required to launch a new vaccine.

This information must be documented and recorded. These decisions caused life changing effects on everyone, vaccinated or not.

In early 2020, following the events in China preceding the declaration of the 'pandemic', a colleague shared newspaper clips going back to the summer of 2019. The National Post Canadian newspaper, along with several international papers and news outlets reported about how two Chinese scientists at the level 4 National Microbiology Laboratory in Winnipeg, and one Chinese scientist at Harvard, were deported to China, labeled as 'spies'. They had been illegally sending coronavirus to the Wuhan lab. Interestingly, when you read these articles today, they do not read as they did back in 2020. Most of these articles appear to have been 'altered'. The current version of these articles does not mention the sending of coronavirus but instead referenced other viral samples. The 'apparently altered' articles even make a point of specifically denying transport of coronavirus to Wuhan. Read the links and listen to the reports. Read between the lines and you will note that one of the scientists from the Level 4 lab in Winnipeg, Canada, was reported to have disappeared in Africa. There are reports of 3 scientists that were to be expert witnesses in a lawsuit. All conveniently vanished/died in unusual circumstances: assassinated, suicide, and heart attack. Naturally, the lawsuit did not proceed.

AUGUST 2019

James Giordano, a neurology professor at Georgetown University and senior fellow in biowarfare at the U.S. Special Operations Command, said this is worrisome on a few fronts.

'China's growing investment in bioscience, looser ethics around gene-editing and other cutting-edge technology and integration between government and academia raise the specter of such pathogens being weaponized', he said.

Bio-warfare experts question why Canada was sending lethal viruses to China

- https://nationalpost.com/health/bio-warfare-experts-question-why-canada-was-sending-lethal-viruses-to-china

China and Viruses: The Case of Dr. Xiangguo Qiu
By Lt. Col. (res.) Dr. Dany Shoham January 29, 2020

The scope of the 2019 incident involving the discovery of a serious security breach at Canada's National Microbiology Laboratory (NML) in Winnipeg is much broader than the group of Chinese virologists who were summarily evicted from their lab. The main culprit behind the breach seems to have been Dr. Xiangguo Qiu, an outstanding Chinese scientist born in Tianjin.

- https://besacenter.org/perspectives-papers/china-biological-warfare/

At any rate, the controversial shipment resulted in the entry of information technology specialists into Qiu's office after hours, in search of her computer. Because of this incident, the security access of Dr. Qiu, her husband, and the Chinese students, were revoked. Her regular trips to China also started being denied.

WUHAN VIROLOGY INSTITUTE, CHINESE BIOLOGICAL WARFARE AND CHINESE-CANADIAN SPY

- https://gews.org/92280/

GreatGameIndia reported on the investigation of Chinese agents involved in a Biological Espionage case at a Canadian lab with alleged links to the recent Coronavirus outbreak, Subsequently, another report on Chinese biowarfare agents at Harvard University caught smuggling deadly viruses from America.

Frank Plummer – Canadian Scientist Key To Coronavirus Investigation Assassinated In Africa? By GreatGameIndia
February 6, 2020 | Last modified on February 14, 2020, at 4:15 am,

In a very strange turn of events, renowned scientist Frank Plummer who received Saudi SARS Coronavirus sample and was working on Coronavirus (HIV) vaccine in the Winnipeg based Canadian lab from where the virus was smuggled by Chinese Biowarfare agents and weaponized as revealed in GreatGameIndia investigation, has died in mysterious conditions.

- https://greatgameindia.com/chinese-researchers-caught-stealing-coronavirus-from-canadian-lab/
- https://greatgameindia.com/coronavirus-bioweapon/

Frank Plummer was the key to the Chinese Biological Espionage case at Winnipeg's National Microbiology Laboratory.

- https://greatgameindia.com/canada-investigates-chinas-biological-espionage/
- https://prime.economictimes.indiatimes.com/news/74068009/economy-and-policy/coronavirus-is-a-bio-weapon-experiment-gone-wrong-suspect-global-experts
- https://www.youtube.com/watch?v=Qjog_2faOz8

In March 2020, when the lockdown was enforced in Canada. The attention on the pandemic created a panic scenario, leaving people in a state of fear. This was unprecedented, and the news media hyped the danger across all channels.

The news about tragic events in China associated with the COVID-19 virus, made its way to North America. The impact of the spreading infections was most profound and shocking among the elderly living in retirement residences and nursing homes. Death rates due to COVID-19 were being reported at a high of 50%, in nursing homes, and particularly in privately run seniors' residences. The scientific community had no answers for the general public other than 'stay home'. Meanwhile, small groups of doctors around the world were earnestly looking at various drugs for possible repurposing, in order to help save lives.

On April 21, 2020, Monash University in Australia released the finding of an in vitro study providing clear evidence that Ivermectin was effective in destroying the COVID-19 virus. This finding led Dr. Jean-Jacques Rajter, an ICU doctor in Florida, to conduct a medical trial. The trial known as the 'ICON (Ivermectin in COVID Nineteen)

Trial' was approved by the Brower Health Medical Centre. It involved the administration of Ivermectin to a cohort of hospitalized ICU COVID-19 patients in his care. A statistically significant improvement in mortality was obtained in the cohort that received this medication. On May 22, 2020, the findings of his research were reported on the live-streamed news channel Newsmax by Dr. Peter Hibberd, the consultant medical expert.

- https://www.newsmax.com/us/ivermectin-drug-virus/2020/05/22/id/968688/

REMARKABLE LIFE-SAVING EFFECT

Following this report, a lady by the name of Nicole Zeigler in Toronto, Canada, contacted me in May 2020. She told me about incredible events that took place at her mother's nursing home in the Greater Toronto area prior to and into the first wave of the pandemic. Nicole had been watching Newsmax and saw the interview with Dr. Peter Hibberd about the very positive report of Ivermectin being used in the Icon Trial. She contacted him to share the events at her mother's nursing home. He recommended that she contact me, his sibling, in Toronto.

Nicole eagerly shared her observations about recent events at the Valleyview Long-Term Care Home located in Greater Toronto where her mother was a resident at the time. According to Nicole, just prior to the announcement of the pandemic, there was a scabies outbreak in the facility and the residents were treated with Ivermectin. This is because Ivermectin is a specific treatment for scabies.

The talk among the staff, about how well the residents did through the first wave of the COVID-19 pandemic, led to Nichole's inquiries at this Long-Term Care Home.

Their survival rate through this first wave of COVID-19 was remarkable. Compared to all reports about the massive deaths &

debilitation from the virus, especially in Nursing Homes & Senior Residences, using Ivermectin appeared to have a remarkable life-saving effect.

I then started researching about Ivermectin.

I spoke with the owner of the Valleyview Residence to explain the significance of the news I received. He was very cooperative, and I was able to confirm the use of Ivermectin and its phenomenal effect on their residents.

All the residents were scheduled to be treated with a series of doses of Ivermectin, as per scabies treatment protocol, between February 19 to March 3, 2020.

COVID-19 was brought into the facility in the first week of April by Personal Care Workers (PCW); in total 7 PCW tested positive for COVID-19. Despite the mandated lockdown orders, the Personal Care Workers (PCW) were free to come and go to Valleyview while also working at any number of other Care Facilities at the time.

Even with the residents of Valleyview being exposed to the COVID-19 positive Personal Care Workers, only 8 out of 170 residents tested positive for COVID-19. All 8 of these elderly residents had significant comorbidities yet only 5 of the 8 patients were symptomatic for COVID-19, and of the 5 symptomatic residents, 3 were posthumously 'labeled' to have died of COVID.

The low infection rate at Valleyview needs to be considered alongside how other Senior Residences were faring during this period. For example, within two weeks of the onset of the COVID-19 infection the Pinecrest Seniors' Residence in Bobcaygeon, Ontario, recorded an alarming number of infected residents; 29 of the 65 residents. The scene would be repeated at long-term care homes across Canada.

Compared to all reports about the massive numbers of deaths and debilitation from the virus, especially in Nursing Homes and Senior

049

Residences, using Ivermectin appeared to have had a remarkable life-saving effect. The findings at the Valleyview Residence certainly highlighted the use of Ivermectin and the phenomenal impact it appeared to have. No doubt about it, this was incredibly important news that I had to share.

I reached out to Canadian news channels, politicians, the offices of the Minster of Health and the Prime Minister's office. I had a network of friends and colleagues who tried to share the experience at Valleyview Residence with politicians and the Health Ministry.

No response came from the Minister's offices, local MPs or the Prime Minister's office. A CTV News journalist that Nicole and I spoke with was very interested in reporting about the possible link between the Ivermectin low infection rate. She was told to drop the story. It appeared that no one in the 'Trusted News Media', Ministry of Health or political circles wanted to touch this story.

If Ivermectin was truly responsible for saving most of the Valleyview residents from contracting the virus, surely it could and would gladly be used to save countless other lives. As a repurposed drug, it is very inexpensive and readily available.

WOW, what a watershed moment! That was a wake-up call, like no other, about the whole pandemic. I instantly experienced a big shift in perception.

I learned very quickly that instead of immediately putting Ivermectin to work to save the day, the World Health Organization (WHO), did not support its use outside of clinical trials, even though the scientists who discovered & developed this 'Wonder Drug' Ivermectin for human use won a Nobel Prize in 2015.

Meanwhile countless people were being intubated and were dying alone in ICU wards.

After wasting precious time trying to engage health professionals

Chapter 3 Canada: 'The Land of the Free'? You Decide

& politicians, I invited Nicole to join me to make a video to post on YouTube. I was determined to get this life saving information out into the world. I was convinced that viewing this video could save lives.

My video rocked the world. It was the first time that Ivermectin was talked about in English, on social media. Comments came flooding in, especially from the South American countries and communities where Ivermectin was a known anti-parasitic and already being successfully used as an antiviral medicine. Thousands of posts were attached to this video talking about how people used Ivermectin and were cured. I listened to South American doctors sharing protocols for treating COVID-19.

Dr. Tom Borody in Australia talked about Ivermectin on Sky News. He saw the video I posted on YouTube & announced that this anecdotal evidence convinced him to study it further. Here's the link for the video:

- https://youtu.be/8XCYzpHBEkI?si=Ylr9NY7lZhCqcrMC

Yet, Canada remained quiet…

News of my video spread fast. I was immediately invited to join the first Ivermectin international discussion group on Facebook, IVERMECTIN MD. Within the group, we shared real time information about what was being reported in our countries. We also shared protocols that doctors and scientists in this group developed. The first Ivermectin therapeutic treatment protocols for COVID-19 were posted on IVERMECTIN MD, and on ResearchGate by Brazilian doctor Gustavo Aguirre in early Spring of 2020. These initial protocols were distributed internationally among medical professionals. Continual updates, refinements and additions were made to the protocols, with the primary drug being Ivermectin. The stages of infection with COVID necessitated different doses and other effective medications to be used in conjunction with Ivermectin.

051

MEDIA CLAMPDOWN ON MEDICAL WARRIORS

At this time, there was limited media available for sharing information. Facebook, YouTube, Instagram, and Twitter made up the entirety of social media. I became a media warrior; I started posting on all sites. I started editing and co-authoring papers. I helped write manuals and books with colleagues. I posted talks on YouTube with doctors from all around the world who were saving lives using Ivermectin. I wanted to share their amazing stories about unique challenges in their countries.

It was just a matter of time before the censors trained their powerful filters on us sharing this lifesaving information. By late 2020, many of us had our YouTube videos blocked and our tweets and posts 'shadowbanned' (blocked for public viewing) on Twitter and Instagram. Yet, we persisted and shared information and supported each other. We realized there were algorithms screening the titles and keywords we used in our posts and videos. We learned to exercise caution with the choice of our written words. The Facebook group, IVERMECTIN MD, having reached over 10,000 participants, was SHUT DOWN with a warning that we had 'violated' community standards.

While Ivermectin was now being vilified in Canada, medical and healthcare regulatory bodies issued stern warnings on treatments for COVID-19 patients. The only approved treatment was "NO TREATMENT. Their advice (to the medical frontline): "Offer Tylenol if needed, but to only seek care at a hospital if you can no longer breathe easily". Healthcare professionals identified for treating COVID patients, using Ivermectin, were reprimanded with disciplinary action through their Regulatory College.

At this time, the eminent cardiologist, Dr. Peter McCollough kept encouraging me to start an alliance in Canada. I told him I needed to find a licensed medical doctor, in order to launch this suggested alliance.

Peter sent me an article about a Canadian doctor who prescribed Ivermectin. This doctor is Dr. Ira Bernstein. One of his patients claimed he saved her life. This was it, I searched for this doctor and, as destiny would have it, his office was in Toronto. We were ready to start this new alliance. Peter then introduced me to another Canadian, an accountant, David Ross. Together we launched Canadian Covid Care Alliance (CCCA), now an internationally recognized group of evidence-based scientists, doctors, lawyers and journalists.

-   https://www.canadiancovidcarealliance.org/

By late summer of 2021, several scientific papers on Ivermectin had been published. I had participated in several medical conferences about the pandemic on different continents. There is no question that engaging with like-minded colleagues across the world brought me in contact with many incredible pioneers for change. Our network of dedicated people grew across the world.

Early in 2021, British medical expert Dr. Tess Lawrie posted her public plea to Prime Minister Boris Johnson, to allow the use of Ivermectin to treat COVID-19 patients. I contacted her and we both agreed that the mainstream scientific messaging lacked crucial evidence-based information and were short on reliable references.

Furthermore, relative to the full spectrum of scientific literature, the mainstream media's reportage was not accurate and was deliberately misleading. While vaccines were being billed as safe and effective, Ivermectin was being mocked and discredited. My colleagues and I had evidence to the contrary. What clearly emerged at the time was the reprehensible fact that the World Health Organization (WHO) was not representing the true needs of the people. As soon as the vaccines became available, the WHO took down their posts on natural immunity. This act spurred Tess and I to launch the World Council for Health.

-   https://worldcouncilforhealth.org

I am on the board of several organizations, working on best strategies to collaborate, and disseminate critical health information. I believe in enabling organizations to grow and take the message of health, sovereignty, and hope for a healthier future to as many people as possible.

Those of us analyzing the true science, free from manipulation by vested interests, realize that we have a role in bringing vital information to light. Each one of us has learned 'the hard way' that we must choose our battles carefully. A critical aspect of the mainstream initiative has been to manage healthcare professionals and keep them from deviating from the prescribed "Emergency Use Authorization (EUA) script". Careers and individual's livelihoods have been cut short with healthcare professionals' lives being disrupted.

Those of us defending truth, freedom of choice without coercion, and personal sovereign rights, are being pressured and shamed in the attempt to silence us. Others surprisingly seem to have become puppets to endorse and enforce a questionable agenda.

Many Canadians did not passively accept the mandates. They spoke out loudly and in large numbers. The Freedom Convoy, a large procession of health advocates, traveled across the country to demand an audience with the Prime Minister to end the restrictive mandates. They came together in Ottawa, the Capital city, and passed through major cities across Canada. Despite the attempted military breakup of the Freedom Convoy in Ottawa, one convoy came through Toronto. I posted a short video showing how the police and the participants were engaged in a community-friendly event.

- https://youtu.be/hlskI464yYY?si=Xf2LoJDvuYtLuaqd

The next morning, my office was raided by the regulatory body, the Royal College of Dental Surgeons' (RCDS). We all realized that the Freedom Convoy was a huge trigger for the forces trying to control the narrative.

I was not in my clinic at the time. These people presented themselves as officers from the college and took over my private office. They searched the clinic, grilled my staff and called me on my phone announcing their presence in my clinic. They told me to check my email to read the charges. The email was sent minutes before they called. The element of surprise was evidently at play. They announced that they had a registrar driven complaint, not a patient complaint, to drive this investigation. Consider for a moment, the unusually rapid timing of the clinic raid and my routine at the time, of not being at the office on a Monday. It's now noteworthy to point out that I had been informed earlier in the pandemic that the 'Five Eyes' were watching me. This raid suspiciously has me considering it was initiated by their sources. The College stated that I was under suspicion of committing acts of professional misconduct by saying the wrong things about COVID-19. They sent my lawyer, Michael Alexander, a laundry list of possible charges, not the least of which was 'not being fit to practice'. After a lengthy period of legal letters being exchanged with the Regulators, I was required to participate in an ethics program and face a disciplinary panel.

Across Canada, the regulatory bodies have placed harsh restrictions on their members. They warned their members on Twitter and posted directives on their college websites that members were not permitted to treat COVID-19 patients with repurposed drugs. Their members were advised to follow only the information and mandates outlined on the regulatory and/or Ministry websites.

Many medical doctors who refused to cooperate have been denied work in hospitals and had their offices invaded by investigators. Many of them facing disciplinary hearings, their licenses suspended while awaiting these proceedings, which could lead to the loss of their license.

Sadly, some healthcare professionals have already given up their Canadian license and moved on to the U.S. or beyond. However, there are others who are standing their ground and seeking justice in the courts.

Several doctors are in disciplinary hearings with the College of Physicians and Surgeons of Ontario (CPSO) are required to complete the college ethics and remediation program, in order to continue their practice. This, along with an accompanying agreement to comply with restrictions on their practice as noted below.

The following is quoted from CPSO official documents; received by a doctor who had his office raided in Toronto and has been continually hounded by his regulators for alleged misinformation.

Practice Restrictions:

- *To not provide medical exemptions in relation to vaccines for COVID-19*
- *To not provide exemptions in relation to mask requirements for COVID-19*
- *To not provide medical exemptions in relation to diagnostic testing for COVID-9*
- *To not provide Ivermectin or hydroxychloroquine in relation to COVID-19*

This doctor was required to participate in authorized professional education programs pertaining to CPSO policies, public health guidance, Ministry of Health directives during a declared pandemic, the prevention and treatment of COVID-19 in an outpatient setting and medical record keeping.

Here are more excerpts from official documents this medical doctor in Ontario received in relation to charges against him:

Chapter 3 Canada: 'The Land of the Free'? You Decide

Lack of judgement in:

1. *Prescribing Ivermectin against the advice from professional and governmental, organizations such as the Ontario Ministry of Health, Health Canada, Ontario College of Family Physicians, Ontario COVID-10 Science Advisory Table, and College of Physicians and Surgeons of Ontario for both immediate and future use, contributing to the overuse and reduction of the already limited supply in Canada.*

2. *Prescribing hydroxychloroquine against advice from professional, governmental, and licensing organizations such as the Ontario Ministry of Health, Health Canada, Ontario College of Family Physicians, Ontario COVID-10 Science Advisory Table, and College of Physicians and Surgeons of Ontario for both immediate and future use, contributing to the which also has some implications of overuse and reduction of the already limited supply in Canada.*

3. *Providing vaccine exemption letters against Ontario Ministry of Health and NACL criteria.*

The Assessor appointed by the CPSO concluded that the Respondent doctor's clinical practice was likely to expose his patients to harm due to:

1. *The (alleged) side effects of Ivermectin*
2. *False reassurance of disease outcome for patients who were prescribed Ivermectin or hydroxychloroquine which may delay the patient seeking further help and*
3. *Potential for the patient to have a higher risk of severe health outcomes from COVID-19 due to inappropriate advice for COVID-19 vaccine exemption.*

This doctor's disciplinary hearings are ongoing.

Let me now present Dr. Charles Hoffe, a medical doctor in British Columbia, Canada. The following is Dr. Hoffe's personal account of events and his positioning, as a medical professional, during this 'pandemic period'. He refers to his ongoing experience as:

PERSEVERANCE' DESPITE PERSECUTION- DR. CHARLES HOFFE

Dr. Charles Hoffe is a South African-born and trained family doctor and emergency room physician, who moved to Canada in 1990. He has worked in the small rural community of Lytton, British Columbia since 1993. About 70% of his patients are Canadian Native Indians.

Early in the pandemic, Dr. Hoffe became a vocal advocate for the use of Ivermectin because of its unique ability to bind the COVID spike protein. The price of prescription Ivermectin in Canada became extraordinarily expensive, with patients paying up to $43.00 a dose, if they could find a doctor to prescribe it. Many doctors and pharmacists were deceived by the barrage of misinformation on Ivermectin, calling it a very dangerous drug, and few would either prescribe or dispense it. In October 2020 the College of Physicians and Surgeons of British Columbia issued a decree forbidding doctors from prescribing Ivermectin for COVID-19. So, the only option for people was to use non-prescription veterinary Ivermectin.

Within three months into the COVID vaccine rollout, there was a significant signal in the form of large life-threatening blood clots from the AstraZeneca vaccine.

By mid-March 2021, 12 countries in Europe had shut down the AstraZeneca vaccines for COVID-19. However, despite the serious safety signals in Europe, Canada continued to administer it. This motivated Dr. Hoffe to send a private email to 18 medical colleagues in his area, directly involved in the vaccine rollout. He questioned the ethics of continuing to administer a treatment that had evidence of serious harm. He informed them that there was a personal liability issue if doctors administered a medical treatment without warning the patients of the risk of harm. One of those colleagues sent the email to the regional health authority. Three days later Dr. Hoffe received a reprimand, warning him not to say anything negative about the COVID-19 vaccines in the course of his work in the emergency room. In addition to this gag order, he was informed that a complaint was being filed at the College of Physicians and Surgeons of British Columbia because he was putting patients at risk by provoking vaccine hesitancy. He was further told that if he had any questions about the vaccines, they must not be addressed to his colleagues, but to the local medical health officer in charge of the vaccine rollout for that area.

Thereafter, Dr. Hoffe began to see serious neurological side-effects in his own patients who received the Moderna vaccine. He sent a letter to the Medical Health Officer to inform her of the evidence of harm. He asked what disease process had been created by this new gene therapy treatment and asked how this new disease should be treated. He received no response. Instead, the letter was sent to the College of Physicians and Surgeons, as a further complaint against him.

Meanwhile, Dr. Hoffe became increasingly alarmed by the number of serious vaccine side-effects he was seeing in his own patients daily. These included a variety of pain syndromes with pain in the head, neck, face, limbs, chest, feet or testicles. They also included odd sensations of tingling, electric shocks or burning along with various cranial nerve palsies including Bell's palsy. Some patients had weakness of limbs, dizziness, light or sound sensitivity and tinnitus.

In early April 2021, Dr. Hoffe sent a letter to the British Columbia provincial health officer, Dr. Bonnie Henry, to ask her the same questions. He also posted it as an open letter to alert the public about the evidence of harm, which was clearly being concealed and denied by both the media and health authorities. The letter went viral on the Internet and was read around the world. Until this time, the Moderna vaccine had not been implicated as causing neurological harm. Clearly, this open letter antagonized the authorities even more. Shortly thereafter, the provincial colleges of physicians and surgeons across Canada issued warnings to all doctors against spreading 'misinformation' and warned that anyone who did so would be investigated and, if necessary, disciplined.

Two weeks later, a vaccine injured patient came into the Lytton emergency room where Dr. Hoffe was the doctor on duty. He knew the patient very well and had been her family doctor for 28 years. She and her family had COVID vaccination five weeks before, with no significant illness. Yet the patient had come into the ER, after being vaccinated for COVID-19 because the COVID vaccine had made her much sicker than her recent COVID infection. Dr. Hoffe stated that the patient did not need her second shot, because she had proven natural immunity to COVID, (evidenced by the fact that her COVID infection had been mild).

He explained groundbreaking scientific evidence on the durability of natural immunity to the SARS virus in the study done at Duke-NUS Medical School in Singapore, published July 2020.

Research scientists recruited people who had recovered from the first SARS virus (2002/2003), analyzed their blood for T-cell immunity, and showed they were still immune to the SARS virus 17 years later. Furthermore, they found this immunity also protected them against SARS CoV-2, even though the two viruses were 20% different. Lastly, they found that approximately 50% of the population in Singapore, who had not encountered any SARS virus, had natural cross-immunity from contact with the other coronaviruses present every flu season. The relevance of this is that Omicron which has about 30 mutations is 3% different from the original Wuhan strain. So, if natural immunity protected against a virus that was 20% different, it would have no difficulty protecting against a variant that was only 3% different. This important research showed SARS T-cell immunity was broad enough to cover every variant currently identified and lasted at least 17 years.

Dr. Hoffe had been practicing emergency medicine for 31 years, without a single patient complaint against him. Yet he was fired from the ER for stating that a person with natural immunity did not need to be vaccinated against a disease to which they were already immune. His work was thereafter restricted to his private practice.

Dr. Hoffe noted that contrary to the claims of Pfizer, it had been revealed, the lipid nano particle delivery system of the gene-based vaccines enabled the vaccine to be distributed in the bloodstream to every part of the body. Furthermore, he noted that because absorption from the bloodstream occurs mostly in capillary networks, micro-clots in capillaries are too small to be seen on a CT or an MRI; they will be scattered throughout the body. So how does one test?

Professor Sucharit Bhakdi suggested doing a d-dimer test on COVID vaccinated people. A blood test before their injection, to get a baseline for that patient, and a blood test 4 to 8 days after the injection to see if clotting had occurred. A d-dimer blood test is a common blood test done in the emergency department, to see if a patient had a recent blood clot. It does not tell you where the clot is, it simply gives you a probability that clotting has occurred somewhere in the body.

Dr. Hoffe started offering this test to his patients to monitor their COVID-19 injections. He expected to see perhaps 5% evidence of clotting. The preliminary results, showed that 62% of people (5 out of 8), had evidence of micro clotting within eight days of their injection.

Dr. Hoffe was so horrified that he could not keep silent. These were people who thought their vaccine had done no harm and was keeping them safe; they were not overtly vaccine injured people. Furthermore, it showed that clots were not rare; they were occurring in more than half of the people vaccinated.

The worst was still to come. About nine days after revealing the micro clotting evidence online, and following a severe heat wave, a fire storm destroyed the village of Lytton where Dr. Hoffe lived and worked; 90% of the town was completely obliterated. The wildfire began on June 30 of 2021 destroyed Dr. Hoffe's medical practice, the entire medical facility, and the lab where the blood tests were being done. This ended Dr. Hoffe's attempts to investigate the disease processes that had been created in his patients by the COVID-19 vaccines.

Dr. Hoffe went on speaking tours around western Canada informing people about the risks of the COVID vaccine injections, and the importance of treating COVID infections with Ivermectin. Trying to safeguard and educate the Canadian public in this way, clearly antagonized the authorities even more. The College of Physicians and Surgeons of BC initiated an investigation with a citation issued for him to stand trial before a disciplinary panel, for his crime of spreading 'misinformation', stating that Ivermectin is an effective treatment for COVID and that the COVID-19 vaccinations have the potential to cause serious life-threatening side effects.

Dr. Hoffe has patients with a great variety of vaccine injuries. Some died, and some remain disabled by COVID-19 vaccines they received over three years ago. Notably, every one of Dr. Hoffe's attempts to report the vaccine injuries in his patients have been blocked by the medical health authorities, who insist that all their new medical problems, which started after the COVID-19 vaccinations, are simply 'coincidental'.

By systematic censorship of vaccine injury, the Canadian health authorities can publish statistics showing that vaccine injuries are exceedingly rare, and that the COVID-19 vaccines are 'safe and effective'. Sadly, most doctors are not even willing to report the injuries for fear of being called anti-vaxxers, so most of the harm goes unreported.

ER physician put out of work for saving three lives with Ivermectin

Another doctor, Dr. Daniel Nagase, an Emergency Room (ER) physician in Western Canada tells a familiar story.

'On September 11, 2021, I was doing a locum in the community of Rimbey, Alberta for the first time. A locum is a fill-in physician who takes over for another doctor on leave or holiday. The province of Alberta Canada has an organized Rural locum program where doctors in small communities can put up a posting for a temporary doctor to cover the community for a weekend or a week. I had been covering small rural Emergency Departments for several years through the Alberta Rural Locum program, prior to arriving in Rimbey. September 11 was my first time in this town in west central Alberta. Prior to working in Rural Emergency Rooms (ERs), I worked in high volume suburban ERs in Vancouver; Canada's third largest metropolis. I always looked forward to working in small towns for the opportunity to share updated skills with the town doctors who may have previously worked in large centers decades ago. The challenge of rural medicine is that specialists are not available; this expanded my knowledge far beyond what I previously had from my big city experiences.

NOTE: A locum is a fill-in physician who takes over for another doctor on leave or holiday. The province of Alberta Canada has an organized Rural locum program where doctors in small communities can put up a posting for a temporary doctor to cover the community for a weekend or a week.

That morning, the charge nurse at Rimbey hospital started the day by informing me that three elderly patients on the COVID ward had deteriorated overnight. My first thought was what did the overnight doctor do about it? Being polite, I asked what was currently being done for the patients. The charge nurse explained that other than high flow oxygen, not much was being given. I confirmed this in the patient's charts, seeing only low dose steroids, no antibiotics and no respiratory medications. It seemed to me that with COVID-19, all the standard therapies doctors would give for any viral pneumonia were suddenly ignored.

NOTE: One basic step with any viral pneumonia is to include an antibiotic to prevent the fluid and phlegm created by the viral inflammation from becoming bacterially infected and turning into bacterial pneumonia. Other basics include the administration of Ventolin (salbutamol) and Flovent (or Pulmicort) to open the airways to improve oxygenation and help the patient cough up fluid and phlegm that might fester and make their pneumonia worse. These basic steps were ignored with the excuse that these interventions did not help with "COVID" pneumonia.

Each of the three COVID patients I was faced with on that Saturday morning was denied standard treatment we are supposed to give for all viral pneumonias. Two patients were in their mid-70's and one in her mid-90's. At these ages any hospitalized illness carries much greater risks than with patients even just a decade younger. And here I had a charge nurse telling me their oxygen saturations were dropping, with a request

Chapter 3   Canada: 'The Land of the Free'? You Decide

that I do something. I examined all three patients. Each had a similar story. They felt like the doctors had just put them away in a corner to die because they had COVID. When I listened to their lungs, all three patients had copious crackles from the bottom of their lungs all the way up to their apices (the top). Audible crackles are a sign of fluid in the lungs. If you take a wet sponge, put it to your ear and let it expand after a gentle squeeze, you too might be able to hear crackles if you listen closely. This is what a doctor is listening for when using the stethoscope.

One patient also had edema in her legs, a sign of fluid overload. I explained to each of these patients that should their oxygen levels continue to deteriorate, they would need mechanical support.

NOTE: Most often this means intubation and a ventilator, but sometimes a less invasive measure such as CPAP or BiPAP can achieve adequate ventilation on a temporary basis through a pressured facemask. The downside to CPAP and BiPAP is that sometimes it ends up inflating the stomach. If this causes vomiting, and the patient accidentally inhales their vomit because of their mouth being blocked by a positive pressure facemask strapped to their face, then they will have gastric acid, with stomach bacteria in their lungs as well as the virus that started their illness.

I explained that unless we try medications to prevent further deterioration, they will need to go to the ICU in Red Deer or Edmonton after being put on life support with a ventilator.

NOTE: Small hospitals generally do not have the staffing or equipment to manage and run an intensive care unit where ventilated patients are usually treated.

I asked each of the patients if they would like to try Ivermectin, a medication that was not recommended by the hospital, but had a large amount of scientific evidence supporting its use. Especially by September 2021, Ivermectin's effectiveness, saving lives in COVID pneumonias, was demonstrated, study after study. The patients all agreed to try everything possible to avoid being put on a ventilator. I prescribed them doses of Vitamin C, Vitamin D, Zinc, Ventolin, Flovent, Pulmicort, high dose dexamethasone, Azithromycin, Hydroxychloroquine and Ivermectin for all three patients.

They received everything except for Ivermectin. Rimbey hospital did not have any, and Red Deer central pharmacy refused to send the medication out from Red Deer. The pharmacist in Red Deer central pharmacy demanded to know why I had ordered Ivermectin. I told him that it was between me and the patients. I suspect this pharmacist had access to my patients' electronic medical records and discovered that they were all hospitalized for COVID pneumonia. What followed were several phone calls, a fax, and a flurry of emails opposing my using Ivermectin. One of the Doctors who sent emails to stop my patients trying Ivermectin was Dr. Gerald Lazarenko, the head of Pharmacy for all of Alberta Health Services. No one could give me a medical reason for their opposition. The best they could manage to say was that "Ivermectin doesn't work." They referred to Alberta Health Sciences Rapid Scientific review of Ivermectin from February 2021.

Since Alberta Health Services refused to send Ivermectin, the charge nurse asked me if I'd like her to contact the local pharmacies and see if they had a supply. A few hours later, one pharmacist from the Value Drug Mart was able to get Ivermectin. I wrote orders to dispense Ivermectin according to weight, but the nurses refused. I had to give the patients syringes with the correct dose of Ivermectin for their weight so that they could take it themselves. It was incredible how these nurses flat out refused to do their job.

Chapter 3   Canada: 'The Land of the Free'? You Decide

Later that day I received a call from the Central Zone Medical Director, Dr. Jennifer Bestard, demanding that I stop offering the patients Ivermectin. She explicitly prohibited the patients from self-administering the Ivermectin I had supplied for them. She gave no clinical reasons, and she seemed completely unaware of the patient's medical history, their deterioration or even their names! I informed Dr. Bestard that her involvement in the care of patients without their consent and without any knowledge of their clinical situation was both dangerous and unethical. She could not offer any medical, scientific or ethical reason for stopping my patients' desired choice of medication and medical care.

I was very concerned that the interference in my medical care by the zone medical director harmed my patients and mentioned this to the Rimbey staff. However, one of the LPN's and one of the RN's subsequently became argumentative. They continued to ignore all the science and insisted that Ivermectin could not be used. The patient's own wish to try Ivermectin did not change her irrational insistence that we were all wrong. The RN took a similar stance, ignoring patient autonomy. The LPN subsequently filed complaints to AHS and the Alberta College about the fact I pointed out her medical qualification was that of an LPN, and her knowledge was insufficient to make medical treatment decisions or take those decisions away from the patients.

The next day, the zone medical director, Jennifer Bestard, tried to remove me from my ER shift with 1 hour notice. When I informed her that it was dangerous to interrupt care on such short notice, she allowed me 2 hours to finish up with my patients. Several of the ER patients were quite ill and, I still had to transfer a number of patients with incomplete diagnoses and treatments to the replacement doctor. Aware that the doctor called in to replace me may not be up to the task, I stayed for a couple hours after handing over the patients to be available if she

067

had any questions or needed any help. She never approached me for help or questions despite knowing that I was next door, in the ward. I subsequently found out this replacement physician canceled all the inhalers, antibiotics and vitamins I had ordered for my elderly patients who had received Ivermectin. Her notes in the patient chart reflected a claim that she did not know why a patient would benefit from a diuretic to relieve fluid congestion in the lungs. She also seemed ignorant of how asthma inhalers can help with oxygen levels in patients with atypical pneumonias. She even wrote a complaint, claiming that I had "missed" a diagnosis of pulmonary embolism even though I was the one who ordered the D-Dimer that looked for the blood clot (but was fired before the result came back). Her complaint to the Alberta college was that the conditions of the emergency patients that I was caring for were 'serious'.

To make sure that I did everything I could to help my patients before they ended up in the hands of doctors who'd rather obey orders from a medical director with no concern as to whether they lived or died, I re-examined my three inpatients prior to leaving. All three had dramatically improved. Their lungs had gone from fluid filled to mostly clear in less than 24 hours. (In the end thanks to reports I received from the freedom community, I heard that all three elderly patients from Rimbey hospital were discharged, even the 95-year-old returned to her nursing home.)

So, I contemplated; where do I go from here? I had given Ivermectin on September 11, 2021, and I was out of a job by the afternoon of September 12. Later that week, I had Emergency Room shifts scheduled for St. Paul, Alberta. This meant driving my travel trailer another 4 hours up north. I called ahead and the chief of the ER said he heard from senior administrators that I had canceled all my shifts last minute. I told him that I did not cancel any shifts. It was incredible that senior administrators, hundreds of kilometers away, had already decided to spread a rumor that I reneged on my work agreements, all because I

Chapter 3   Canada: 'The Land of the Free'? You Decide

saved three elderly patients from the ICU.

After explaining to the ER chief at St. Paul that I was available to work all week just as I had previously scheduled, I asked him if I should make the drive. He said that I should show up in St. Paul Alberta for work, because if I did not show up, the senior administrators would charge that against me. Could they have been planning a defamatory narrative in advance? Spreading rumors that my shifts were cancelled, and then blaming me for not showing up and leaving a busy ER unstaffed? There was only one way to stop this.

I traveled 4 hours from Rimbey to St. Paul. I went to the ER before my shift to chat with the day physician who was a friend of mine. I stayed in the ER ready to work my shift at 7pm waiting for something official. I had no plan to let them slander me with accusations that I 'quit' my shift.

Upon hearing that I was present in the hospital, the Alberta Health Services North Zone medical director, Dr. Brian Muir, came down to the ER. He walked into the doctors' area and told me that I was not to work my scheduled shift. I told him that just telling me not to work my shift was not enough. He would have to put something in writing. Dr. Brian Muir refused. I gave him a pen and a piece of paper and instructed him to write that he had cancelled my shift. If not, I'd instruct the doctor he called in from Edmonton that night to go home, as I was scheduled to work that evening. Dr. Muir still refused to put anything in writing. He sat in one of the ER doctor chairs and called someone saying that I would not leave the Emergency Department. I then repeated to him that I was staying in the ER unless the medical director could put in writing that I was removed from my scheduled shift. Dr. Muir stubbornly stayed in the ER, despite having no patients or business there. It appeared to me that it was his attempt to physically threaten me into not working my shift.

At 7pm, Dr. Brian Muir told me to check my work email, saying that I now had written notice to stop working. There was nothing. He got on

069

his cell phone again. Shortly after his second call, an email from a medical administration secretary arrived saying all my shifts had been 'rescheduled'. However, my work in St. Paul's was never rescheduled to any other date, and all my work assignments for the rest of the year were canceled.

Hearing what happened, a friend of mine, (the chief of Athabasca hospital) invited me to come to work that weekend in Athabasca, since my St. Paul's work was canceled. They were in desperate need of a doctor for the weekend and were facing an ER closure. However, a day later after inviting me to drive up to Athabasca, he phoned to apologize because the zone medical director had threatened him as well, saying if he scheduled me to work in Athabasca hospital there would be 'consequences'. The chief at Athabasca hospital complained to me that he had thought Dr. Muir was a good guy. They went golfing together. He thought they were friends.

With all my work assignments for the rest of the year 'reassigned', I tried to pick up shifts in other rural communities on the waitlist for an emergency physician. All my offers to cover shifts in understaffed communities were rejected. Again, no explanations were given. Since then, there have been several ER closures in Alberta, despite my repeated offers to work in communities that posted the need for doctors.

The Alberta College imposed restrictions on my practice making it impossible for me to work in December of 2021. Their restrictions stated that I was prohibited from seeing any COVID or suspected COVID patients, I was prohibited from writing vaccine exemptions, and that I had to preface any public speeches with a statement that my views were not in line with the practice of medicine. I have not worked in or renewed my Alberta medical license, My British Columbia medical license was suspended in January 2022. Despite having retired from the British Columbia Medical College due to suspension of my license, the British Columbia College is still conducting a disciplinary "investigation" over a speech I made my treatment success with Ivermectin and warning about *the dangers of the mRNA vaccine.*

Little has changed in Canada despite the trucker's Freedom Convoy and two years of advocacy on my part. As an ER doctor, my standard was always to get to the source of the problem as much as humanly possible in the Emergency Room. The source of the problem lies far deeper than mRNA injection mandates, lockdowns, and the healthcare system.

Dr. Nagase concludes…

It has become very clear that the medical censorship is an integral part of this agenda. Doctors and scientists who question the mandates set in place are targeted and punished. The sharing of evidence-based information and engagement in healthy debate is being continually blocked and dismissed. Patients have been denied the fundamental right of informed consent when presented with the experimental COVID-19 injections. People are blocked from obtaining the information necessary to understand the risks and benefits of the current 'vaccines', and any alternatives, because of the widespread censorship by the medical community and public health officials.

Dr. Nagase's disciplinary investigation is ongoing.

As Dr. Daniel Nagase ultimately came to realize, his personal experiences as a physician, at this time, reflects a much broader issue. The damage to our medical system and the medical profession is so broad that full recovery does not appear possible.

The greatest influence for the public is the controlled messaging set in place by the organized 'Trusted News Initiative'. It became evident very early in the 'pandemic' that lockstep messaging had been set in place by the 'Mass Media'. Journalists across the world were delivering the same statements. Most statements were inciting fear to drive individuals to follow their directives; a psychological maneuver called 'nudging' and a form of neurolinguistic programming.

The integrity of our most prestigious medical societies, journals and institutions has been seriously compromised. Real-time data is being censored while unscientific claims are being advanced and published. Access to vaccine injury data reporting sites has been made so complicated that it is common to hear that many doctors often do not even bother to process a report. Physicians, scientists, and all health professionals started being intimidated early in the first wave of the pandemic. Many, like myself, have been formally threatened in regulatory hearings. Others had their licenses revoked for providing exemptions.

Why do innocent people suffer the effects of these catastrophic decisions when at the onset of this pandemic we had evidence of effective treatments such as Ivermectin? All people should have the opportunity to be informed about these treatments.

CONSIDER THE FOLLOWING:

We now know that the National Institute of Health (NIH), Food and Drug Administration (FDA), Centers for Disease Control (CDC), National Institute of Allergy and Infectious Diseases (NIAID), United Nations (UN), World Health Organization (WHO) and World Economic Forum (WEF) are heavily funded by the pharmaceutical industry and public-private partnerships, notably the Bill and Melinda Gates Foundation and GAVI. These previously esteemed institutions can no longer be trusted. They have lost their scientific credibility.

The pressures put on healthcare providers to follow have been so smoothly orchestrated that the majority of healthcare providers in Canada and worldwide, withholding early treatment and endorsing unproven 'vaccines' and 'boosters', without proof of their safety and effectiveness. There are many stories about how doctors refused to treat sick patients if they were not vaccinated. Some unvaccinated patients were taken off transplant lists. The media ran with the damning of the vaccine hesitant with powerful endorsements from Canada's Prime Minister Justin Trudeau:

"They are extremists who don't believe in science, they're often misogynists, also often racists," said Trudeau. "It's a small group that muscles in, and we have to make a choice in terms of leaders, in terms of the country. Do we tolerate these people?"

NATIONAL NEWSPAPER HEADLINES:

'Trudeau says people who are not fully vaccinated won't be able to travel on domestic planes or trains.'

"It seems that the PM's motto, 'diversity is our strength' only applies to those who are diverse in the ways he supports," Dr. Leslyn Lewis tweeted on the article. "Instead of his hateful and divisive language toward fellow Canadians, he should treat others with dignity and respect and work to heal and unite our country."

Dr. Leslyn Lewis is a Conservative MP for the Constituency of Norfolk in Ontario.

On very rare occasions, concerns peek out from behind the censorship screen in the mainstream media. For instance,

'The prime minister has a long way to go to heal the rifts that the unvaccinated feel he has introduced into the Canadian narrative. The only way Trudeau will walk back his concerning comments is if opposition leaders hold him accountable. Their silence is as alarming as

Trudeau's disturbing tirades".
Posted by Joe Warmington of Postmedia, Jan 7, 2022.

- https://torontosun.com/opinion/columnists/warmington-opposition-shockingly-silent-on-pms-hatred-of-unvaccinated-canadians

Examples of media posts that erroneously warned the public about the use of Ivermectin.

Health Canada issues warning against using Ivermectin dewormer to treat COVID-19

Sean Boynton Global News August 21, 2021

Health Canada is warning the public not to use the deworming drug Ivermectin to treat COVID-19, particularly the version that is used for animals.

The health agency said Tuesday that it has "received concerning reports of the use of veterinary Ivermectin to prevent or treat" the novel coronavirus.

"Canadians should never consume health products intended for animals because of the potential serious health dangers posed by them," the agency said.

Health Canada doesn't want COVID-19 patients to use the human version of the drug either, which is only authorized to treat parasitic worm infections in people.

But it came out particularly strong against the use of the more highly concentrated veterinary version, which is often used to deworm livestock like horses and pigs.

The agency said veterinary Ivermectin can cause serious health problems — especially when ingested at high doses — including "vomiting, diarrhea, low blood pressure, allergic reactions, dizziness, seizures, coma and even death."

Health Canada did not say how many reports it has received or where in Canada the reports originated from.

But Global News found this week that demand appears to have gone up in Calgary, where at least one feed shop has been forced to remove veterinary Ivermectin from its shelves.

The increased demand for Ivermectin comes as the deworming drug is being seized on by anti-vaccination critics, Republican politicians and members of right-wing media in the United States as a possible cure or preventative treatment for COVID-19.

Earlier this month in Mississippi, the state health department said at least one person had been hospitalized after taking Ivermectin. Officials said about 70 per cent of recent calls to poison control were due to ingestion of the veterinary drug.

The U.S. Food and Drug Administration was forced to issue statements urging people not to take the drug, including on social media. "You are not a horse. You are not a cow. Seriously, y'all. Stop it," the agency's tweet read.

Health Canada has issued an advisory against using the anti-parasitic drug, Ivermectin to treat COVID-19. Then the Canadian Broadcasting Corporation (CBC) reported the following on September 3, 2021.

Ivermectin is a wonder drug but not for COVID — and misinformation is causing a shortage

Health Canada has issued an advisory against using the anti-parasitic drug to treat COVID-19

Sarah Rieger

Ivermectin is a Nobel Prize-winning anti-parasitic drug that has improved the health of millions and has helped to eradicate diseases like river blindness in multiple countries.

But there's a shortage of the drug in Canada, as global demand surges due to unproven claims that the medicine can be used to treat COVID-19.

That shortage could put people who actually need it for treatment are at risk, including those who are more susceptible to illness from parasites due to COVID-19.

"The use of this medication for COVID is really putting people who are already in a difficult situation in an even worse situation," said Barry Power of the Canadian Pharmacists Association. "I would really urge people to think twice before trying to access this medication that has been proven to do nothing in the case of COVID."

Quantities of the drug have been limited in Canada since January due to global demand, and the shortage is expected to continue until the end of this year.

On Tuesday, Health Canada issued an advisory asking people not to take the drug to treat COVID-19 after reports that some people were taking the veterinary form of the medicine intended for livestock.

"There is no evidence that Ivermectin in either [the human or veterinary] formulation is safe or effective when used for those purpose," the federal agency warned.

'People were trying everything'

Demand for Ivermectin started to rise in December last year.

Early, limited and lower-quality studies suggested the drug might show promise as an anti-viral as well as an anti-parasitic — with hope that further study could prove it inhibits the growth of the novel coronavirus in human cells and improve patient's outcomes.

Dr. Lynora Saxinger, an infectious disease specialist at the University of Alberta, explained that those early studies did not consist of high-quality data.

Chapter 3   Canada: 'The Land of the Free'? You Decide

That's either because in initial positive reports patients were receiving multiple medications, so the effect of Ivermectin couldn't be parsed out, or because high doses that showed promise in test tubes didn't translate to human subjects.

That didn't stop the drug from being used widely in an attempt to treat patients in some countries like Colombia, because it was easily available and inexpensive, Saxinger said.

If you're a doctor faced with a hospital full of patients sick with a new virus, it makes sense to get creative.

"In the beginning [of the pandemic] people were trying everything in a sense of, I think, desperation," she said.

"Really, the only way to tell if something is truly helping is to do a randomized controlled trial … the higher-quality trials, by and large, have not shown any benefit whatsoever."

Media targeted doctors using Ivermectin to treat COVID. This has not let up since early in the pandemics.

Canada's Toronto Star reported the following as an investigative report by Lex Harvey on January 27, 2022.

A covert network of Canadian doctors is prescribing Ivermectin to treat COVID

Science and medicine dismiss the drug as a COVID treatment. But for the misguided or desperate, there are those in Canada willing to supply it.

On the same day another heading appeared in Global News which is also Canadian media.

COVID-19: Ontario doctor banned from prescribing Ivermectin now director of company offering drug

An Ontario doctor prohibited from prescribing Ivermectin to treat

077

COVID-19 has launched a telehealth service offering the unapproved treatment to Ontarians to treat the virus, Global News can reveal.

Dr. Patrick Phillips, a family doctor who is the subject of several investigations by the College of Physicians and Surgeons of Ontario (CPSO), is the director of a new telehealth service based in Ontario that is offering Ivermectin, an antiparasitic treatment not approved by Health Canada to treat COVID-19.

The service, called Canadian Covid TeleHealth Inc (CCTH), was launched by members of the Canadian Covid Care Alliance (CCCA), a website promoting information at odds with public health advice, which also features new initiatives from at least two other Ontario health professionals with COVID-related license restrictions.

But Phillips' involvement, as well as the existence of the service, is not breaking any provincial laws.

CBC also reported on the same day.

Doctors face sanctions for prescribing unproven COVID-19 drugs to friends and family, regulators warn

Medical regulators in Canada suspect some doctors have been stockpiling drugs that are being tested as potential treatments for COVID-19 and are now warning them they can be sanctioned if they prescribe the drugs to themselves or friends and family.

The drugs in question — hydroxychloroquine and azithromycin — are among a number of medications being studied as part of a global effort to fight COVID-19. So far, experts say evidence of their effectiveness in treating the disease is thin.

Hydroxychloroquine is currently used to treat malaria, rheumatoid arthritis and lupus, while azithromycin is an antibiotic for infections caused by bacteria and can be used in treating bacterial pneumonia...

This has left a majority of healthcare providers; medical doctors, nurses, dentists, naturopaths along with all alternative health providers, hospital staff, scientists and all educators in a 'trance state', following orders to comply without question. Many educated people took it upon themselves to enforce these mandates, refuse lifesaving treatments, therapies and transplants.

We have reached the stage of our journey within which we must understand fully what occurred during the dreaded COVID years.

How have the forces at work been so successful at ruling our lives and usurping our freedoms? Someday it will become common knowledge that in the COVID years, the fundamental PRINCIPLE : **do no harm**... was abandoned. The world was strewn with the wounded and dead, victimized by medical crimes against humanity.

One might wonder, was this perhaps a relatively successful experiment in mass manipulation? Fear and hysteria make us exquisitely vulnerable to persuasion. Despite there being simple solutions as Ivermectin, readily available and safety-certified, they were outlawed, to ensure the emergency use authorization (EUA) could be authorized and kept in place. The profits associated with these vaccines that proved to be neither safe nor effective are so high, they are off the scale. While the regulators and governments have coerced so many practitioners into obeying their directives and have threatened others, we must find new ways to protect our victimized colleagues and to embolden those who have cowered and stepped away from their professional ethics. May more and more healthcare workers stand bravely in their truth and serve others.

As Canadians, may our national anthem speak the truth:

. . *With glowing hearts we see thee rise,*
The true north strong and free'...

Oh Canada, we stand on guard for thee.
God keep our land glorious and free...'

May we all stand on guard for humanity, at peace, united and strong, to achieve the power of self-actualization across Canada and the world.

Jennifer Hibberd, BSc, DDS, DDPD, MRCDC

Dr. Hibberd is a dental surgeon, a specialist in paediatric dentistry and a university educator with extensive clinical and academic experience. She attended University of Toronto for her undergraduate and graduate degrees and attended Albert Einstein College of Medicine for her post graduate degree in Paediatric Dentistry.

Prior to the pandemic, she ran a large paediatric dental practice in Toronto, Canada.

Dr. Hibberd co-founded several important organizations disseminating evidence-based scientific information & resources.

She is also a freelance editor & has written several papers with leading Drs & scientists, notably during this pandemic period.

Caribbean

Chapter

4

Saint Lucia

Dr. M. Gilberta St. Rose

Ivermectin Endangered and Recovering

Saint Lucia is one of the islands in the Caribbean Sea, 27 miles long and 14 miles wide, with a total area of 238 square miles. The country has a population of 180,000 and is proud of its two Nobel Prize winners for literature and economics, and has one of the fastest female runners in the world. Saint Lucia is the world's top-rated honeymoon destination, home of the majestic Pitons, formed from a dormant volcano that is also a major tourist attraction.

In March 2020, when the World Health Organization (WHO) declared the COVID-19 pandemic, I thought it timely to encourage our people to adopt healthy lifestyles and augment their immune systems with vitamin-rich foods, supplements, and herbs. To my astonishment and dismay, this message was not forthcoming from our health authorities. Instead, preparations for administering COVID-19 vaccinations were touted as the only way out of the pandemic.

I was convinced from the outset that giving a biological agent against COVID-19 was not the best way, hence I delved into more research.

I escalated my message to the health professionals and the public and included the importance of personal hygiene, social hygiene and lifestyle adjustments in terms of what is consumed, fasting, elimination, detoxification, optimal breathing, rest, exercise, relaxation, adequate water intake, sunshine, supplements, herbals, steaming, absence of inner conflict, good relationships, good emotional health, optimum spiritual health. I specifically recommended:

- Supplements, as needed: Vitamin C, Vitamin D3, Quercetin, Melatonin, Zinc, Magnesium, garlic, onions, propolis.

Chapter 4   Ivermectin Endangered and Recovering

- The beneficial effect of grounding and avoidance or limitation in the use of electronic and smart gadgets.
- Utilization of Saint Lucia's sunshine and beaches.

Here in Saint Lucia, we have very easy access to herbs that support the following: detoxifying, anti-inflammatory, nutritional, mucus clearing, immune boosting, immune-modulating, anti-bacterial, antiviral, broncho-dilating, decongestant, appetite stimulating, anti-anxiety, sleep inducing, nerve restoration, energizing and adrenal stimulating, to be dispensed and/or used as per the need of the patient.

In keeping with the dictates and conveniences of efficacious allopathic and integrative medicine, I used some pharmaceuticals effectively in the early stages of the COVID symptomatology (e.g., antihistamines, if the patients presented symptoms of rhinitis …itchy, running nose, sneezing). The use of corticosteroids has been shown to be effective with early severe symptoms and even the use of antibiotics on occasions of purulent sputum with fever and chest pain and of course with pneumonia.

People were advised to monitor their oxygen saturation, but only a few patients had oximeters.

I also needed a more acceptable treatment for the medical community, as some practitioners were not fully convinced of the efficacy of certain supplements and herbs and required more evidence.

I was happy to discover evidence of the effective use of Ivermectin and was elated to share this treatment and prevention with my colleagues, staff, patients, and our health authority.

INITIAL RESEARCH FINDINGS REGARDING IVERMECTIN

My Initial Research Findings on Ivermectin and COVID-19 infection are as follows:

087

1. Ivermectin is a U.S. Food and Drug Administration (FDA)-approved antiparasitic drug that is used to treat several neglected tropical diseases, including onchocerciasis, helminthiases, intestinal worms, lice, mites and scabies.

2. Ivermectin has been taken safely by over 4 billion people over the past 40 years.
   It is documented by the World Health Organization (WHO) and in the Uppsala Center's VigiAccess database for pharmacovigilance or drug safety from 1992 to 2021.

3. Ivermectin can be repurposed for use against COVID-19 infection.

4. Ivermectin prevents transmission of the COVID-19 infection when taken either pre or post exposure.

5. Ivermectin hastens recovery and decreases hospitalization and mortality in patients with COVID-19 infection.

6. Ivermectin is on the WHO list of essential and most important medicines.

7. Ivermectin is effective against all strains of the COVID-19 virus.

8. Ivermectin can be taken safely by children weighing 15kg or more.

9. Several countries have already made Ivermectin available to their citizens.

10. Ivermectin is anti-inflammatory and protects against organ damage post COVID-19.

11. Ivermectin can be taken by persons who have taken the COVID-19 vaccine injection.

12. Ivermectin's recommended dose is 0.2mg – 0.6mg per kg body weight.

13. Ivermectin can be taken with all medications and by patients with underlying health issues.

14. Not to be taken during pregnancy or the first 6 months of breastfeeding. To be taken only under medical supervision if

Chapter 4   Ivermectin Endangered and Recovering

you are on anticoagulant drugs. Safe to take, if you are on blood thinners.

15. To be taken only under medical supervision if you are on anticoagulant drugs. Safe to take, if you are on blood thinners.

I believe our people need to come out of health damaging lockdowns, curfews and restrictions. Due consideration must be given to making Ivermectin available immediately as a medication to prevent and treat COVID-19 infection to save lives and reduce the strain on the hospitals and health care professionals.

These figures below show the number of COVID-19 cases between the periods of January 1, 2020, to September 22, 2023.

Ivermectin was studied by the National Institute of Health of the United States of America along with some other drugs for usefulness against the COVID-19 virus. In an ironic turn of events, when it

	2020	2021	2022	2023	Grand Total
January	0	2,031	7,479	174	9,684
February	1	1,419	1,310	87	2,817
March	16	474	211	43	744
April	1	297	560	15	873
May	1	532	2,588	55	3,176
June	3	226	1,032	21	1,282
July	3	335	977	38	1,353
August	1	3,256	807	56	4,120
September	1	2,784	596	16	3,397
October	100	926	140	0	1,166
November	142	373	57	0	572
December	109	942	34	0	1,085
Grand Total	378	13,595	15,791	505	30,269

F gure1. COVID-19 case in Saint Lucia Sources: Case Notifications, Epidemiology Databases, Ministry of Health (MOH) Saint Lucia

became necessary to use it, its use and distribution were blocked in many countries.

I continue to be thankful for the clinical guidance from Front Line COVID-19 Critical Care (FLCCC) Alliance, the group in the United States of America led by Drs. Paul Marik and Pierre Kory. Praise God for their perseverance and continuing advocacy in the ethical practice of Medicine. I am also cognizant of those doctors from the countries including Japan, Slovakia, Bulgaria, India, Egypt, South Africa, Zimbabwe, Bolivia, Brazil, Peru, and Argentina who campaigned valiantly to make Ivermectin readily available to their people.

In Saint Lucia, the then Minister of Health, Honorable Mary Isaac, and I had a good relationship. At that time, I was a volunteer with on the local cannabis commission, and we had agreed on the need for educating our people on cannabis.

I continued to research the use of Ivermectin to cure and prevent COVID-19 infection. I apprised the Minister of Health and Wellness, on the usefulness of Ivermectin in a letter dated February 2021. But she responded that the Ministry of Health and Wellness does not recommend the use of the drug for conditions other than what was approved by the FDA. It appeared that the off-label use and repurposing of a drug or repurposing the drug Ivermectin for new usage was not under consideration.

PERMISSION TO TRAVEL WITH IVERMECTIN DOSE

A clinical trial is any research study that prospectively assigns human participants or groups of humans to one or more health-related interventions to evaluate the effects on health outcomes.

We already had the anecdotal evidence from my local practice and the regional and international communities that Ivermectin not only cured COVID-19 but could also offer prophylaxis by taking a dose once or twice a week depending on the persons' level of exposure to the virus.

It was suggested that if a traveler could show evidence of being on prophylactic Ivermectin, this could convey the evidence to the immigration authorities that the traveler does not have the COVID-19 infection. Moreover, our research had also shown that Ivermectin also prevented transmission of the virus.

The Medical and Dental Council (Saint Lucia, W.I, MDC), had never asked me about my conducting a clinical trial. I ascertained from my staff that no one from the Council had come into my office physically or asked about our execution of a clinical trial. If they had come in or asked, we would have told them or allowed them to look at our documentation of names and addresses of patients. We recorded the names, addresses, telephone numbers, doses of Ivermectin given whether for prevention or treatment and the doses prescribed for each patient. This was to form the basis for initial data collection and in the event that an approved clinical trial was to be undertaken, we would already have some names of potential respondents. The letter below, on my letterhead and with my signature and office stamp, was given to 5 patients in the hope that it would satisfy the authorities that the person does not have and will not be able to transmit COVID infection.

This letter was used by the MDC as the basis for accusing me of carrying out a clinical trial and charging of EC$10,000.00 for doing so.

To: Whom it may concern
Date..

*RE: Observational Clinical Trial of Ivermectin as treatment and prevention against the **SARS-CoV-2 virus***
This is to hereby certify that:

Patient:

Date of birth:

Is currently registered in a clinical trial and study of effectiveness of Ivermectin against the SARS-CoV-2 virus.

Patient started on ….and is currently taking a dose of Ivermectin every 7 days.

The above subject is therefore exempt from taking the Covid vaccine for the duration of the clinical trial.

Sincerely,

This above letter misinformed and/or blinded the MDC into their false accusation.

The MDC should be aware that I first spoke of conducting a clinical trial on the use of Ivermectin with Dr. Sharon Belmar-George, Chief Medical Officer (CMO), on Timothy Poleon's television program on May 19, 2021. The CMO at that time said that she would not subject our people to a clinical trial with Ivermectin.

Initially, I did not bother to apply to the Research and Ethics Committee of the MDC, as is the required procedure. I proceeded with my off-label use of Ivermectin supplying information and getting agreement as to the off-label use of Ivermectin.

At that time there was a rise in cases. There were lockdowns and a shortage in the Saint Lucia police force as officers, if not sick, were in quarantine.

We were speaking publicly and giving guidance and recommendations on how to end the pandemic. Or at least we were treating those infected and giving prophylaxis with Ivermectin to avoid the unnecessary quarantines. We advised people to take Ivermectin if they needed to attend important gatherings like weddings and funerals.

My therapeutic regimen was based on FLCCC's protocol - 0.2 mg per kg body weight, daily after meals, on Day 1 and Day 3. If the person was proved to be infected or still had symptoms, another dose on Day 6 and 8.

In August 2021 when the deadly Delta variant emerged, we followed the increased dose recommended by FLCCC. I was then prescribing 0.4 mg per kg body weight. When infections abated, I gave between 0.2 mg to 0.6 mg depending on the clinical presentation of the patient. I also began using a daily dose for 5 days.

This synchronized with the dosage recommendation published in the National Institute of Health (NIH) USA's website.

The Clinic staff and I initially took 1 dose of Ivermectin weekly as prophylaxis in early 2021. Personally I took a 5-day course of Ivermectin when I experienced symptoms of COVID-19 infection.

Some of my patients who were on prophylaxis with Ivermectin claim that they were not infected by their officemates who were sick with COVID-19.

I also received a lot of phone consultations. We documented the names of patients given Ivermectin for treatment or prophylaxis. Some persons called specifically asking for Ivermectin. For some, I would recommend it, at all times reminding them that the Ivermectin was being prescribed off-label. Many persons thanked me for having saved their lives or cured their illnesses by having Ivermectin available for them.

The push back was very real from our health authorities. But I exercised my professional autonomy, I was happy to provide hope and have testimonies of healing and prevention of the COVID-19 infection with the use of Ivermectin.

The Saint Lucia Ministry of Health issued a press release on February 19, 2021, announcing that "Ivermectin is not approved for the treatment of COVID-19 and does not prevent COVID-19 infection".

The Ministry of Health sent me a letter from the Minister of Health, Mary Isaacs, dated February 23, 2021, and other correspondence. In response, I repeated my request to allow the use of Ivermectin in a letter to Health Minister Isaacs dated February 26, a letter to the Government of Saint Lucia and health authorities dated March 29, and a petition.

THE BAN ON IMPORTING IVERMECTIN

It was never communicated to me that the status of Ivermectin was changed and that it would not be allowed to be imported into Saint Lucia.

As an independent private practitioner, I proceeded to order the Ivermectin for our use.

On April 13, 2021, I submitted the required application for importation to the drug inspector, Ms. Astrid Mondesir.

However, Ivermectin never arrived. I realized that refusal of importation was stamped by the drug inspector on April 16, 2021. This was communicated to me by letter from the Chief Medical Officer (CMO) dated May 7, 2021, after the medication arrived on May 6, 2021. There was ample time to respectfully inform me of the unlawful refusal, so we could make a decision about our expenditure for the fight.

I wrote again to the CMO on May 10, appealing for the release of Ivermectin and asking to be advised of the legal basis for this extreme and arbitrary action taken by the Ministry of Health. I had written three letters requesting clarification from CMO. She did not give me any clarification.

On May 18, 2021, I wrote to the Minister of Health appealing for the release of Ivermectin. But I did not receive a response or positive action following my letter.

On May 19, 2021, during an episode of News Maker Live television show on Daher Broadcasting Service (DBS), on which the Chief Medical Officer (CMO), Dr. Sharon Belmar-George, was a guest, I took the opportunity to announce my opposition to the COVID-19 'vaccine' and to proclaim that Ivermectin gave "fantastic results" and was "exemplary" in the treatment of COVID-19 infections. I insisted "Having researched it and having used it on over 300 patients from January 2021, including myself and my staff, I have proceeded to import so persons who do not want the vaccine or want to take Ivermectin in addition to the vaccine…" can benefit.

I asked Dr. Belmar-George, "…this drug, can it be used in Saint Lucia for the treatment of COVID-19?" The CMO answered "No." Dr. Belmar-George explained her position and emphatically stated that "we are not authorized to utilize a drug against what its approved purpose is, and that it is what it is for the Ivermectin". Indeed, this was a new era in medicine where off-label prescribing was banned for Ivermectin.

Timothy Poleon further questioned the CMO and asked her what would happen if persons took the Ivermectin and she answered that it would make them sick.

The CMO, on the said public television program warned the public that taking Ivermectin would make them sick and that she would not subject the public to a clinical trial with Ivermectin. This statement was made by the CMO at a time when leading clinicians were getting excellent results with the use of Ivermectin for COVID-19 infection, preventing illnesses, getting miraculous recoveries and minimizing hospitalizations and deaths in many countries. This was being announced at a time when persons in my practice too, were experiencing the miraculous healings from taking Ivermectin and confidently maintaining good health with a preventative weekly dose regime.

In response to the CMO saying that we are not authorized to use Ivermectin, I suggested to her that we can use Ivermectin to treat and prevent COVID-19 infection as part of a clinical trial. The CMO stated that she would not subject the public to a clinical trial with Ivermectin.

When one wants to carry out a clinical trial in Saint Lucia, an application is submitted to the Research and Ethics Committee of the MDC, of which CMO is NOT a committee member. Even the CMO is just a member of the MDC.

The use of Ivermectin was totally highjacked. The CMO spoke against its off-label use in spite of it being an approved drug. We Clinicians have used and continue to use approved drugs off label and the FDA has encouraged such use.

Our efforts to publicly encourage the use of Ivermectin in the prevention and treatment of COVID-19 contrary to the advice of health authorities were consistent and persevering.

I teamed up with Humans Are Free group, created by Krysta Sylvester-Anthony and we took to the streets to spread the truth. Humans Are Free is a group of persons who got together to discuss, educate, protest and support those who wanted to maintain and spread the truth of the COVID-19.

I proceeded to import the Ivermectin labeled for human use and to my astonishment, the Ministry of Health and Wellness here continued to refuse to authorize the clearance from customs. Dermatologists and other doctors too, have used Ivermectin for scabies, head lice and parasitic infections in patients and the drug had been imported into Saint Lucia for years. There is no new legislation prohibiting the importation or use of Ivermectin; the shipment of Ivermectin was retained by customs, who said that they needed authorization for

Chapter 4   Ivermectin Endangered and Recovering

release by the Ministry of Health.

On May 27, in a letter to the CMO, I expressed to her my great concern regarding her statements on Ivermectin made on the national televised interview on May 19, 2021.

I wrote the following in the letter.

"Given your position where it is expected that you honestly inform the populace, I was quite surprised at your gross inaccuracies on the issue of the use of Ivermectin. As a consequence of these gross inaccuracies, as well as non-observance of medical protocol, I am forced to speak out with a view to protecting the health of the nation. To this effect I wish to call for a rectification of your statements."

"I have labeled your statement as gross inaccuracies and breakdown of protocol on three counts:

1. Your false statement that only 26 clinical trials have been done on Ivermectin and none showed benefits...
   ...at least 56 clinical trials have been done and at least 88% showed benefits for prevention and/or treatment of COVID-19 infection.
2. Your statement that if people take Ivermectin "they will get sick" ...You may imagine what this false information will do to patients who are currently taking the Ivermectin or considering the use of it.... quick healings from COVID-19 infection has been documented with Ivermectin, and side effects from use of Ivermectin at recommended doses are nil or minimal. Ivermectin has been taken by 4 billion persons over 40 years for treating parasitic infections in humans. For the prevention and treatment of COVID-19 infections the same dosage recommendation is used.
3. Your statement that you will not allow our people to undergo

097

clinical trials with the approved drug Ivermectin, all the while ignoring required protocols with this new biological agent called a vaccine, now under stage 3 clinical trial".

I received only acknowledgement of receipt of the 3 letters written to Dr. Belmar-George.

I filed a complaint against the CMO with the MDC on June 7, 2021.

MDC responded on August 4, 2021, to inform me of their inability to process the complaint *"on the premise that Health Practitioners Act Cap 11.06, does not give the Council jurisdiction to hear complaints of this nature."*

On August 6, 2021, my 8-year service on the MDC expired. I had served as board member, then was appointed as Deputy Chair and had acted as Acting Executive Director when the Executive Director was on leave.

MEETING WITH MOH AND CMO

The Saint Lucia Labor Party (SLP) replaced the United Workers Party at an overwhelming victory at the polls in July 2021. The new Minister of Health, Wellness and Elderly Affairs was appointed. The CMO was kept in her post.

I requested a meeting with the new MOH, Honorable Moses Jn Baptiste, which he accepted. He asked me whether we should ask the CMO to be in attendance. In retrospect I should not have said yes to invite her.

I recall CMO looking at me with ...was it disdain? And mostly remained quiet during the meeting. It made more sense to me when, during our discourse, the Minister asked to CMO about the use of Ivermectin after I had announced its benefits and that it could get us

Chapter 4   Ivermectin Endangered and Recovering

out of lockdowns and curfews and get us back to normal living.

CMO promptly responded that we were not allowed to use it.

I was astounded and I questioned why, and it slipped out of the CMO that Pfizer had instructed that Ivermectin should not be used. I was taken aback that a pharmaceutical company would be the one making such a mandate or recommendation which our CMO was acting on. I quickly checked whether the usual off-label use of drugs no longer applied and later confirmed that the FDA was in fact advocating for more off-label use of approved drugs.

We got to know that Pfizer was bringing Paxlovid onto the market. This was a patentable, expensive, synthetic modern version of the now off-patent Ivermectin. According to the U.S. Department of Health and Human Services, Paxlovid costs US\$530 - US\$700 for a 5-day course per person, distribution is also managed by the federal government. Ivermectin is typically sold at US\$1 to US\$2 per 12mg tablet – An average 5-day course would cost US\$5 to US\$10.

We now know that Paxlovid does not match the high efficacy of Ivermectin, and we have yet to gather evidence of Paxlovid's safety.

This mention of Pfizer as being on top of the chain of command, brought me back to a day when I visited the Ministry to drop off the required application for importation of Ivermectin. I heard a very jubilant and excited Officer who oversaw the vaccination program announce that an email had just arrived from Pfizer. …it was like Christmas had come early.

I fully explained to our Minister how I used the Ivermectin and emphasized how its use could put a stop to this pandemic with its curfews and lockdowns.

I left the meeting with some amount of despondency, knowing that our Minister was misinformed by an international narrative which was being touted by his chief technical officer, the CMO. The Minister did

099

suggest we should have another meeting. Should I have persevered and reached out more to him…. this is for discussion.

Was the CMO's advice to the Minister lawful, and from where did the CMO get her authority? Certainly not from the FDA! In August 2023, the U.S. FDA stated that it had no legal power to prevent doctors from prescribing Ivermectin and that, in a sense, the agency was just "joking" when it issued the advice/suggestion.

In early October 2021, the Medical and Dental Council (MDC) filed a complaint against me.

In the Complaint it was alleged that I committed acts of professional misconducts between February 8, 2021, and August 2021 and continuing by performing my duties as a Medical Practitioner in a negligent and incompetent manner by:

1. *"Prescribing and supplying Ivermectin to her patients as a treatment for COVID-19 in the absence of authorization for such use by the Ministry of Health or the Chief Medical Officer (CMO).*
2. *Contrary to the express advice of the CMO publicly encouraging the use of Ivermectin as a treatment for COVID-19.*
3. *Conducting an 'Observational Clinical Trial of Ivermectin as treatment and prevention against the SARS-CoV-2 virus' without the approval and/or monitoring of any local entity or organization authorized to oversee such clinical trials in the interest of public health safety."*

The complaint further stated the following demands.

1. *"Required Dr. St. Rose to appear before the Council to show cause why disciplinary action, including the suspension or cancellation of her registration should not be taken against her; and*

Chapter 4   Ivermectin Endangered and Recovering

2. *Stated that Dr. St. Rose may be assisted by another person including an attorney-at-law, for advisory only, when appearing before the Council; and*

3. *Stated that the appearance before the relevant Council was not open to the public; and*

4. *Specified that the Hearing would be held on October 1, 2021, at 2pm via the Microsoft Teams virtual platform."*

Negligence is a term that we medical practitioners work to avoid. The mention of negligence implies that something went wrong and usually the outcome is catastrophic. I wondered where this emanated from. No specific complaints were detailed as is customary and required according to the Health Practitioners' Act.

IVERMECTIN FINALLY CLEARS CUSTOMS BUT...

On September 1, 2021, after change of government in July 2021, the shipment of Ivermectin was released by the same Ministry of Health. This amount of Ivermectin was quickly consumed through the pharmacy system with prescriptions. We proceeded to reorder, but this shipment of Ivermectin was illegally withheld from release by customs at the direction of the Ministry of Health.

Notwithstanding the legal action being taken against me, I need to ensure the continuous supply of Ivermectin for our people. I got it from reliable sources. Early in the pandemic, the French government donated hundreds of dosages of Ivermectin to Saint Lucia as part of good relations. The use of the Ivermectin was discontinued in Martinique, French territory and maybe never commenced here in the hospitals in Saint Lucia as our health authorities probably obeyed the advice from Caribbean Public Health Agency (CARPHA), based in Trinidad and Tobago and also Pan American Health Organization

101

(PAHO).

Saint Lucia is signatory to the International Health Regulations (IHR) of the PAHO, which is the division of the WHO responsible for Latin America and the Caribbean. CARPHA is responsible for looking after the affairs of the Caribbean. Each country however is allowed to follow its own dictates, do its own research, and seek to treat and protect their people for optimal health. Doctors who work in public health institutions are constrained in following the protocols and directives from this institution. As a private medical practitioner registered and licensed by the MDC and Allied Health Council as a Herbalist, I need to follow the codes of good medical practice and a Doctor's oath of doing no harm. I follow the advice of the FDA to use approved drugs off-label as the research guides and shows efficacy and continued safety.

On September 7, 2021, I wrote to Honorable Philip J. Pierre, Prime Minister of Saint Lucia, congratulating him on his victory at the polls and for gaining the confidence of the people to lead us. I commended him on his statements…. *"Follow the science……. take responsibility for your health"*. I told him that I was happy that he intends to facilitate the use of the effective tools at our disposal as we fight this surge of COVID-19 infections. I asked him if he knew of my saga in getting Ivermectin landed in Saint Lucia on May 6, 2021, finally released on September 1, 2021. I told him that the 5,000 x 12mg tablets which were finally released will be completely dispensed in a few days.

I also told the Prime Minister about the donation of Ivermectin by the Government of Martinique to the people of Saint Lucia earlier this year that had not been utilized and is presently in storage here.

I suggested that the government sell all or part of this stored Ivermectin to Island Pharmacy so we can continue to supply our people with this essential drug. This did not occur.

Chapter 4   Ivermectin Endangered and Recovering

In fact, my next shipment of Ivermectin, which landed here on October 27 was not released from customs by the Drug inspector.

The MDC invited me to a hearing set for October 2021. At this 4-hour exhausting hearing I believe I was able to convince the Council of my intention to continue to use and advocate for Ivermectin.

My daughter, Amanda, Biomedical Engineer, flew from London where she works to be with me. I was so very thankful to have her with me and also to drive me home and keep me company that night after the hearing.

It was the Creole weekend, and we visited my brother and I danced to Creole music, which Amanda recorded and broadcasted. This dance served to show and console my people that I was remaining strong and cheerful in spite of my persecutors.

While traveling through the countryside and interacting with my patients, staff, colleagues, friends, and some family members, I have been encouraged and thanked for standing up for our freedom and truth. They sometimes expressed remorse and resentment for the way the MDC had treated me. I always implored, cautioned and consoled them with the assurance that justice will prevail. *"Let not your heart be troubled, God is in charge...forgive them who know not what they do and even those who know what they do"*.

On September 27, 2021, I wrote to the CMO about clinical trial with Ivermectin.

"This attached incomplete application which I will be submitting to the Medical Council for clinical trial requires the participation of the Ministry of Health, Wellness and the Elderly Affairs. Accompanying documents are being prepared. Please advise if your Ministry will agree to participate in this collaborative effort. If you agree, please advise when a meeting can be convened to discuss further and lead to

implementation."

In an email response on October 14, the CMO replied to my request for participation of the Ministry in the clinical trial.

However, her email refused to allow clinical trials on the grounds that 'the draft Clinical Trials Act needs to be edited, reviewed and updated' and that 'there is currently no legal framework for human clinical trials'.

At one of the 2 HUMANS ARE FREE public sessions at Constitution Park in Castries on October 8, 2021, "Group of Supporters of Dr. Mary Gilberta St. Rose", led by Fremont Lawrence gave me a copy of a letter sent to Moses Jn. Baptiste, Minister of Health, Wellness and Elderly Affairs. The letter stated that :

"It is with a heavy heart and concern for the health and safety of our citizenry that we write this letter to you in the expectation that what is contained herein will allow good sense to prevail in dealing with this unpresented COVID-19 pandemic, with the potential to decimate our population and do incalculable and possible irreparable damage to our fragile economy. In spite of the current modus operandi currently being employed by the government to stem the COVID-19 infection rate through vaccination, (more onerous protocols and restrictive lockdowns), the virus continues to spread with no end in sight. .... We are aware Hon. Minister, of alternative treatments for patients infected with COVID-19 such as Ivermectin and Hydroxychloroquine. .... "

"Two distinguished doctors namely, Doctor Tess Laurie (world-class researcher and consultant to the WHO) and Dr. Pierre Kory (intensive care specialist physician) both well qualified in their respective fields, have lectured extensively in support of Ivermectin.

However, the WHO, Centre for Disease Control and Prevention

(CDC) and FDA continue to strenuously oppose the use of Ivermectin as a treatment for COVID-19…. We are opposed to mandatory vaccination and believe that an individual has the right to decide on an alternative treatment to the 'vaccine' such as Ivermectin after consulting with his or her doctor.

Furthermore, the Medical and Dental Council of St. Lucia recently served Dr. M. Gilberta St. Rose with Complaint No. 3 threatening disciplinary action against me for successfully treating a COVID-19 patient with Ivermectin in accordance with the Hippocratic Oath, which states, 'According to my ability and judgment, I will choose the treatment I think will benefit the patient and never the treatment I know will do harm.'"

"We believe that the Government of Saint Lucia should be open minded and ready to weigh scientific information from all sides in a fair and impartial process that would lead to a balanced approach to the treatment of the COVID-19 virus.

It is unfair and a gross travesty of justice for the Council to attempt to penalize Dr. St. Rose and by extension, members of the public for exercising their right of choice.

Against this background and in light of the potential catastrophic situation we all will face as a country if we do not change direction and stop running towards the 'pandemic cliff', we trust that you will use your influence among your colleagues, as well as the Medical and Dental Council to let good sense prevail and make the best decisions (even if difficult), in the health interest of our beloved Saint Lucia. We stand ready in whatever way possible to assist in this regard."

This caused the birth of FREEDOM COALITION SLU. We continue to advocate for Freedom, justice, love and truth.

In a document dated December 7, 2021, MDC decided to suspend my license to practice medicine and also issued a fine of EC$ 10,000.00 for carrying out an unauthorized clinical trial; a trial which I did not carry out.

I am a registered and licensed herbalist and so I continued to practice as an herbalist.

I am appreciative of a letter written by Dr. Sonia Roach, Family Medical Practitioner in Trinidad and Executive Director of Caribbean College of Family Physicians, on December 15, 2021, to The President & Members of MDC:

…"It was with a sense of deep sadness and a certain amount of outrage that I received the news of the suspension of Dr. Gilberta St. Rose by your esteemed organization. I do not know all the facts, and as a member of the Committee appointed by PAHO/CARICOM to form CAMC, the Caribbean Association of Medical Councils, I value and appreciate the autonomy of each individual Medical Council within CARICOM, but equally I have noted over the years, the devotion and dedication that Dr. St. Rose has shown to the discipline of Medicine in her beloved country and yours, as well as her ethical and reasoned behavior towards her patients and the delivery of her craft. I know as well that she is not only a qualified allopathic doctor but a leader in her field as a licensed and duly qualified Alternative Medical Practitioner and Herbalist. She therefore has always been committed to her patients, believing that whatever she does brings them no harm, whether this method of treatment is accepted 100% or not by her peers. But this has always been the case for us as doctors-accustomed as we should be to controversies, hypotheses, clinical trials and peer reviews.

The Controversy seems to center around Ivermectin and Vaccination against the SARS-Co-V2 virus.

There has always been the concept of re-purposing of drugs or

Members of the MDC Board-November 2022

Name	Position
Dr. Natasha Innocent - Thomas	Chairperson - Medical Practitioner
Dr. Curlyn Phillips - Jordan	Deputy Chairperson - Dental Practitioner
Dr. Sharon Belmar - George	Chief Medical Officer - Ex-officio member
Dr. Samantha Mathurin	Member - Medical Practitioner
Dr. Sherry Ephraim - Le Compte	Member - Dental Practitioner
Mr. Dexter Theodore	Member - Attorney -at-Law
Ms. Debra Charles	Member - Allied Health Council nominee
Mr. Sibi Gopalakrishnan	Member - Lay Person

Figure2. Members of the MDC Board- November 2022

dispensing them off label without being penalized. I can remember for instance using Propranolol for migraine, Tofranil for nocturnal enuresis, Amitriptyline for nerve pain, and now Metformin for metabolic syndrome or cancer prophylaxis.

I ask myself- in the same way that our CARICOM Medical Councils value their individual autonomy, where have we placed our individual sense of inquiry and independence of thought?

Re Ivermectin- WHO has authorized the use of Ivermectin in COVID-19 in clinical trials only and the jury is still out, since results of all Clinical trials being done are still to be published. Yet doctors like Dr.

St Rose in our CARICOM Region have applied for permission to carry out clinical trials and are yet to receive approval......I can understand the position of the Council since Dr. St Rose has been so open with her opinions and behavior- this may appear to you as hostility and disrespect but I think she has just been deeply convicted, honest and above board. To my mind, your best rebuttal would have been the results of a properly conducted Clinical Trial- prospective or retrospective. If you are so sure that Ivermectin is useless, what do you have to lose...I am writing as an older doctor.......I write to you most respectfully......"

Dr. Roache's advice went unheeded by MDC.

The response from the Ministry of Health about importation of Ivermectin stated that *"The Department of Health and Wellness informs you that out of an abundance caution for the public you will not be allowed to import Ivermectin for use in COVID-19 patients to treat or to prevent COVID-19 in St. Lucia".*

On December 16, 2021, I wrote to Ms. Jenny Daniel, Acting Permanent Secretary, Ministry of Health, Wellness and Elderly Affairs about the release of my second shipment of Ivermectin held at FedEx since October 27, 2021. My letter stated:

"I have looked through the Pharmacy Act and note that only narcotics can be detained by customs.

It has been acknowledged by the Saint Lucia Government that there is currently no legislative framework for the regulation / importation of medications. This was officially recorded in 2012 Saint Lucia Pharmaceutical Country Profile produced by the Ministry of Health in collaboration with the PAHO/WHO. As far as we are aware, there have been no amendments made to the associated pieces of legislation.

Your ministry has erred in law, notwithstanding your policy and are illegally preventing our people from benefiting from the use of Ivermectin. Your ministry is acting in excess of its jurisdiction for whatever reason[s].

From the foregoing it is clear that there is no legal reason or authority to detain the shipment of Ivermectin."

I also sought the expertise of Nigel Edwin, Trade and Customs Adviser, who wrote to Ms. Daniel on December 24, 2021, as follows:

"I wish to challenge your authority and that of the Ministry of Health to deny the importation of a consignment of Ivermectin imported ex FedEx on October 27, 2021, strictly on the grounds of Customs and International Trade law."

Speaking of the Pharmacy Act he cited that it:

"Provides a list of all controlled drugs which includes Ivermectin which can be imported and is imported by other importers under no conditional release.... As I cannot cite any legislative authority, I consider the control measures previously stipulated and administered by your Ministry for Dr. St. Rose and the relevant decision not to release the current consignment, arbitrary and discriminatory from the perspective of International Trade. I am therefore convinced that the action taken by you, or your Ministry is unfair and may be illegal in the circumstances and not in keeping with international standards of practice. In that vein, I submit that your decision not to release the consignment of Ivermectin is inconsistent to the principles of predictability and Transparency as stipulated by Articles 1,2, 5 and 7 of the WTO agreement on Trade Facilitation, an agreement that Saint Lucia ratified by Cabinet Conclusion #634 of 2015. In fact, Article 7 of the said agreement, mandates 'the application of common customs

procedures and uniform documentation requirements for release and clearance of goods throughout its territory'. I am therefore requesting that you review your decision or otherwise I will be requesting that my client seeks judicial review of your actions and that of your ministry......."

The COVID-19 vaccine injection was being rolled out under Emergency Use Authorization (EUA). EUA can continue, if it is shown that no other substance or drug can do that which the substance given EUA does. Use of inexpensive Ivermectin was a threat to the EUA hastily bestowed on the COVID-19 injections.

On February 11, 2022, there was a hearing about the reinstatement of my practice. The MDC claimed that they did not know of the hearing. Another hearing was set for February 18, 2022. MDC did not show up for the hearing. Justice Rohan A Phillip granted leave for me to file for Judicial Review in respect of the MDC's decision against me On December 7, 2021.

The decision of the MDC against me was temporarily stayed until the final determination of the matter before the Court. My registration and license to practice were reinstated with immediate effect and I thank my lawyer David Moyston for making that happen.

I joined my colleagues and friends at the World Council for Health conference in May 2022 in Bath, UK. and I made a presentation.

The experience was educational and uplifting and I was able to make physical contact with friends and like-minded colleagues.

In the meantime, Ivermectin became available in the local private Tapion hospital at an astronomical cost with the increasing evidence of efficacy of Ivermectin. My shipment of Ivermectin was still not released.

We celebrated the 3rd World Ivermectin day 2023 on 29 July, as spearheaded by the World Council for Health. I did a press release

Chapter 4   Ivermectin Endangered and Recovering

and commissioned a short video portraying the PAHO actively suppressing the use of Ivermectin while persons were dying or being long term injured and COVID injections being pushed.

I am thankful for the experience. It has helped me to find my inner strength, deeper Faith in God, experience the love and support of family, friends, my staff, some colleagues, patients and so many other well-wishers who are awake to the depth and breadth of these occurrences…and that we are in this together.

I am also thankful for the diligent and successful work done by my lawyer.

I am grateful for the many individuals, and associations that I have become a part of, for spiritual, social, and professional advancement. I will be continually grateful.

Most importantly it is encouraging and edifying to be a part of World Council for Health as we forge a better way together.

- www.worldcouncilforhealth.org

On a matter of principle these injustices must be arrested and reversed and allow freedom with truth to prevail.

And so, it will be …by the Graces of GOD

SOME NEWLY DISCOVERED OFF-LABEL USES OF IVERMECTIN

- Ivermectin is a semisynthetic, highly active, approved, broad spectrum, anti-parasitic agent.
- Ivermectin can be repurposed for use against DENGUE infection.
- Ivermectin can prevent you from getting sick or dying from the DENGUE infection.
- Ivermectin is effective against all strains of the DENGUE virus.
- Ivermectin can be taken as part of effective treatment for malaria.
- Ivermectin can be effective in the treatment of certain types of cancers.
- A course of treatment for COVID-19 infection and also respiratory syncytial virus [RSV] or other respiratory viral infections is your calculated dose, daily with food for 5 days.
- Ivermectin has been shown to be effective for or as part of the treatment of long haul COVID, caused either by COVID infection or adverse effects from COVID vaccine. Daily doses should be taken for 2 to 3 weeks or longer depending on patient response. Continuing treatment can be 1 dose weekly.

I offered voluntary service to the Ministry via the CMO. She referred me to someone whom I could assist with contact tracing and would promptly want to give 2 to 5 doses of Ivermectin, which would satisfy the need for no quarantine as our research was showing.

It has never been proper for the Ministry of Health or the Chief Medical Officer to interfere with the essential part of the practice of medicine which is the clinical evaluation of a patient and the prescription of safe and effective medications. There have been instances of recommending treatments for some illnesses and sometimes a protocol for treatment is documented for physicians in the public health sector.

It is highly unusual that the health authorities engaged in a dogged interference with the proper use of Ivermectin, which has long been approved as fully safe for human use.

I feel fulfilled that I researched, educated, and used Ivermectin off-label for the benefit of my patients and I know that I saved lives and livelihoods.

I believe I served my patients to the best of my ability and in keeping with my sacred oath as a physician by the Grace of God.

M. Gilberta St. Rose
Dermatologist, Herbalist, Integrative Health Care Specialist

M.B.: B.S. [UWI] ; Dip. [Derm]; MNIMH.
Managing Director - Eden Herbs
Managing Director - Creative Health Centre
3 Reduit Road, Rodney Bay, Gros Islet, PO Box L 3132, Castries, Saint Lucia
Tel/Fax: (758) 452 7308; Tel: (758) 454 8737; Mobile: (758) 460 2967; (758) 286 6191
Email: gsrgstrose@gmail.com; Website; edenherbs.com; Facebook.com/edenherbs

I am a 71 year old widowed, mother of 4, grandmother of 7. I am born in Saint Lucia, West Indies. In 1979, I successfully graduated from the University of the West Indies. [UWI] , Jamaica and Barbados, with a Bachelors Degree in Medicine, and a Bachelors Degree in Surgery- M.B;B.S. In 1971 In January 1972, based on my success in the UWI open exams, I was able to pursue and complete my medical career, having received scholarships from the Canadian and Saint Lucia governments.

I returned home to serve, then got a Commonwealth Scholarship in 1985, to pursue training in General Practice at St. Georges University School of Medicine in London, England. I took the opportunity to complete short courses in Homeopathy, Acupuncture, Hypnosis and Nutrition.

I again returned home to Saint Lucia then returned back to United Kingdom [UK] and self financed my post graduate studies in Dermatology and Phytotherapy [Herbal Medicine] as well as working in the National Health Service in London, England.

From 1994 to present day I live and practice Dermatology, Integrative Medicine and Phytotherapy at our Creative health center, Rodney Bay, Gros Islet in Saint Lucia. From 1996 I started developing my own line of products, Eden Herbs to serve my practice and also to sell at pharmacies and major supermarkets locally, regionally and internationally . You may view my range of 55 products at www.edenherbs.com and interact on my Facebook page www.facebook.com/edenherbs .

I spearheaded and participated in various herbal organizations over the years. I am a founding member of the 42 year old Traditional Medicines of the Islands [TRAMI] Project – www.tramil.net and Caribbean Association for Plant Science, Industry, Commerce and Use in Medicine [CAPSICUM]

Our overall objective has been to educate, propagate and cultivate our Caribbean herbs and encourage persons to make use of those. Integration of herbal medicine into our health care system has been an un-relentless goal.

South America

Chapter
5

Brazil

Dr. Flávio A. Cadegiani

Ivermectin and Brazil
A Love-hate Story in COVID-19

INTRODUCTION

I was one of the few medical doctors who kept on the use of Ivermectin despite all the discouraging actions and threats to our reputation. I firmly believe that our experience with its use has drawn out these vital human traits:

1. Intelligence: to understand the mechanism of action of Ivermectin; why and how it works against the COVID-19 virus in different individuals and
2. Integrity, to avoid succumbing to the highly tempting narrative that killed millions; and
3. Bravery, to confront all the obstacles to my clinical practice, like defamation, loss of employment.

The majority of Brazilian doctors, when facing the worldwide health emergency, have shown to present all these three characteristics. Throughout this chapter, readers will learn a little bit about the Brazilian reality and peculiarities.

HOW BRAZIL PREPARED FOR THE DEADLIEST OF COVID-19 VARIANT

Before we reveal the specific measures that clearly saved thousands of Brazilian lives in, we will first discuss the general situation in Brazil at the time.

Brazil did not experience any significant delay in the distribution of COVID-19 vaccines among the populace. While it was not the very first country to offer a nationwide immunization, Brazil was ahead of many countries with a similar economic rank and status. Brazil did not fight against the vaccines. Some legal impediments may have caused some delays in the emergency use approval of the vaccines but the government accelerated the pace of vaccination.

The medical community in Brazil wanted to save as many lives as they could by employing all the tools that were proven safe and potentially beneficial for COVID-19 patients. And Ivermectin was one of the most powerful tools.

CONTRASTING STUDIES CONDUCTED IN BRAZIL

Brazil held one of the randomized clinical trials on Ivermectin for COVID-19, and it was seemingly designed to fail. Several flaws were encountered in the protocols, including the absolute lack of any adverse effect in the Ivermectin trials, when compared to the placebo effect. It is known that Ivermectin may cause diarrhea, so the absence of data on adverse effects is implausible. It makes us wonder if Ivermectin was ever used in any of the groups, OR in both groups, Also, investigators were unable to explain the source of the Ivermectin, which is another red flag. Curiously, the principal investigator of the trial has a history of collaborating with Big Pharma in conducting studies on expensive drugs for patent. These facts beg the question, is this really an authentic study or an attempt to totally discredit the efficacy of Ivermectin?

On the other hand, Brazil also held the largest observational study on Ivermectin, with more than 220,000 persons, in the Southern state of Santa Catarina. In July 2020, a few months after the outbreak of the pandemic, the city of Itajaí, Santa Catarina, offered a citywide program of protection for its citizens. Under the program, Dr. Lucy Kerr and her team, started recommending and providing free Ivermectin on a schedule of two consecutive days, every 15 days as prophylaxis. When results of this period were analyzed, the efficacy of Ivermectin as prophylaxis for COVID-19 was as high as 90%, when used regularly.

While the neighboring cities experienced case-fatality rates increasing more than 50%, Itajaí presented a rate of 22% fatality even though the majority of its population did not use Ivermectin in the long run. Effects would have been better if at least 10% of the population had continued in the program.

To corroborate the findings of Itajaí, a deeper analysis was conducted. Tests on regular Ivermectin users showed a reduction in COVID-19 infection rates (Figure 1), in the first 15-day cycle. The findings also showed a reduction in deaths from COVID-19, which previously was as high as 98% (Figure 2). Different angles were even used to analyze the data, and which consistently provided positive results (Figure 3). When accumulated doses in the previous cycles reached 240mg to 300mg (more than 50 tablets of 6mg), the chance of dying from COVID-19 basically dropped to zero, as seen in Figures 4, 5, and 6.[1]

Despite these encouraging results, we observed a pattern of coordinated destruction of the image of repurposed drugs used as therapies for COVID-19. Mainstream Media and social media bombarded the public with disinformation to discredit and disqualify Ivermectin as an effective protection measure against COVID-19. The anti-Ivermectin campaign hit hard in Itajaí, which made people more afraid of Ivermectin than COVID-19 itself.

We had prepared a thorough research project to conduct a trial with high doses of Ivermectin. Named H(DIVA)-CoV (High Dose Ivermectin Administration – COVID-19), it can be found in clinicaltrials.gov. Unfortunately, we failed to obtain a budget for this trial, thus its premature demise.

APPLYING BIOETHICAL PRINCIPLES IN THE USE OF IVERMECTIN

The program used in the city of Itajai, in the state of Santa Catarina, fully supports the basic human principles of bioethics which are respect

Chapter 5   Ivermectin and Brazil

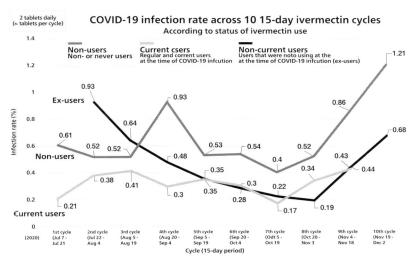

Figure1. COVID-19 infection rate in non-Ivermectin users, current users, and previous users, throughout the Itajai Ivermectin program.

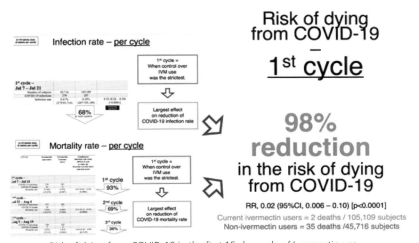

Figure2. Risk of dying from COVID-19 in the first 15-day cycle of Ivermectin use.

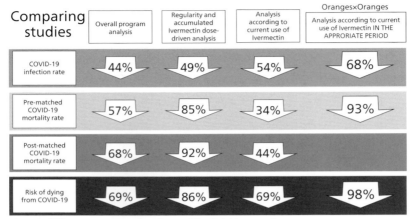

Figure 3. Different manners of analyses of the Itajai Ivermectin program.

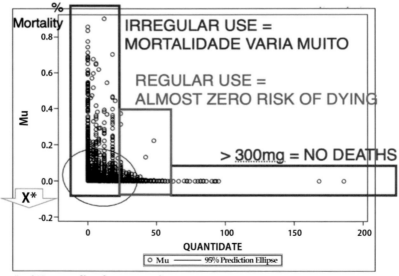

*< 0% mortality does not exist

Figure 4. Comparing regularity and the total of Ivermectin use and COVID-19 mortality rate.

Chapter 5 Ivermectin and Brazil

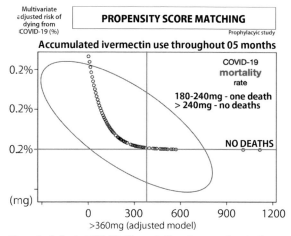

Figure5. Adjusted COVID-19 mortality rate according to the accumulated Ivermectin use.

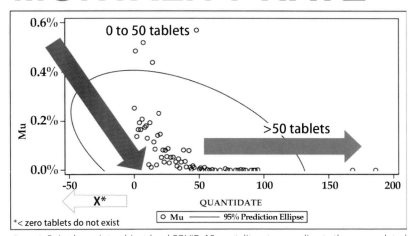

Figure6. Point-by-point, subject-level COVID-19 mortality rate according to the accumulated number of Ivermectin tablets used.

for persons, nonmaleficence, beneficence and justice. The principle of beneficence, which supports the use of emergency medicine in the absence of effective therapeutic alternatives – was the key argument for the emergency use approval of the COVID-19 vaccines. In a similar vein, Ivermectin which is known to be extremely safe is now shown to also be effective against COVID-19. Its potential benefits, combined with its proven safety and cost-effectiveness all reinforced the importance of the drug in ending the pandemic.

Medical societies and health organizations acknowledged the safe use of Ivermectin but deemed it too 'mild'-- insufficient for the treatment of COVID-19. The pharmaceutical companies justified the emergency use of the vaccines by citing the surmounting deaths caused by COVID-19. To increase the confidence of the public to the new treatment, they underplayed the long-term safety profile of these prematurely tested vaccines. When the vaccines were approved, they were still in Phase 3 trials and untested in humans.

A single-drug therapy is unlikely to be 100% effective against a complex disease such as COVID-19. Clinical trials on Ivermectin done early in the pandemic, required the drug to be offered as monotherapy, and introduced in the 4th to 5th days after the appearance of the symptoms. This was in complete contrast with what we learned about testing for interventions against COVID-19. The window to test drugs was almost always within 72 hours and testing was done with a combination of drugs such as Paxlovid.

Ivermectin sales and statistics reveal that approximately 80% of the Brazilian population used Ivermectin or nitazoxanide in their first episode of COVID-19. In contrast, only 16% of the Brazilian population had received the bivalent COVID-19 vaccines (as of November 2023). The 2022 national elections in Brazil were theoretically split 50/50 between right and left political orientations. Yet the majority of leftists, who supported COVID-19 vaccines and were against early treatments, were employing protocols that did the exact opposite. A significant majority of the population were afraid to express their actual opinions. Talking to patients with different political orientations, I believe that opinions held in private were far from positions shown in public.

As doctors in a low-to-middle income country, it is our duty to provide affordable treatment options. Likewise, it is the government's duty to determine the most cost-effective medical technologies for its population. It was thus unusual that the Brazilian government favored a drug like Paxlovid, which not only cost billions of dollars but also failed to reduce or eliminate mortality rates for long COVID.

Braving coordinated attempts to silence us, we published an observational study of 585 patients in mid-2020, comparing the effects of Ivermectin, hydroxychloroquine, and nitazoxanide, and to compare their results with those untreated subjects. We wanted to identify the most promising option among these three repurposed drugs.

Surprisingly, the difference between treated and untreated subjects was significant, in a manner that opened some ethical issues. We saw that we needed to conduct randomized clinical trials with a pure placebo in one of the arms just to confirm the results of our RCTs. Our solution was to follow a Standard of Care (SOC) accordingly, with at least one of the three drugs used as an 'active' SOC. The drug to be tested would be administered as an add-on therapy, instead of single drug therapy. (Figure 7) [2]

Cities that adopted early treatments for COVID-19 are coincidentally the areas with the lowest case-fatality ratios. These include the States of Santa Catarina and Distrito Federal, and the city of Porto Feliz, in the state of São Paulo. In Figure 8, are three examples of cities that adopted early treatment with Ivermectin. They were compared to cities with similar access to healthcare and levels of

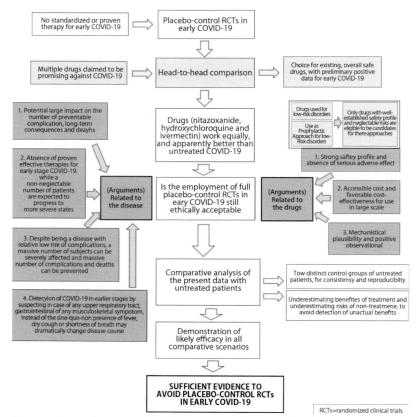

Figure7. Conclusions regarding the observational study that compared treated to untreated subjects for COVID-19.

human development that did not adopt early treatment, showing an alarming difference of more than 50% in their case-fatality ratios.

When the Gamma variant surged, we promptly noticed that none of the treatments were being sufficiently effective: Ivermectin, hydroxychloroquine, nitazoxanide, anti-androgens, and even glucocorticoids and anticoagulants in the later stages. Using our past learnings, we found an urgent solution. By increasing the dose of

Chapter 5   Ivermectin and Brazil

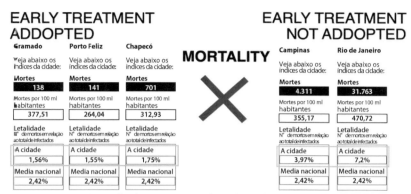

Figure 8. COVID-19 case-fatality rate in cities that adopted early treatment (left) compared to similar cities that did not adopt early treatment (right).

Ivermectin to doses as high as 1.0mg/kg/day for 05 days, and combining it with 5 to 8 other drugs, we observed a dramatic improvement. I created and named this protocol COVID-21 BRA and shared it with medical practitioners throughout the country. This treatment has since then been widely used and has saved hundreds of thousands of lives.

THE IMPRESSIVE STORY OF THE AMAZONIAN CITY THAT SURVIVED THE MOST LETHAL COVID-19 VARIANT

One critical evidence of the efficacy of Ivermectin in COVID-19 as a prophylaxis, was the happy lack of patients in the middle of the Amazon.

This is a shocking story that occurred during our trial of hospitalized patients, for another drug for COVID-19 at the height of the Gamma variant transmission. This true story happened in a number of cities in the state of Amazonas, in Central Amazon. All cities in that region had no available hospital beds, leaving thousands of ill people lined up along hospital aisles, suffering from dyspnea or difficulty in breathing.

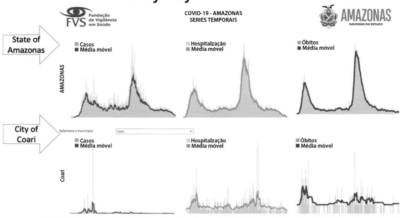

Figure9. COVID-19 cases (left), hospitalizations (middle), and deaths (right) in the whole state of Amazonas (top) and in the city of Coari (bottom).

Each of these patients also required high oxygen flow – which was typical of the Gamma variant outbreak.

When we arrived in the city of Coari, we were welcomed by its city mayor and secretary of health. They immediately took us to the main city's hospital. Surprisingly, the hospital was empty, with just a few hospitalized patients, and even fewer requiring oxygen use. That scenario contrasted dramatically with all the other cities we had visited previously. It was worth noting that the city of Coari was surrounded by cities that were facing the most severe health outbreak in their history. As I tried to understand this stunning discrepancy, I had to discreetly investigate what may be keeping the number of hospitalized patients very low. Because the City's Secretary of Health was reluctant to divulge the reason why, I then invited her to talk privately. I discreetly asked her whether they had used any medication as a prophylaxis. She answered rather emotionally that they distributed

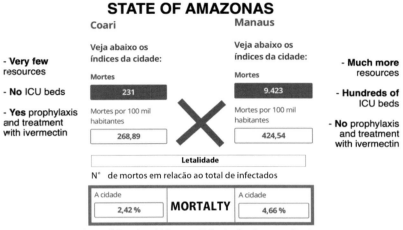

Figure10. Comparison of Coari and Manaus Cities in the Amazon Region

dozens of thousands of Ivermectin tablets throughout the city of Coari as soon as the Gamma wave struck. It is estimated that between 60% to 70% of the city population took Ivermectin both prophylactically, and upon the appearance of the first symptoms of COVID-19 (where patients did not wait for a medical diagnosis).

Figure 9 shows the cases, hospitalizations and deaths due to COVID-19 in the city of Coari (bottom), compared with the entire Amazonas – top). In Figure 10 we compare the capital city of Manaus, and Coari, a city with fewer resources. Despite the scarcity of resources, Coari had half of the mortality rate of Manaus.

MORTALITY RATES IN THE PLACEBO ARMS BETWEEN DIFFERENT HOSPITALS

Following my Hippocratic oath, I served as the principal investigator for double-blind, randomized clinical trials on different drugs. One of these drugs was called proxalutamide, a very strong non-steroidal anti-androgen for prostate and breast cancer. Although patented, it was relatively inexpensive.

In the first trials, early stage COVID-19 outpatients who received proxalutamide experienced spontaneous improvements in inflammatory and thrombotic markers, without requiring the use of steroid glucocorticoids and anticoagulants. As a result, we tested proxalutamide in hospitalized COVID-19 patients.

The trials were conducted on later-stage, moderate-to-severe,oxygen-using patients with very low oxygen levels. When the Gamma variant hit Brazil. Gamma (P.1), as said before, was the most pathogenic variant we ever faced, and even high-dose Ivermectin therapies were insufficient in containing the progression of the illness. Interestingly, the aggressive Gamma variant spared regular Ivermectin users.

Proxalutamide led to reductions of almost 80% in the mortality rate as compared to the placebo arm.

However, what called our attention was the heterogeneity of the mortality rate in the placebo arms.

As a double-blind, randomized clinical trial, proxalutamide or placebo were provided as an add-on to the standard-of-care (SOC) therapy. Consequently, the SOC of each hospital was different as it was not established by the investigators. Rather, the medical directors and the hospital medical staff decided on the SOC.

The hospitals commonly used high-dose glucocorticoids, full anticoagulation therapy, and broad-spectrum antibiotics, as they all observed that these agents did prevent deaths at the height of the COVID-19 pandemic.

The mortality rate among those who received the placebo (instead of proxalutamide) and avoided Ivermectin was 50%, whereas those in the placebo arm that used Ivermectin had a mortality rate below 35%. The combination of Ivermectin and proxalutamide led to an almost-zero death rate in severely ill patients with extremely low oxygen levels.

THE (HIDDEN) WIDE IVERMECTIN USE IN BRAZILIAN COMPANIES AND INDUSTRIES

In a developing country like Brazil, laws protecting employees against employers are very strong in order to prevent exploitation and slave labor.

However, these laws may also prevent some good intentions, when they do not conform with regulations.

One company from the region of Brasilia, in the Brazilian Savannah (termed as 'Cerrado'), provided Ivermectin to their 3,000 workers weekly (or biweekly) basis. For these workers, working from home during the lockdown was not an option.

Of the 3,000 employees, 2,700 regularly took Ivermectin. As of January 2022, less than 30 workers got COVID-19 with only 1 hospitalization. Of the 300 that did not take Ivermectin regularly, 150 contracted COVID-19. Of the 150 cases, 100 took Ivermectin for treatment, with 2 hospitalizations. Of the 50 who did not take Ivermectin, there were 7 hospitalizations and 3 deaths. These are statistically significant differences. Unfortunately, this company's case is considered anecdotal since it was not designed to be a study, and controls were not strictly in place.

Another company from Southern Brazil that provided Ivermectin both prophylactically and as early therapy for COVID-19 for its 1,500 employees did not have a single death.

A third company with 120 employees had a full agreement between employers, employees, and the company doctor in charge that all employees would take Ivermectin on a regular basis. The company provided critical services to infected subjects from June 2020 until December 2021. Not a single case of COVID-19 infection was reported despite the prolonged exposure. This could be considered a 'single-arm study', that shows how Ivermectin had protected the laborers.

BRAZILIAN DOCTORS VERSUS BRAZILIAN DOCTORS: WHEN NUMBERS SPEAK FOR THEMSELVES

As observed throughout the world, there were Brazilian doctors who fought against the use of Ivermectin, hydroxychloroquine, or any early treatment for COVID-19 and were quoted in the mainstream media. Conversely, there were highly respected doctors who defended treatments with repurposed drugs but were unfortunately silenced and persecuted.

The doctors who treated COVID-19 patients with a variety of drugs including Ivermectin reported a zero or below 0.5% mortality rate. The rare deaths occurred in patients that had sought treatments after the 4th to 5th day of appearance of symptoms.

Conversely, doctors that only provided treatments whenever the person became severely ill and needed oxygen or hospitalization, had mortality rates varying between 1.5% to 3.0%.

Since each of these doctors treated thousands of patients, the differences resulting from the comparisons were brutal.

IVERMECTIN BEYOND COVID-19

I have witnessed an astonishing case where Ivermectin has produced pleiotropic effects. Here is a case of a couple in their 70s who first visited me at the beginning of the pandemic. Both had type 2 diabetes with glycated hemoglobin (HbA1c) of 9.9% and 8.7%, respectively, as well as severe and mild fatty liver disease (Non-Alcoholic Fatty Liver Disease – NAFLD). They could not visit their doctors during 2020 and 2021 due to the risk of COVID-19– but continued taking their medications and maintained their diets. They were given a daily dose of Ivermectin: 0.2mg/kg/day for 2 consecutive years. Considering their age and the natural progression of type 2 diabetes, NAFLD, I was expecting a deterioration in their health. Surprisingly, they were not only asymptomatic but were feeling very well, with no decrease in their cognitive function. They did not receive any vaccination, yet they had not experienced any COVID-19 infection. The man's results revealed substantial improvements, from 9.9% to 6.3% in his HbA1c, disappearance of the NAFLD, and improvement of his alanine transferase (ALT) levels, from 87 to 22 U/L. High ALT levels in the blood are indicative of liver injury or disease. His wife improved from 8.7% to 6.6% HbA1c, was fully remitted to the NAFLD, and her ALT decreased from 37 to 17 U/L. I dare to attribute these improvements mainly to Ivermectin.

In a secondary analysis of the Itajai program, it was observed that hospitalized patients given Ivermectin, had significantly lower levels of creatinine (Figure 11), highly sensitive C-reactive protein (hs-CRP) (Figure 12), and alanine transferase (ALT) (Figure 13), compared to age-

KIDNEYS IN HOSPITALIZED PATIENTS

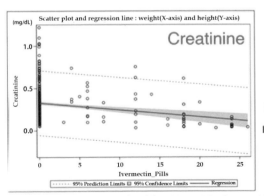

Figure 11. Patients hospitalized for COVID-19 who used Ivermectin prior to their illness exhibited zero incidence of kidney damage

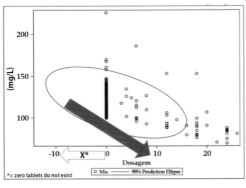

Figure 12. Inflammatory marker hs-CRP in hospitalized COVID-19 patients.

, sex-, and comorbidity-matched subjects who did not use Ivermectin prophylactically. This only means that, while these were a group of people that did not respond to Ivermectin for COVID-19 treatment, they still demonstrated long-term and residual liver and kidney protection, as well as the anti-inflammatory properties of Ivermectin.

THE LACK OF EFFECTIVE TREATMENTS AS A SINE-QUA-NON FOR 'COVID-19 VACCINES'

The Brazilian Health Regulatory Agency (Anvisa – Agência Nacional de Vigilância Sanitária) became a member of the International Council for Harmonization of Technical Requirements for Pharmaceuticals for Human Use (ICH). By becoming a member of ICH, Anvisa adopted international standards in their decision-making and protocols.

If the strict criteria of efficacy and safety had been followed, it would have taken two to three years of rigorous testing before the vaccines could be approved. The lack of effective therapies for worsening COVID-19 epidemic became a condition for the emergency

LIVER IN HOSPITALIZED PATIENTS

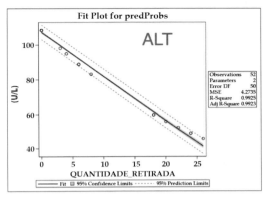

Figure 13. Patients hospitalized for COVID19 who used Ivermectin showed significantly low ALT (alanine transaminase) levels. The present of ALT cells in the blood is a sign of liver damage

use authorization of the vaccines.

It is not surprising that an orchestrated campaign against inexpensive COVID treatments began at the same time as the clinical trials for COVID-19 vaccines. Due to the massive investments in accelerated research for a COVID-19 vaccine, the pharmaceutical industry needed a 'guarantee' that the resulting product would be used widely. This meant that other medicines or repurposed drugs would no longer be promoted as effective therapies for COVID-19. This could be why Pfizer discontinued clinical research for Paxlovid (as part of a treatment protocol for COVID-19), despite its strong 'biological plausibility'. Their own vaccines were approved in major countries.

In an extreme health emergency with surmounting fatalities, all available treatment remedies should have been made accessible. Many have questioned why the supposed "lack of effective alternatives" was being pushed as a basis for the approval of the COVID-19 vaccines.

Brazil has served as a major test country for many of the COVID-19 vaccine trials, as well as for "designed-to-fail" trials of repurposed drugs. Despite being a low-to-middle, peripheral country, Brazil's Ministry of Health, acting on the recommendation of the 'Scientific Council' (Conitec – Comissão Nacional de Incorporação de Tecnologias no Sistema Único de Saúde) and with approval from Anvisa, spent billions of dollars on COVID-19 vaccines for its 215 million citizens.

This same council – which I was a part of, recommended against repurposed drugs, after conducting masked standardized tests with an uncharacteristic rigor that was absent in the COVID-19 vaccine trials. Interestingly, at the end of 2022, the International Council for Harmonisation of Technical Requirements for Pharmaceuticals for Human Use (ICH), together with the US Food and Drug Administration (FDA), the European Medicines Agency (EMA), and Health Canada published a paper on the importance of integrating real-world evidence into regulatory decisions. If this paper had been released earlier in the pandemic without the suppression of evidence on the efficacy of repurposed drugs, we would have received official approval and access to non-patented, low-cost, indisputably safe and effective medicines for COVID-19.

In February 2023, the FDA mentioned in a report that it a 'long history' of using 'real-world data' (RWD) and 'real-world evidence' (RWE). I am curious to know if they had indeed employed RWD and RWE when assessing the therapeutic alternatives, such as repurposed drugs. These have been conveniently 'forgotten' so the vaccines could be approved 'without risks' to the investors.[3]

THE FIGHT AGAINST PROHIBITION OF IVERMECTIN USE IN BRAZIL

In any business, risks must be minimized. In the pharmaceutical industry where millions are invested in research, risks must likewise be minimized.

In the first trimester of 2020, the early stages of the pandemic, medical doctors and the mainstream media said that repurposed drugs could be helpful in selected cases and were undoubtedly safe. The health authorities, following the principle of bioethics, announced that while the development and approval of COVID-19 vaccines should be accelerated, their efficacy and safety should not be overlooked, for these new treatments like the mRNA vaccines (Pfizer and Moderna).

With the increase in spending on the development of the COVID-19 vaccines, one observed a growing coordinated campaign versus early treatments and their proponents who were presenting real-world, frontline evidence of the effectiveness of safe repurposed drugs.

Since the Brazilian President, Mr. Bolsonaro, supported the use of these drugs like Ivermectin, hydroxychloroquine nitazoxanide, albendazole, he became the target of a smear campaign.

The Brazilian Board of Medical Doctors or Conselho Federal de Medicina (CFM) was the authority in charge of inspecting medical prescriptions. CFM was pressured to control or prohibit the prescription of Ivermectin. It is interesting to note that, the acceleration of the vaccination program in Brazil was parallel to the sharp rise in the number of deaths per day, due to the most deadly variant, P.1 (Gamma). These vaccines may only have mildly helped the elderly population.

THE ESSENTIAL ROLE OF THE BRAZILIAN BOARD OF MEDICAL DOCTORS

The Brazilian Board of Medical Doctors or CFM has historically protected doctors' autonomy to prescribe the most effective treatments for each patient. I recall Hungarian physician Semmelweis and his anti-infection protocols and the destruction of his reputation as a valuable lesson in the history of medicine. Semmelweis was a pioneer in hand washing and other disinfectant methods but was continually criticized by the medical community in 19th century Europe.

It is essential to remember that medical autonomy must be balanced with patient safety and regulatory guidelines to prevent malpractice.

Evidence has shown that repurposed drugs are safe and have been used to treat a growing number of diseases. As such, their therapeutic benefits are yet to be fully determined. Prompt solutions are needed when lives are being lost is the justification that was used for the emergency approval of COVID-19 vaccines. It was also used as the reason why repurposed drugs like Ivermectin were shunned as effective treatment for COVID-19.

Allowing patients access to potentially beneficial therapies, as well as providing them with full information on these therapies, is based on the equity and justice principles of bioethics.

The strong biological plausibility combined with the positive preliminary evidence and positive response observed in the medical frontline, is more than sufficient proof to adopt these therapies, since no other therapies were available for the treatment of COVID-19.

Despite the attempt to blame Ivermectin on liver injuries by using fabricated data and invented stories, not one single case of hepatitis or kidney injury could be attributed to Ivermectin, providing further obvious evidence of its safety.

Our initial observations to determine whether Ivermectin, nitazoxanide, and hydroxychloroquine had any reaction (between treated and untreated subjects) was quite encouraging. Because the outcomes showed positive signs of patient progress, we decided that it would be unethical to employ full placebos without an active standard-of-care in the following randomized clinical trials. At the onset of the pandemic, patients were facing potential harm due to the lack of an effective treatment.

Chapter 5   Ivermectin and Brazil

Any attempts to restrict or prohibit any sort of safe intervention or treatment would be in conflict with the principles of the Brazilian Ethical Medical Code. Thankfully, the Brazilian Board of Medical Doctors remained solid in their ethical principles and chose to let our doctors be doctors.

ENTRANCE INTO FLCCC AND THE CONTRIBUTION OF BRAZIL TO THE WORLD

The Front-Line COVID-19 Critical Care (FLCCC) Alliance started in 2020 with two world renowned doctors, Dr. Paul Marik and Dr. Pierre Kory, who were unsatisfied with the censorship of clearly effective interventions against COVID-19. FLCCC became famous worldwide among those of us who remained faithful to our ethical principles of healthcare. COVID-19 treatment was heavily based on moderate doses of Ivermectin combined with vitamins for early exposure, and later, Ivermectin with anticoagulants and glucocorticoids in the inflammatory phase.

In early 2021, Brazil was invaded by the deadliest SARS-CoV-2 variant, Gamma (P.1). which originated in the Amazon region. Doctors that were successfully treating their patients noticed that the usual treatment, that included Ivermectin, was losing its effectiveness.

Studying the pathophysiology of the Gamma variant, I proposed a high-dose Ivermectin treatment regimen combined with drugs like nitazoxanide and antiandrogens and increased the doses of glucocorticoids. In the later stages of the disease, we added large-spectrum antibiotics. This protocol, which was introduced within 48 hours from onset of symptoms, rapidly changed the course of the disease. We have learned and improved the level of care of these patients, and those who followed this updated protocol were no longer requiring hospitalizations, with few exceptions.

141

When the Delta (the second most lethal SARS-CoV-2 variant) manifested in the USA, Pierre and Paul reached me to discuss options to improve the treatment protocols because the previous FLCCC protocol was not as effective as before. I then joined this great organization, hoping to contribute what I had learned from my experiences in Brazil. We introduced more options such as nitazoxanide and antiandrogens, recommended even more molecules to be used as treatment and introduced higher doses of Ivermectin. These recommendations were extremely helpful to the thousands of doctors that followed the FLCCC guidelines and their patients. Thus, making Brazil a major contributor of new information about high-quality COVID-19 treatments that would spread to different parts of the world.

TESTIMONIALS FROM BRAZILIAN DOCTORS AND SCIENTISTS – A MUST-READ

We had the honor of receiving testimonials from leading doctors and scientists in Brazil who raised their voices in defense of Ivermectin. These testimonials may be heartbreaking, but they are based on well-documented procedures that follow the scientific requirements. While some of the testimonials may seem to be redundant, they actually demonstrate the consistency of observations from many doctors and scientists widely distributed across a large country.

1. WHAT IS IVERMECTIN

Tribute to Dr.Satoshi Omura

Lucy Kerr, MD

Ultrassound Specialist, Head of the Itajaí Ivermectin Study

Ivermectin comes from nature and is a semi-synthetic derivative belonging to a group of avermectins from Streptomyces avermectinius. Avermectins are a group of chemical compounds that were found to treat a number of parasitic infections. Discovered by Satoshi Omura in 1973 in a Japanese golf course soil sample, it is formed by two avermectins in the following proportion:

- 80% 22.23 - dihydroavermectin B1a
- 20% 22.23 - dihydroavermectin B1b

What is most remarkable to me are its wonderful effects in curing countless diseases and pathologies, which have affected large populations. It is a multi-target and multi-action drug, proven to inhibit the replication of 22 viruses, including SARS-CoV-2.

Ivermectin binds to the host's tissues in several ways:
It was found to have an ionophoric effect on gram-positive bacteria, which means it is able to block the virus as it circulates in the blood (before the virus reaches the cell membrane). When it is three levels deep in the cell membrane, Ivermectin prevents the cell receptors from allowing the virus to enter the (cell) nucleus.

It thwarts the SARS-CoV-2 virus mRNA strand from occupying the Golgi apparatus and also prevents inactive viral microproteins from becoming harmful to its host.

It neutralizes alpha and beta importins, which transport molecules through the pores of the nuclear membrane, that would halt the formation of the virus and inhibit its spread throughout the body.

There are countless (yet untold) stories of people who were saved from COVID-19 by Ivermectin's multiple actions in all phases of the disease. Thank you, Dr. Satoshi Omura, for your discovery!

We have mentioned earlier the multiple therapeutic properties of this medicine which has been on the WHO list of essential medicines since 1981. Ivermectin is shown to prevent inflammation of the heart, kidneys, and liver without causing any damage to these organs.

It also is worth noting that Ivermectin is a potent treatment for type 2 diabetes as it acts on the FarnezoidX receptor in the liver. This receptor controls the metabolism of glucose, insulin, cholesterol, triglycerides and bile salts. It is also shown to reduce liver fibrosis.

Ivermectin's remarkable immunomodulatory properties which stimulate or suppress the immune system, may be useful in the body's response to cancer.

It was discovered that Ivermectin has potent antineoplastic (cancer-fighting) properties. Ivermectin is the only drug that acts on triple negative breast cancer, which is known to be resistant to all traditional forms of oncological treatment.

Ivermectin is also the only one that acts against the Multidrug Resistance gene (MDR), which is responsible for the recurrence and metastasis of cancers by targeting cancer cells that have resisted even the most potent chemotherapy drugs.

For this and much more, we are deeply grateful to Prof. Dr. Satoshi Omura for his very important discovery of the bacterium Streptomyces avermectinius.

2.ADDITIONAL EFFECTS OF IVERMECTIN

Ellen Guimarães, MD
Board Certified Cardiologist

I was surprised and dismayed by the response of the medical and scientific community to the COVID-19 pandemic. Instead of looking for solutions that could quickly restore normality and reduce the panic spreading among people, we went exactly the other way. A glaring example of this is the repositioning of Ivermectin.

At the beginning of the pandemic, my colleagues and I studied intently the promising preclinical studies that showed the biological plausibility of Ivermectin's antiviral action against coronavirus. We were disappointed to see how some medical authorities downplayed this information and even created obstacles to its mainstream use by overestimating side effects of a drug with a known safety profile.

Despite these countering efforts, we read encouraging results from the first observational studies and randomized clinical trials. The studies showed anti-inflammatory and immunomodulatory actions of Ivermectin in both phase 1 (viral) and phase 2 (inflammatory) of COVID-19. We also learned about its effective pre- and post-exposure prophylaxis properties.

As we were in a global emergency, we did not hesitate to prescribe the drug, knowing its safety profile. We observed the excellent results in treatment and in pre- and post-exposure prophylaxis. We realized that, if prescribed very early, it alleviated symptoms thereby reducing the number of patients who progressed to stage 2.

While it is true that we did not use it as monotherapy, there was undoubtedly synergy when used in association with some repositioned drugs.

Here is an inspiring success story. At the beginning of the pandemic, a patient from another city contacted me remotely with symptoms of the advanced inflammatory phase of COVID-19. In our initial consultation, his inflammatory markers already were significantly altered with 50% lung involvement, indicating severity of the disease. Ivermectin had been prescribed to him before the results of the laboratory imaging tests were released. Subsequently, I had lost contact with this patient, who did not respond to our calls.

A week later, after continuous search of his family members, I finally found the patient. He expressed concern that he had not been prescribed corticosteroids or anticoagulants (which was given to severe cases at the time). I commented that the patient looked much better than when he initially came to see me. The only treatment he used was the Ivermectin that I had prescribed. From then on, I became even more confident in using Ivermectin and did so extensively with excellent results. It is a shame how the medical community bypassed an accessible and safe treatment, which could certainly have changed the course of so many cases.

3.MY INSTINCT PROVES CORRECT

RICARDO ZIMERMAN, MD
Infectious Disease Doctor, Board Certified
Former consultant at World Health Organization (WHO)
Former consultant at the Ministry of Health of Brazil (MS)
Former consultant at the National Agency for Sanitary Surveillance (ANVISA)
Former Expert ad Honorum in Biosafety at Organization of American States (OAS)

My long-term experience with Ivermectin started in the treatment of disseminated parasitic infections in transplant patients. Therefore, when the COVID-19 pandemic began, we already knew about the excellent safety profile of the drug. Our main concern was whether to consider the use of repositioned agents until significant scientific evidence emerged. However, its multiple mechanisms of action made

Chapter 5   Ivermectin and Brazil

sense from the medical and historical perspective. After all, microbial products thrive throughout natural evolution if they are advantageous and beneficial to other organisms.

My instinct proved correct when numerous studies, initially in silico, and then in vitro, confirmed its potent and versatile action against COVID. The crucial role the drug would play in managing the pandemic quickly became clear. In addition to the safety profile and the extensive tablet supply, Ivermectin has shown action in both phases of the disease, exhibiting not only a multifaceted antiviral action that showed resilience against viral attack, but also an anti-inflammatory and immunomodulatory effects, which are crucial for the thrombo-inflammatory phase of the disease. Therefore, my clinical experience and the extensive body of evidence that was accumulating would prove the effectiveness of the medicine in treating COVID-19.

The field experiences were impressive. During a multicenter randomized clinical trial we conducted, we could not believe that we were unable to register a single case of COVID-19, amid the height of the calamity, in just a single city. The health secretary called us to talk and confessed, strangely embarrassed: "Here, we use prophylactic Ivermectin for our entire population". Ivermectin is the most impressive postbiotic evolution has ever given us. Every time we administer it, we are administering more than just a medication. In fact, we are managing millions of years of natural selection and evolutionary advantage.

4.REMARKABLE POSITIVE OUTCOME

Francisco Eduardo Cardoso Alves, MD
Infectious Disease Doctor, Board Certified
ICU Attending Physician, Emílio Ribas Infectiology Institute - São

Paulo, Brazil
Federal Medical Expert, Ministry of Social Security.
President Director (2015-2020) and Vice-President Director (since 2020) of the National Association of Federal Medical Experts (ANMP)
Expert ad Honorum in Biosafety, SSM/OAS (2021-2022)

During the COVID-19 pandemic, I experienced remarkably positive outcomes while treating patients with Ivermectin. In the first half of 2020, I accessed pioneering studies on the use of this medication to fight the SARS-CoV-2 virus. The observed results were encouraging, showing a rapid and effective response to treatment. When I faced COVID-19 myself, I turned to Ivermectin and experienced a quick clinical recovery.

My experience was not isolated. Fellow medical colleagues who opted for Ivermectin in their treatments reported similar successes. Incorporating Ivermectin into my therapeutic arsenal was a decision based on direct observation and meticulous analysis of available data. Despite numerous published studies questioning the efficacy of this medication, a thorough review of the data and meta-analyses reinforced my conviction about its primary role in combating SARS-CoV-2.

I continue to use Ivermectin in my medical practice, as my use is grounded in my clinical experience and the real-life evidence. Choosing this medication for the treatment of COVID-19 turned out to be one of the best decisions I have ever made in my career. This is not only positively reflected in clinical outcomes but also strengthened my conviction in the power of evidence-based medicine and the importance of always being open to new therapeutic approaches, especially in times of crisis.

5.FINALY WE KNOW

Roberta Lacerda, MD
Board Certified Infectious Disease Doctor

Quoting the eminent Dr. Fernando Antônio Brandão Suassuna on using Ivermectin during the COVID-19 pandemic:

"The first study that caught our attention was a drug repositioning study, where 15 drugs including Ivermectin, and hydroxychloroquine showed an antiviral effect against SARS-CoV-2.

Then came the work from Australia by Caly, et al that showed the efficacy of viral clearing of SARS-CoV-2 in vitro within 48 hours of using Ivermectin with a virucidal effect."

Therefore, two facts were presented with biological plausibility: drug repositioning could be a therapeutic alternative in COVID-19, and Ivermectin had a proven virucidal effect in vitro.

In 2020, we also began to observe a phenomenon that bolsters the power of Ivermectin. For context, Ivermectin was given as prophylaxis for scabies in nursing homes. Both caregivers and residents were administered the drug.

In a home of 27 elderly people, prophylaxis was carried out starting February 2020. On May 18, 2020, the first outbreak of COVID-19 occurred. 5 elderly people in the home tested positive, while some were asymptomatic. Thankfully there were no hospitalizations or deaths among our senior patients.

Likewise, in the 600 inmate Alcaçuz prison, Ivermectin was being administered as early as January 2017 as a prophylactic. None of the inmates presented any cases that required hospitalization or death. In contrast, other long-term care facilities that did not do such prophylaxis had outbreaks of severe COVID among the elderly.

In the first outbreak of the Alpha variant, the predominant groups with severe symptoms were the elderly, obese, diabetic, and hypertensive. All of these patients had morbid conditions associated with the metabolic syndrome, a set of factors associated with heart disease. Metabolic syndrome is also the precursor to all chronic non-communicable diseases.

Another outstanding feature of Ivermectin is its anti-inflammatory action. There was a reduction in the inflammatory lesions in the eyeball that indicate suppression of the inflammasomes that can cause or contribute to the progression of some diseases, such as the inflammatory storm of interleukin and prothrombotic components found in severe COVID-19 cases.

We now are more certain about how the disease affects the body's innate immune response. With the evidence pointing to its the anti-inflammatory and anti-viral action, we can surmise that Ivermectin, with other drugs, can control the patient's worsening condition.

In 2016 the Nobel Prize went to Yoshinori Ohsumi for his research on intermittent fasting and autophagy. Autophagy is the process of recycling damaged or diseased cells that could reduce inflammation. The study cites that intermittent fasting would cause non-selective autophagy - destroying both damaged and healthy cells. Furthermore, this study cited that Ivermectin promoted selective autophagy (mitophagy, pyroptosis, and the destruction of old organelles, such as mitochondria), thus countering the harmful effects of intermittent fasting. This, for me, was the highlight of this study, that would serve to guide all our actions a posteriori.

The CD47 protein, also known as the "don't eat me" protein is produced by SARS-CoV-2 stimulation. This protein can cause a malfunction of the body's innate immune response, since it prevents macrophages from being recognized as infected cells by rearranging the outer membrane of said cells. Ivermectin's immunomodulatory action strengthened the patient's innate immune response.

This was later corroborated by the understanding that the long-lasting COVID immune response was not due to the adaptive immune response of T lymphocytes, B lymphocytes, antibodies or NK lymphocytes but rather it was from the improved innate immune response.

Numerous studies have confirmed the pleiotropic action of Ivermectin. In the first week of November 2023, a work was published on CD47 and cancer cells with the same mechanism as COVID-19, showing the importance of this protein's effect on macrophages. The study's results confirm that the biggest virulence factor in COVID-19 was not its prothrombotic and proinflammatory effect alone, but that the immunodeficiency is linked to the loss of macrophage action and the increased inflammasomes generated from patients with metabolic syndrome (i.e. obesity, diabetes, and hepatic steatosis).

Another important study we found was about the CD147 protein, which works to prevent red blood cells from adhering to platelets, and those platelets to the endothelium, causing microthrombosis. Since Ivermectin could inhibit this protein, it was shown to have anticoagulant action.

Subsequently, other studies showed that Ivermectin reduced inflammation in COVID-19 by reducing the levels of IL6 and IL10, which is typical of the inflammatory storm that caused injury and thrombosis in critically ill patients. There have also been studies proving the action of Ivermectin in reducing oxidative stress, including reducing the synthesis of fatty acids (by inhibiting the farnesoid X receptor in the liver), as well as reducing hepatic steatosis in an animal.

In terms of proposals for action, I always thought that pandemics should be fought first through chemoprophylaxis rather than through immunoprophylaxis - especially because of the well- documented the safety of chemoprophylaxis with Ivermectin. What a disappointment and surprise we had when we learned that one of the safest medicines recognized worldwide for its prophylactic use, and included in the WHO list of essential medicines was being proscribed, defamed, and criminalized in this recent COVID-19 pandemic. What absurdity!

In this context of disinformation, we very cautiously, followed the dosage used in global standards of care (SOCs). We never exceeded a dose of 105 mg daily, which is well tolerated in human use.

Our results from 528 patients treated by telemedicine showed a mortality rate of less than 5%. All of these patients were with comorbidities and had already passed the 7th day of illness without early treatment.

It was during this period that I, an infectious disease specialist trained at UFRN, became a participant in this large study group that, included researchers, infectious disease specialists, epidemiologists, immunologists, and clinicians. By March 2020, there was a terrible schism.

On the one hand, there were those who advocated the need to continue with randomized, placebo-controlled clinical trials in order to analyze the level of evidence and only then suggested that Ivermectin be used as prophylaxis and treatment.

On the other hand, our group, led by Dr. Fernando Suassuna, Dr. Luiz Alberto Carneiro Marinho, Dr. Iara Marques Carrilho, Dr. Rosângela Morais, among many others, stood behind our belief, that the creation of a prophylaxis and treatment protocol for COVID-19 with Ivermectin, HQC, colchicine, corticosteroids, heparin, doxycycline, azithromycin, Bromhexine and in the sequence antiandrogens was the only possible response to save the greatest number of lives during an unprecedented humanitarian crisis in the face of a new and unknown disease. We were driven by the Hippocratic oath, bioethics of non-maleficence, and sufficient evidence of safety, and efficacy in vitro and in animal models. We believe that the most vulnerable, were saved through the prophylactic use of Ivermectin. We started in nursing homes and facilitated the direct purchases from the general public. As a result, we witnessed an abrupt drop in the number of infections and hospitalizations in May/June 2020, coincided with the highest consumption of Ivermectin.

And for this reason, we were persecuted, censored, ridiculed, even prevented from treating our patients in certain private hospitals with these repositioned medicines.

As Dr. Fernando Suassuna has taught us, Ivermectin has an anti-inflammatory and metabolic effect on the body's innate immune response. It is not an antibody-based medicine, where long- lasting immunity to COVID-19 necessitates the use of (vaccine) boosters. For this reason, BCG would be the best vaccine candidate versus COVID-19 because it elicits a much more important immune response through macrophages.

Regarding post-COVID, Dr. Fernando Suassuna once again brings us good news that post-COVID symptoms are related to the inflammasome or autoimmune injury. This explains why even after viral clearance, the pro-inflammatory effects remain with the D-dimer helping as a marker of both inflammatory and prothrombotic conditions.

We began to see an excellent anti-inflammatory response with Ivermectin and improved immune response (with recovery of T, B and NK lymphocyte populations) in post-COVID patients.

Even in psoriasis cases, we also see an important anti-inflammatory action of Ivermectin.

But the most promising aspect of Ivermectin is the recent studies of its selective autophagic action in reducing the breast cancer cell population in vitro.

Unfortunately, this was not what happened in the COVID-19 pandemic, where the evidence pyramid was inverted and doctors were made to wait for randomized clinical trials to be completed before they could be permitted to treat their patients, in a clear violation of the code of medical ethics, and the Declaration of Helsinki on vaccine mandates.

Concluding with a message from Professor Fernando Suassuna:

"In my opinion, Ivermectin will be considered the drug of the century, and it will dominate the field of oncology as it remains undisputed that the problem of the treacherous evolution of (cancer) cells and tumors lies in compromising the innate immune response and inflammation with perennial oxidative stress."

To which I humbly add: This could be true, if the pharmaceutical industry continues spending billions to downplay this clear evidence at our bedsides.

As Sir William Osler would say: *"Do not allow your conceptions of the manifestations of disease to originate from words heard...or read. Observe and then reason, compare and judge. But initially observe. Two eyes never see equally, nor do two mirrors reflect the same image. Let the word be your slave, not your master. Live in the words."*

6.USEFUL AND VERY SAFE

Michelle Chechter, MD
Board Certified Gynecologist

My perception as a doctor is that Ivermectin reduces viremia, or viruses found in the bloodstream including COVID-19. It considerably diminishes the symptoms of inflammation, such as fever, body pain, and headache, and helps with lung recovery when used in conjunction with other necessary vitamins and medications. It is a useful and very safe drug and can be used in several clinical illnesses in addition to COVID-19.

7.NEGATIVE STUDIES ARE OFTEN REMOTE STUDIES

Daniel Victor Tausk, PhD
Ph.D. in pure mathematics in 2000
Associate professor - Mathematics Department - University of São Paulo

My perception is that the totality of randomized controlled trials supports the conclusion that Ivermectin has clinically relevant efficacy, even if a modest one, for the early treatment or prophylaxis of COVID as well as in the reduction of viral load. Earlier results, available at the beginning of 2021, seemed to point towards a large efficacy, but later results, most notably of trials conducted in the United States (such as COVID-OUT and ACTIVE-6), suggest little to no effect. The considerable heterogeneity of trial results, which in my view is not satisfactorily explained, makes it challenging to obtain clear estimates of effect. It should be noted that the effect size could depend significantly on factors such as the number of days between symptom onset and the beginning of treatment, on daily dosage, on whether the drug is taken on an empty stomach, and the duration of treatment.

Randomized controlled trials are usually underpowered, especially in combined meta-analyses, with multiple variables such as hospitalization and mortality. These events have a low frequency among population studies. However, for the reduction of viral load, where statistical power is not a problem, efficacy is more evident. Attempts to explain positive results on viral load reduction by claiming them to be mere products of publication bias (unconfirmed claims of funnel plot asymmetry created by poor choices of small study measures and disregard of between-study heterogeneity) were found to be incorrect. Meta-analyses with "no effect" findings often use one of the following "tricks":

1. focusing on endpoints for which there is little statistical power and then confusing "no statistical significance" with "no effect",
2. discriminate study selection based on questionable criteria,
3. not combining results to reduce statistical power.

There have been rumors that all of the positive studies are either frauds or highly biased. There is absolutely no serious foundation for such rumors. Although one of the positive studies seems to be a fraud and some studies have early exaggerated efficacy estimates, it is crucial to note that the negative studies also have issues. These are often remote studies in which the drug is delivered by mail, and patients were not adequately monitored. Moreover, treatment did not usually start early enough, and adherence to medication was unknown. Authors of such negative studies have never shared any of their raw data.

There have also been attempts to explain positive results by the so-called "worms' hypothesis". According to this hypothesis, what Ivermectin is really doing is just treating worm infections, and without worm infections, patients have better COVID outcomes. In my view, there is no good evidence supporting such a hypothesis, and it doesn't adequately explain the effects on the reduction of viral load. In fact, the existence of such a hypothesis only underscores that positive results

Chapter 5   Ivermectin and Brazil

from randomized clinical trials are undeniable.

At the end of the day, even with uncertainties about the effect size, Ivermectin is clearly a safe and inexpensive drug with few side effects. Therefore, the risk-benefit analysis is certainly in favor of using Ivermectin.

8.NO COVID-19 PATIENT THAT I TREATED DIED

Vinícius Nunes Azevedo, MD

Ivermectin was a fundamental part of my prophylactic and therapeutic arsenal.
Prescribing the medicine at the appropriate times, in the right doses to achieve a therapeutic index, was very relevant aspects in my clinical experience.

My COVID-19 experience is best told through this case: I had a single male patient admitted to Intensive care and under Orotracheal Intubation (OTI). He was an elderly man with extreme health conditions. Finally, the proven safety of Ivermectin provided immeasurable relief to my patient. These emergency medicines and the numerous science-based evidence supporting them, enabled advising doctors to use their professional autonomy to treat their patients. As a patient myself, using Ivermectin for prophylactic and therapeutic purposes, I only lost my sense of taste for 3 weeks and did not have any further consequences.

I am thankful to my physician in the COVID ICU in Brasilia when I contracted the Manaus variant.

Currently, I have been treating shingles and vaccinated patients with autoimmune conditions with monthly doses of Ivermectin and continuous doses of hydroxychloroquine with very interesting and successful results. I eagerly look forward to more studies in this context.

9.ON THE FALLACY OF AUTHORITY

Regis Bruni Andriolo, PhD

As an enthusiast and supporter of the search for the truth about phenomena related to the natural sciences, particularly in the fields of health and the environment, I have witnessed the repetition of historical errors in the use of scientific instruments, which have been replaced by "scientism". I saw, for example, the overestimation of statistical technicalities to the detriment of the empirical and manifest minimization of suffering and death associated with certain choices - an error once pointed out by Austin Bradford Hill in 1965 in his postulate of causality.

I also saw the repetition of the error of placing non-religious faith in institutional authorities (fallacy of authority), including the press - something also highlighted more than a century ago by Monsignor de Segur in the book Revolution Taught to Young People. In it, the author warned us of the unholy efforts of impious newspapers as veritable machines for training the unwary and the ignoble flatterers; what some informally call the clique syndrome.

10.CENSORED TRUTHS ABOUT IVERMECTIN
The drug that scares the pharmaceutical industry

Jandir Loureiro, MD

At the beginning of the pandemic, I was still at a period in my career where I was performing mostly imaging diagnosis in private clinics and in SUS hospitals as a certified radiologist. However, I also had a strong background in emergency medicine, and periodically practiced life support training. Eventually I returned to active duty in emergency rooms because I wanted to reduce the incidence of administering contrast media in the examination room. Shortly after my return in 2020, I started receiving a high number of chest CT scans with suspicious COVID-19 infection. I instantly realized that we were facing a different disease.

At that time, I was already participating in COVID-19 study groups on WhatsApp, communicating with colleagues who did not understand the direction taken by the WHO, especially on early intubation, which we viewed as a dangerous measure that cost many lives. This is why doctors began to consult other colleagues. In one of these groups, we were guided by Dr. Marina Bucar, a Brazilian doctor with roots in Piauí who was practicing in Madrid. She passed on her guidance to fellow doctors from her hometown, who naturally shared the knowledge with the public. Unfortunately, she was defamed for this. Thus, the Médicos Pela Vida group was born, made official by Dr. Antônio Jordão and Dr. Cristiana Altino de Almeida.

I also contributed information on medical practices to combat COVID-19 to the Médicos Pela Vida group. There was already an outpatient, pre-hospital protocol that I used successfully for my wife, an oncology hospital nurse, when she tested positive for COVID-19. I became a doctor for my family, friends, and friends of friends, which enabled me to help many sick people and thus, honor my Hippocratic oath. Soon after, I became an emergency doctor at the Pólo Gripal de Silva Jardim, a municipality that ranked 7th (among the 92 municipalities in the state of Rio de Janeiro) in the COVID-19 death rate. I treated around 900 patients with the flu syndrome from November 2020 to April 2022, with the data available at the Municipal Health Department of that municipality.

The truth about COVID-19 is emerging. We know that it is not just a flu with pneumonia complications, or even an acute respiratory syndrome. It is a systemic disease (affecting the whole body) that has an initial viral phase which may evolve into an inflammatory, pulmonary, and immunothrombotic conditions (bruising and bleeding). The best way to approach the disease is to divide it into phases and treat it quickly, during the initial viral phase. Treatment must be continued in the succeeding phases. Today, we are aware of post-COVID syndrome or long COVID, where pulmonary and thromboembolic sequelae arise. This may be due to the viral load or the vaccine spike protein. What we now have to contend with is that at least 80% of the world's population received at least one dose of the inoculant.

The medication that will make a difference in all phases of COVID-19 is Ivermectin. I will present some data below, based on my clinical experience during the pandemic.

After controversy over whether or not the FDA would release Ivermectin for COVID-19, North American professor Dr. Paul Marik, one of the founders of the FLCCC, spoke about this agency: "The FDA is not a doctor. It has the authority to inform and announce – but not to endorse or advise…" Following this line, both North American and Brazilian doctors can make use of their medical autonomy based on scientific articles and prescribe the drug.

"The FDA suggested that Ivermectin would be a medicine for horses, but it never prohibited American doctors from prescribing it for COVID-19" said São Paulo immunologist, Dr. Roberto Zeballos in yet another censored video on castration platforms. And he's right, Ivermectin wasn't banned in the USA, but the publication on that

Chapter 5　Ivermectin and Brazil

Why You Should Not Use Ivermectin to Treat or Prevent COVID-19

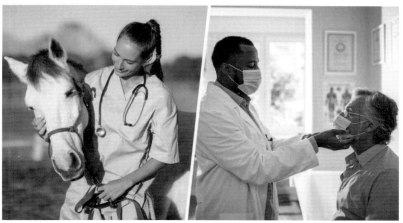

Figure 14. Despite Ivermectin's development from an animal drug and its track record of saving billions of humans from tropical diseases, the US Food and Drug Administration warned against Ivermectin use, calling it "You are not horse. you are not cow." on Twitter.

agency's official Twitter was shocking.

Zeballos, who helped Belém do Pará overcome the first wave of COVID-19 in that capital, recognized the importance of Ivermectin for this disease. He also breaks the silence of Brazilian medical entities who insist that Ivermectin is proven to be ineffective for COVID-19 and uses it when necessary.

Still in June 2020, a few months after the pandemic began, the drug showed inhibitory activity against SARS-CoV-2 in vitro by interacting with importins α/β1. In March 2021, infectious disease specialist Roberta Lacerda said in a memorable radio interview and reproduced the speech of IBRD leader Dr. Tess Lawrie: "Ivermectin has the power to stop the pandemic". They were right, today with 99 studies in 27 countries, the evidence for Ivermectin for patients with COVID-19 continues to accumulate.

For prophylaxis, there are at least 16 studies with the highest levels of evidence, both for pre-exposure and post-exposure. Of these, we highlight one carried out by a North American company in Bulgarian patients, which was multicenter, randomized, double-blind, placebo-controlled and with an independent data monitoring committee. This study meets the most rigorous criteria to classify it as a "gold standard" and should not be ignored. There are many others, and their evolution can be consulted in real time.

And if this drug weren't wonderful, it wouldn't be so attacked by the pharmaceutical industry, and it would never earn its discoverers, biochemists Satoshi Omura and William Campbell, the Nobel Prize in 2005. Furthermore, the award-winning drug belongs to the hall of essential medicines of the WHO and not only that, it changed the lives of thousands of inhabitants of tropical countries suffering from infectious and parasitic diseases. For this reason, African countries that apply parasite prophylaxis with multiple drugs have not had major problems with COVID-19. Nigeria, for example, which is a fan of deworming distribution programs, has a population close to that of Brazil and, throughout the pandemic, reported only 3,155 deaths from COVID-19.

Ivermectin, in addition to preventing mutilating parasites such as onchocerciasis (river blindness) and lymphatic filariasis (elephantiasis), showed favorable evidence in the treatment of 18 RNA and 4 DNA viruses. From that point on, this powerful medicine became a major concern for the multibillion-dollar pharmaceutical industry. The pharmaceutical company Merck denied the antiviral application of Ivermectin, even with increasingly robust studies backing the application.

Dr. Omura discovered the molecule, after noticing a bacteriium with fungal characteristics, Streptomyces avermectinius. He then extracted the "wonder drug" from its substrate. Campbell, linked to Merck, purified the molecule and registered its patent in 1981. Six years later, in a rare gesture of altruism, he released Ivermectin to combat Neglected Tropical Diseases. This changed the natural history of disease in Africa, Asia, and Oceania.

As for the safety of the drug, here is a story of a failed suicide attempt using an overdose of Ivermectin. Even though the African woman used more than 100 times the recommended dose, she only had moderate side effects, and recovered after simple measures.

Another interesting story is of a group of researchers from the University of Alfenas (MG) who conducted a study to relate Ivermectin with elevated liver enzymes. Even with overdoses, they were unable to prove this. Saying that Ivermectin is hepatotoxic is a huge mistake, as it can be prescribed to patients with liver failure. The study certainly confirmed the safety of Ivermectin.

Contrary to what is reported in mainstream media, scientific studies are being published about the hepatoprotective effect of Ivermectin. Yang, S.Y.; et al demonstrate that Ivermectin acts favorably on the liver X receptor and the farnesoid X receptor with multiple potential metabolic benefits. This effect was confirmed by Jin, L et al. Other studies show promising results in protecting against liver fibrosis in mice and possibly humans.

The most recent attempt, also frustrated, was against the observational study from Itajaí (SC) on 220 thousand patients evaluated under the E-SUS primary care system which cannot be tampered. Roberta Lacerda classified the attempt as the "Tupiniquim Surgisphere" because it involved a Brazilian doctor. Surgisphere is a data analytics company known for providing flawed and questionable research data for respected scientific journals.

The results of prophylaxis with Ivermectin in Itajaí were so 'disturbing' to naysayers that, in an attempt to defame the study, the doctor and her team added 245 (fake) deaths (as confirmed with the city's official epidemiological bulletin). This is a shameful attempt at fraud– made worse, by releasing the results in the Medrxiv platform.

Fortunately, Doctors for Life are "vaccinated" against fraudulent scientific journals.

Throughout the pandemic, this pattern of deception was repeated. Whenever a repositioned drug (being cheap, generic, and low-cost) was tested, there was always a reason for checking its efficacy. They just could not explain the disparity in death rates between Brazilian municipalities, where the lowest fatalities were in those places that adopted some form of early treatment, mainly with Ivermectin.

There is no room for arguments against facts and figures. I cite the example of Porto Feliz (SP) which, in addition to using Ivermectin in treatment, also used it in the severely affected neighborhoods as post-exposure prophylaxis. I had the opportunity to carry out a technical visit in August 2020.

In Silva Jardim at Polo Gripal, a part of Rio de Janeiro, Ivermectin was officially recommended at the beginning of the pandemic in 2020 until July 6, 2021, according to the print of the Polo's official protocol. The health department provided free supplies to patients with a doctor's prescription (despite not officially remaining in the protocol), as a result, the municipality maintained 1.4 % fatality rates. When compared with the other 91 municipalities in the state, Silva Jardim remained in 7th place in the COVID-19 death rate (CIEVS-RJ bulletin from the State Health Department of Rio de Janeiro, last update 09/11/2023. See figures 7 and 8). I attribute the low death rate to the fact that an ICU unit was not available in that municipality. This situation postponed patient intubation and non-invasive ventilatory support was provided as the alternative.

Finally, when ANVISA restricted the sale of Ivermectin and nitazoxanide from April to September 2020 (as shown in figure 7) there was an explosion in pediculosis cases, mainly in schools and daycare centers in more remote places in the country where medical access was problematic.

The old slander: "Ivermectin is a medicine for lice" was the strongest reason for the medication to be widely released again without restrictions. Ivermectin is the molecule of life, and every Hippocratic doctor must fight for it. Don't be ashamed of saving lives!

I want to leave a message of hope and solidarity for fellow doctors in the frontlines of the COVID-19 pandemic:

Do not let anyone think for you or make the decision for you. The responsibility to save the patient will be yours alone and is non-transferable.

11. THE GREATEST STORY OF HUMANITY IN THE LAST 80 YEARS

Filipe Rafaeli

Filipe is a Brazilian who has written about the pandemic and published articles in France Soir from France, Brownstone Institute from the USA, and Trial Site News, also from the USA.

In my view, the COVID-19 pandemic represents the most significant event in human history since World War II. Since then, nothing has instilled such terror and fear across the global population.

This pandemic has completely halted the world's activities.

The Cuban Missile Crisis in 1962, when the Soviet Union placed nuclear missiles in Cuba during the Cold War, instilled genuine fear in many, leading some U.S. families to build nuclear bunkers in their homes. However, this episode does not come close to the magnitude of COVID-19.

From the Cold War era, the sense that the world could end with nuclear explosions gave rise to a remarkable culture. Woodstock emerged from this context, as did iconic bands like the Beatles, the Rolling Stones, and Pink Floyd. From the fear of the world's end came the birth control pill and the miniskirt. Global protests in 1968 witnessed young people worldwide seeking protagonism after overcoming their fears—they wanted to live fully.

However, even though COVID-19 instilled panic on a global scale, it is slowly losing relevance. Few people discuss it, and even fewer look back to recount the story.

I understand the reason for this. The official narrative is fragile, susceptible to collapse with any new information. The untold aspect of this story is that there has always been a treatment from the beginning, and one of the main medications is Ivermectin.

The shocking truth is that cheap, generic, and unpatented but effective treatments were sabotaged by a well-orchestrated corporate machinery, resulting in the death of millions. This is hard to believe, even though it echoes the plot of the 2014 Oscar-winning film "Dallas Buyers Club" about AIDS patients who opted for unconventional treatments that were shunned by the medical community."

Since the mid-80s, doctors who chose generic, affordable, and unpatented treatments have been persecuted, humiliated, and fired.

The same pattern repeated itself in COVID-19. Those who prescribed Ivermectin were persecuted, dismissed, and humiliated, but their patients did not succumb. In Brazil, Dr. Cadegiani treated over 4.000 COVID-19 patients with no fatalities. In the U.S., Drs. George Fareed and Brian Tyson treated 3,962 outpatient COVID patients, and none of them died. All those who embraced these treatments (furthering replicating the efficacy of Ivermectin) achieved similar results.

In November 2023, there were 16 studies dedicated to prophylaxis using Ivermectin. Without exception, all these studies presented positive results, including four considered "gold standard" randomized studies.

I started taking Ivermectin regularly since the first prophylaxis study by Shouman came out in Egypt. I began taking it every week. Clearly, in the risk-benefit calculation, taking Ivermectin is already worth it. The medical community has continued to ignore the amazing findings from the 16 studies.

From the moment I started taking Ivermectin, my fear of the disease disappeared. And I continued to see the world as completely crazy, engaged in an insane war against solutions. When I tried to tell as many people as possible about my experience: I was ridiculed, insulted, and censored.

We must keep telling the truth. Sooner or later, people will realize the absurdity of denying the facts, to protect the interests of the giant pharmaceutical companies who are pushing for the vaccines.

In time, people will understand the pandemic, brought out and best and worst in human nature. All we have to do is wait for many people wanting to change the world and, as a result, spark a new Woodstock. I wouldn't miss that for anything.

CONCLUSION:
BRAZIL AS A KEY PLAYER IN EXPOSING THE TRUTH ABOUT IVERMECTIN AND THE PANDEMICS 'GAME' BEHIND THE SCENES

Brazil is a country of contrasts. We endured one of the strongest campaigns to coerce our brave doctors against keeping their Hippocratic Oath throughout the pandemic. Several prestigious institutions and medical 'experts' were pressured to destroy the reputation of Ivermectin and discredit anyone who dared to use it to treat COVID-19. On the other hand, we also had amongst us the greatest support for doctors (by the national medical board of doctors, and the vast majority of our citizens). An overwhelming 80% of the population used Ivermectin when they were infected by COVID-19. We were able to show how Ivermectin and other repurposed drugs could overcome political barriers. Considering the severity of disease and its variants that infected Brazilians, we can clearly say that the bravery of Brazilian doctors and the Brazilian population saved more than 1,000,000 lives by using Ivermectin at different levels. [4]

All figures in this chapter, with the exception of the FDA tweet diagram, are ©Flávio A. Cadegiani.

Chapter 5   Ivermectin and Brazil

Références

1. Kerr L, Cadegiani FA, Baldi F, Lobo RB, Assagra WLO, Proença FC, Kory P, Hibberd JA, Chamie-Quintero JJ. Ivermectin Prophylaxis Used for COVID-19: A Citywide, Prospective, Observational Study of 223,128 Subjects Using Propensity Score Matching. Cureus. 2022 Jan 15;14(1): e21272. doi: 10.7759/cureus.21272.

2. Cadegiani FA, Goren A, Wambier CG, McCoy J. Early COVID-19 therapy with azithromycin plus nitazoxanide, Ivermectin or hydroxychloroquine in outpatient settings significantly improved COVID-19 outcomes compared to known outcomes in untreated patients. New Microbes New Infect. 2021 Sep; 43:100915. doi: 10.1016/j.nmni.2021.100915.

3. https://www.gov.br/anvisa/pt-br/english/international-position
https://www.icmra.info/drupal/en/news/ich_reflection_paper
https://www.fda.gov/science-research/science-and-research-special-topics/real-world-evidence

4. https://www.nature.com/articles/s41591-022-02185-4#Sec2

Flávio A. Cadegiani, MD, MSc, PhD

Board Certified Endocrinologist (Médico Endocrinologista com Título de Especialista em Endocrinologia e Metabologia pela SBEM - RQE 12.398)

Master of Sciences (MSc) degree in Clinical Endocrinology at Federal University of São Paulo (Mestre em Endocrinologia Clínica pela Universidade Federal de São Paulo / Escola Paulista de Medicina (Unifesp/EPM))

PhD degree in Clinical Endocrinology at Federal University of São Paulo (Doutor em Endocrinologia Clínica pela Universidade Federal de São Paulo / Escola Paulista de Medicina (Unifesp/EPM)

Residência Médica em Endocrinologia e Metabologia / Fellowship in Endocrinology and Metabolism

Medical residency in Internal Medicine (Residência Médica em Medicina Interna - RQE 12.397)

Brazilian Medical Registration - CRM/DF 16.219 and CREMESP 160.400

Chapter

6

Argentina

Dr. Héctor E. Carvallo and
Dr. Roberto R. Hirsch

Ivermectin on COVID-19 in Argentina

A TIMELINE OF EVENTS

SARS-CoV-2 outbreak started in Wuhan, Hubei, China, in November 2019 (There are several discrepancies on the exact, initial moment of the outbreak).

First imported case in Buenos Aires: 3 March 2020 (The first case was an Italian tourist, who died two days after hospital admission).

Héctor Carvallo and Roberto Hirsch performed the first in vivo trials on Ivermectin on SARS-CoV-2: *The associated use of Ivermectin, aspirin, dexamethasone, and enoxaparin (in different combinations and doses) reduces the impact of COVID infection 19, the need of admission to the intensive care unit, and mortality. The I.D.E.A. Protocol*
Start: 2020-05-01 Completion: 2020-08-30
ClinicalTrials.gov ID NCT04425863
Later published as: *Safety and Efficacy of the Combined Use of Ivermectin, Dexamethasone, Enoxaparin and Aspirin against COVID-19*

J Clin Trials, Vol.11 Iss.3 No:1000459. March 31, 2021
Usefulness of Topical Ivermectin and Carrageenan to Prevent Contagion of COVID-19 (IVERCAR)
ClinicalTrials.gov ID NCT04425850
Start: 2020-06-01 Completion: 2020-08-10
Later published as: *Study of the Efficacy and Safety of Topical Ivermectin + Iota-Carrageenan in the Prophylaxis against COVID-19 in Health Personnel*
November 17, 2020. DOI: https://doi.org/10.31546/2633-8653.1007

Journal of Biomedical Research and Clinical Investigation Volume 2
Issue 1.1007

***Ivermectin as Prophylaxis Against COVID-19 Retrospective Cases
Evaluation IVERPREV***

Hirsch R, Carvallo, Héctor. Ivermectin as Prophylaxis Against
COVID-19 Retrospective Cases Evaluation. Microbiol Infect Dis.
2020; 4(4): 1-8.

CLINICAL USE AND EVALUATION OF IVERMECTIN IN ARGENTINA

After the results of above-mentioned first studies were published,
Ivermectin was then recognized publicly as the "most promising
compound to treat COVID-19" by the Director of ANMAT (the
Argentinian version of American FDA), Dr. Limeres.

Despite these findings, however, Ivermectin was still not authorized
for use throughout the entire country of Argentina.

The following provinces that used it officially were:
- Jujuy
- Salta
- Corrientes
- La Pampa
- Tucumán
- Misiones

This implied that only 6 out of 23 provinces represented the whole
country in the use of Ivermectin as treatment for COVID-19.

However, the following 6 other Provinces also used it extensively (albeit unofficially):

- Buenos Aires (both BA Province and BA Federal District)
- Santa Fe
- Córdoba
- Chaco
- Entre Ríos

In the remaining eleven provinces, users were able to obtain Ivermectin over the counter, without medical prescription. There are reports that even veterinary Ivermectin was also consumed by individuals.

JUJUY

The Province of Jujuy has 800,000 inhabitants.

During the first wave of the pandemic, Jujuy's healthcare system was quickly overwhelmed by a large influx of patients who had to be admitted for severe dyspnea.

The Provincial Government, at the request of Dr. Wilmer Bracho Colina, issued a decree by which all outpatients with a positive PCR result for COVID-19 should receive Ivermectin, while moderate cases, which were at risk of hospital admission, were prescribed Ivermectin and Corticosteroids (prednisolone 40 mg/day for 5 days).

As a result, the health system of Jujuy was decompressed in less than a fortnight, thanks to a sharp drop in admissions and deaths.

SALTA

In the Province of Salta (1,440,000 inhabitants), Ivermectin was used by doctors and hospitals both for prophylaxis and early treatment.

Dr. Carolina Alveró obtained authorization for its preventive use in the health personnel of the San Bernardo Hospital, whose staff was

Chapter 6 Ivermectin on COVID-19 in Argentina

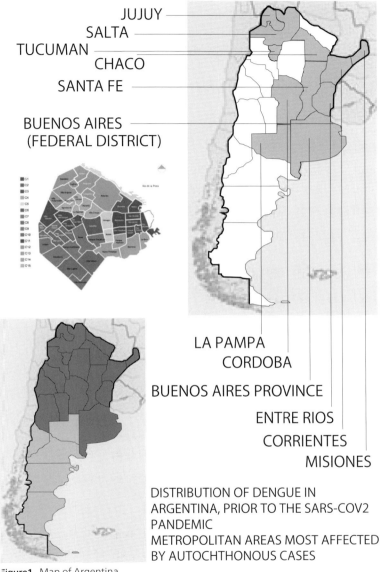

Figure1. Map of Argentina

being decimated by infections.

In as little as ten days, absenteeism at the hospital was reduced to less than 5%. Meanwhile, Dr. Antonio Salgado used Ivermectin as early treatment for all outpatient cases with positive PCR.

Out of 1,200 patients treated with Ivermectin, none required admission.

CORRIENTES

The Government of the Province of Corrientes (1,197,000 inhabitants) had authorized the sale of Ivermectin without a medical prescription, during the first wave of the COVID-19 pandemic.

Although no official survey of results was collected, the general response to Ivermectin was very satisfactory.

A clinical trial was held by private researchers, who conceded that "…it was almost impossible to recruit a placebo group, since everybody is buying Ivermectin at pharmacies…"

LA PAMPA

After an initial refusal to use Ivermectin, the Ministry of Health of the Province of La Pampa (360,000 inhabitants), through Dr. Mario Kohan, later determined the early use of Ivermectin in confirmed cases of COVID.

Official statistics showed a 44% reduction in hospitalizations, as well as a 42% reduction in deaths due to COVID.

TUCUMAN

The Ministry of Health of the Province of Tucumán (1,610,000 inhabitants) - through Dr. Rossana Chala and the Provincial Faculty of Medicine requested advice from the Authors of this chapter to replicate the IDEA and IVERCAR protocols thus creating their equivalents

IDEA-TUC and IVER-TUC, whose use led to the reduction of the number of COVID cases by 62%, and the number of deaths by 53%.

This effectively ended the quarantine in Tucuman that was imposed at the beginning of the pandemic.

MISIONES

The Province of Misiones made a massive purchase of Ivermectin for the prophylactic use by health personnel.

The data from that Province reveals a contagion reduction of 49%.

BUENOS AIRES (FEDERAL DISTRICT)

The Federal District of Argentina is called Buenos Aires City (3,121,000 inhabitants).

One of our trials (IVERPREV) was performed there, at the largest Argentinian hospital dedicated exclusively to infectious diseases (F.J. Muñiz Hospital).

After the trial, the use of Ivermectin both for prophylaxis and treatment spread within the City. Since Ivermectin was available for purchase over the counter at any pharmacy.

Being an unofficial move, there is no official recorded data of results.

BUENOS AIRES PROVINCE

This is the most populated region of Argentina, with 17,500,000 inhabitants.

Dr. Aroldo del Franco held an extensive study (with the Authors of this chapter) on the beneficial effect of Ivermectin on Long Covid, at Mercante Public Hospital.

Results were very satisfactory as it was observed that long COVID symptoms were dramatically shortened.

The use of Ivermectin for prophylaxis and treatment skyrocketed after that, surpassing one hundred times the usual sales. As it was happening at Buenos Aires City, people purchased Ivermectin without prescription, in most cases.

In the rural areas, people used oral fractions of veterinary Ivermectin.

We strongly refused to endorse that form, since polyethylene glycol (used in veterinary) may provoke neurological symptoms. Yet, no case of side effects was reported.

SANTA FE

Prof. Carlos Alonso took a sabbatical year at his job as Professor of Legal Medicine at Rosario School of Medicine and moved back to his birthplace. He led a vigorous campaign on the use of Ivermectin for early treatment of COVID-19. He treated over 1,800 cases with only one fatality.

Later on, use of Ivermectin spread rapidly, but as its uses was not officialized, there is no recorded data.

CORDOBA

The Province of Córdoba (4,000,000 inhabitants) showed a spontaneous move towards the use of Ivermectin, with no official data available.

CHACO

The same thing happened at this Province (with 1,143,000 inhabitants).

Ivermectin was "unofficially" prescribed at the two largest hospitals, and its use later spread to the rest of the province.

Chapter 6   Ivermectin on COVID-19 in Argentina

ENTRE RIOS

Gustavo Bordet, the Governor of the Province of Entre Ríos (with 1,425,000 inhabitants) unsuccessfully tried to pass a law for the official use of Ivermectin for COVID-19.

During his opening speech for a second period in office, he stated: *"…I am here thanks to you (the voters) and to Ivermectin…."*

Though the drug was not accepted by Congress, he personally addressed the population, encouraging them to use Ivermectin.

CONCLUSIONS

In spite of the fact that Big Pharma, Big Media, and the National Government colluded to undermine the use of Ivermectin, its use was not officially prohibited.

Thus, patients could still purchase it easily at most pharmacies, and without the need of a prescription.

Some dedicated MDs (many mentioned above) and Veterinarians challenged the "official story" regarding the safety of Ivermectin use, and encouraged their patients to use Ivermectin, both as prophylaxis and early treatment for COVID-19.

Sadly, lockdown policies and the official decision to prioritize the distribution and administration of experimental vaccines over early treatments may have added to the numbers of severe (and sometimes, even fatal) COVID-19 cases than during the pandemic itself.

EFFECTIVE IN THE TREATMENT OF DENGUE FEVER - FUTURE PERSPECTIVES OF IVERMECTIN

Ivermectin's anti-viral properties had already been successfully studied against dengue fever, Zika, Chikungunya, and malaria, long before onset of the COVID-19 pandemic.

In fact, dengue is already a re-emerging disease in Argentina, and

179

it is already entering the endemic category.

In 1916, the first known dengue outbreak occurred in Argentina, which was introduced through a case imported from Paraguay.

The control campaigns carried out by the Pan American Health Organization in the Americas around the middle of the 20th century led to a decline in the spread of the virus in the areas colonized by A. aegypti.

In the 1970s, cases became confined only within the insular sector of Central America and in the extreme north of South America.

A decade later however, a reinvasion of the vector to the south occurred, which led to the disease reaching the territory of Argentina once again.

Ivermectin has already demonstrated its efficacy in reducing dengue viral load, in a dose-dependent manner.

Ivermectin also has a proven antiviral effect against other single-stranded RNA viruses such as dengue or yellow fever, against which it has succeeded in inhibiting their replication in vitro.

In addition, it has an immunomodulatory role that is interesting to evaluate, since it has been seen that one of the great problems of the dengue virus is immunoamplification.

When it is administered early, the disappearance of the clinical picture occurs in less than 72 hours.

Likewise, subjects receiving prophylactic doses of Ivermectin will not contract dengue, even when inoculated through the bite of Aedes mosquitoes, which confirms the virucidal effect of the compound.

This was observed in farm animals, who are given Ivermectin to prevent mosquito-borne diseases (Culex, Anopheles, Aedes, etc.).
Given this finding, the effect was replicated in human volunteers, with equal success.

Yang S et al., identified that the Ivermectin molecule can prevent important factors of the viral replication cycle from entering the nucleus; for example, in the case of HIV, it was observed that Ivermectin inhibits the entry of integrase into the cell nucleus.

In dengue, Ivermectin could inhibit the entry of the dengue NS5 protein into the host nucleus.

DENGUE AND VACCINES

As we already explained, immunoamplification is the cause of cases of complicated/severe dengue (dengue shock and dengue hemorrhagic fever).

It occurs when an individual, with Ac. against a dengue serotype, comes into contact with one of the other serotypes.

The risk of multivalent experimental vaccines was observed when Sanofi tested the Dengvaxia vaccine.

The phase III study of the Dengvaxia vaccine was heavily criticized as the report failed to mention the potential risks and even excluded them from the list of serious side effects.

Despite these risks, the vaccine was accepted by the WHO as "theoretically promising", and its use was even approved in the Philippines (2019).

Unfortunately, more than six hundred children died after receiving the vaccine, which is why it was permanently banned in that country, with the case still being investigated by the Public Prosecutor's Office.

PROPHYLAXIS SCHEME WITH IVERMECTIN IN ARBOVIRUSES

IVM, 0.3 mg per kilo of weight, after a high	fat meal, twice a week

PROPHYLAXIS SCHEME WITH IVERMECTIN IN ARBOVIRUSES

CASES	DOSE	FREQUENCY	DURATION
Mild	0.4 mg/Kg	once a day	5 days
Severe	0.6 mg/kg	once a day	7 days

IVERMECTIN IN ONCOLOGY

Ivermectin has powerful antitumor effects, including the inhibition of proliferation (spread), metastasis (growth), and angiogenic activity (formation of new blood cells), in a variety of cancer cells.

This is related to the regulation of multiple signaling pathways by Ivermectin through the enzyme PAK1 kinase.

Ivermectin also promotes programmed cancer cell death, including apoptosis, autophagy, and pyro ptosis. Ivermectin induces apoptosis, and autophagy is mutually regulated.

Ivermectin can also inhibit tumor stem cells and reverse multidrug resistance and exerts the optimal effect when used in combination with other chemotherapy drugs.

IVERMECTIN IN AUTO-IMMUNE DISEASES

Several research studies have concentrated on the impact of Ivermectin on T-cell-mediated autoimmune illnesses, which include Multiple Sclerosis (MS), rheumatoid arthritis, type 1 diabetes, inflammatory bowel diseases (IBD), Sjogren's syndrome, systemic lupus erythematosus, and psoriasis.

Case reports have displayed the protective effect of Ivermectin on systemic lupus erythematosus and psoriasis.

Other authors have also reported that Ivermectin can directly attenuate Experimental Autoimmune Encephalomyelitis (EAE) clinical symptoms by altering T-cell responses and CD4+ T cell subsets.

Chapter 6   Ivermectin on COVID-19 in Argentina

References

1. Hirsch Roberto, Carvallo Héctor: SARS-CoV2, Emerging, Reemerging and Potentially Emerging Diseases in Argentina J Virol Infect Dis. (2021), Volume 2 Issue 1, pp 13-17.

2. Del Franco, A., Carvallo H. and Hirsch, R.: Ivermectin in Long-Covid Patients: A Retrospective Study. Journal of Biomedical Research and Clinical Investigation, doi:10.31546/2633-8653.1008 Mar 2021

3. Carvallo, H., et al: IVERMECTIN Multicenter Study. January 2021
   DOI: 10.13140/RG.2.2.19384.57603

4. Hortal M. Emerging and re-emerging infectious diseases: updated information. Rev Méd Urug. 2016; 32:1.

5. Morens DM, Folkers G.: The challenge of emerging and re-emerging infectious diseases. Nature. 2004; 430:242-249.

6. Rogiervan Doorn H. Emerging infectious diseases. Medicine. 2014;42(1):60-63.

7. Mayer J. Geography, ecology and emerging infectious diseases. Soc Sci Med. 2000; 50(7-8):937-952.

8. Corteguera RR. Emerging and re-emerging diseases: a challenge for the 21st century. Rev Cubana Pediatr. 2002; 74:1.

9. https://www.researchgate.net/publication/270901162_BIOENSAYO_DE_IVERMECTINA_CONTRA_LARVAS_DE_AEDES_AEGYPTI_ALTERNATIVA_PARA_CONTROL_DEL_DENGUE_EN_ECUADOR

10. file:///C:/Users/dinfeccionesas/Documents/Downloads/admin,+Efectos_de_la_ivermectina_sobre_Aedes_aegypti_despu%C3%A9s_de_la_administraci%C3%B3n_oral_en_humanos.pdf

11. https://www.bibliotecasdelecuador.com/Record/oai:localhost:28000-2702/Description

12. https://coe.tucuman.gov.ar/novedades/ver/653

13. Heidary F, Gharebaghi R (2020), Ivermectin: a systematic review from antiviral effects to COVID-19 complementary regimen, J Antibiot (Tokyo). Jun 12:1-10. doi: 10.1038/s41429-020-0336-z

14. Guzzo CA, Furtek CI, Porras AG, Chen C, Tipping R, Clineschmidt CM et al. (2002), Safety, Tolerability, and Pharmacokinetics of Escalating High Doses of Ivermectin in Healthy Adult Subjects. J Clin Pharmacol. 2002 Oct;42(10):1122-33. doi: 10.1177/009127002401382731

15. Levy M, Martin L, Bursztein AC, Chiaverini C, Miquel J, Mahé E et al. (2019), Ivermectin safety in infants and children under 15 kg treated for scabies: a multicentric observational study British Journal of Dermatology, doi: 10.1111/bjd.18369

16. Baraka OZ, Mahmoud BM, Marschke CK, Geary TG, Homeida MMA, Williams JF (1996), Ivermectin Distribution in the Plasma and Tissues of Patients Infected with Onchocerca Volvulus, Eur J Clin Pharmacol (1996) 50: 407–410, doi: 10.1007/s002280050131

17. González Canga A, Sahagún Prieto AM, Diez Liébana MJ, Fernández Martínez N, Sierra Vega M, García Vieitez JJ (2008), The Pharmacokinetics and Interactions of Ivermectin in Humans—A Mini-review, The AAPS Journal, Vol. 10, No. 1, March, doi: 10.1208/s12248-007-9000-9

18. Simmons C Farrar J van Vih Chau N. Dengue. N Engl J Med. 2012; 36: 1423-1432 2.

WHO. Dengue and severe dengue. Descriptive note No. 117. 2015. Available at http://www.who.int/mediacentre/factsheets/f s117/es/

19. González M. Data from serological analyzes and circulating serotypes of Dengue Costa Rica, January-December, 2014. INCENSE. 2015: 1-10. Available at http://www.inciensa.sa.cr

20. Islam R Salahuddin M Salahuddin MA et al. Dengue epidemiology and pathogenesis: images of the future viewed through a mirror of the past. Sinic Virology. 2015; 30(5): 326-343

21. Mustafa MS Rasotgi V Jain S Gupta V. Discovery of fifth serotype of dengue virus (DENV-5): A new public health dilemma in dengue control. Medical Journal Armed Forces India. 2015; 71:67-70

22. Velandia ML Castellanos JE. Dengue Virus: Structure and Viral Cycle. Infectio. 2011; 15(1):33-43

23. Murphy B Whitehead S. Immune Response to Dengue Virus and Prospects for a Vaccine. Annu Rev Immunol. 2011; 29:587-619

24. Simon A Sutherland M Pryzdial E. Dengue virus binding and replication by platelets. Blood. 2015; 126(3):378-385

25. Mortina B Koraka P Osterhaus A. Dengue Virus Pathogenesis: an Integrated view. Clinical Microbiology Reviews. 2009; 22(4):564-581

26. Chuang Y Wang S Lin Y Chen H Yeh T. Re-evaluation of the pathogenic roles of Nonstructural protein 1 and its antibodies during dengue virus infection. Journal of Biomedical Science. 2013; 20:42

27. Montes de Oca M Martín P Monsalvo M Ruiz E. Endemic viral infections: dengue, Nile fever, others. Medicine. 2014; 11(50): 2965-2972

28. Sosothikul D Seksarn P Pongsewalak S Thisyakorn U Lusher J. Activation of endothelial cells, coagulation and fibrinolysis in children with Dengue virus infection. Thromb Haemostasis 2007, 97:627–634.

29. Ooi E Ganesananthan S Anil R Kwok FY Sinniah M. Gastrointestinal Manifestations of Dengue Infection in Adults. Med J Malaysia. 2008; 63(5):401-405

30. Ramos A Remes J González M et al. Abdominal and gastrointestinal symptoms of dengue. Analysis of a cohort of 8,559 patients. Gastroenterol Hepatol. 2011; 3. 4(4): 245-247

31. Puccioni-Sohler M, Rosadas C, Cabral-Castro MJ. Neurological complications in dengue infection: a review for clinical practice. Arch Neuropsychiatrist 2013; 71:667-671.

32. Bordignon J Strottmann D Mosimann A et al. Dengue neurovirulence in mice: identification of molecular signatures in the E and NS3 helicase domains. J Med Virol 2007; 79:1506-1517.

33. Verma R, Sharma P, Garg RK, Atam V, Singh MK, Mehrotra HS. Neurological complications of dengue fever: Experience from a tertiary center of north India. Annals of Indian Academy of Neurology. 2011;14(4):272-278

34. Discovery of berberine, abamectin and ivermectin as antivirals against chikungunya and other alphaviruses. Finny S. Varghese a 1, Pasi Kaukinen a 1, Sabine Gläsker b, Maxim Bespalov c, Leena Hanski d, Krister Wennerberg c, Beate M. Kümmerer b, Tero Ahola Antiviral Research Volume 126, February 2016, Pages 117-124

35. Ivermectin, a potential anticancer drug derived from an antiparasitic drug Mingyang Tang,a,b,1 Xiaodong Hu,c,1 Yi Wang,a,d Xin Yao,a,d Wei Zhang,a,b Chenying Yu,a,b Fuying Cheng,a,b Jiangyan Li,a,d and Qiang Fanga,d,e: Pharmacol Res. 2021 Jan; 163: 105207. Published online 2020 Sep 21. doi: 10.1016/j.phrs.2020.105207 PMCID: PMC7505114 PMID: 32971268

35. Juarez M., Schcolnik-Cabrera A., Duenas-Gonzalez A. The multitargeted drug ivermectin: from an antiparasitic agent to a repositioned cancer drug. Am J Cancer Res. 2018;8(2):317–331. [PMC free article] [PubMed]

37. Liu J., Zhang K., Cheng L., Zhu H., Xu T. Progress in Understanding the Molecular Mechanisms Underlying the Antitumour Effects of Ivermectin. Drug Des Devel Ther. 2020;14:285–296. doi: 10.2147/dddt.S237393. [PMC free article] [PubMed] [CrossRef]

33. Antoszczak M., Markowska A., Markowska J., Huczynski A. Old wine in new bottles: Drug repurposing in oncology. Eur J Pharmacol. 2020;866:172784. doi: 10.1016/j.ejphar.2019.172784.

39. Kobayashi Y., Banno K., Kunitomi H., Tominaga E., Aoki D. Current state and outlook for drug repositioning anticipated in the field of ovarian cancer. J Gynecol Oncol. 2019;30(1):e10. doi: 10.3802/jgo.2019.30.e10.

40. Yoshida G.J. Therapeutic strategies of drug repositioning targeting autophagy to induce cancer cell death: from pathophysiology to treatment. J Hematol Oncol. 2017;10(1):67. doi: 10.1186/s13045-017-0436-9.

41. Yu Xie,#1,2 Chaolei Jin,#1 Hongzhen Sang,1 Wenhua Liu,1 and Junpeng Wang PMCID: Ivermectin Protects Against Experimental Autoimmune Encephalomyelitis in Mice by Modulating the Th17/Treg Balance Involved in the IL-2/STAT5 Pathway. Inflammation. 2023 May 25 : 1–13. doi: 10.1007/s10753-023-01829-y PMC10209955 PMID: 37227550

Héctor E. Carvallo, Ph.D.

Former Professor of Internal Medicine, University of Buenos Aires, Argentina. Former Director of Ezeiza´s Public Hospital, Argentina. Professor of Internal Medicine, Universidad Abierta Interamericana, Argentina.

Roberto R. Hirsch, Ph.D.

Former Professor of Infectology, University of Buenos Aires, Argentina. Director Career for Infectology Specialist, Hospital F. J. Muñíz, Argentina. Director Department of Infectious Diseases, Hospital F. J. Muñíz, Argentina.

East Asia

Chapter

7

Japan

Dr. Kazuhiro NAGAO

Encounter and Experience
with Ivermectin

I am a 65-year-old physician, M.D., born in 1958.

I specialize in gastroenterology and am a member of the Society of Gastrointestinal Endoscopy. I had been practicing as a general practitioner and primary care physician for 28 years in Amagasaki City, Hyogo Prefecture, adjacent to Osaka, providing routine medical care and home care. My Nagao Clinic was a community-based clinic operated by 115 staff, including 20 registered physicians.

I have treated more than 10,000 patients with fever, more than 3,000 with COVID-19, and more than 200 with post-vaccine sequelae, and retired on my 65th birthday in June 2023. In this article, I review my experience with Ivermectin (IVM) during the 3.5 years of the COVID-19 pandemic.

EARLY DIAGNOSIS AND IMMEDIATE TREATMENT OF INFECTIONS

On the first Monday in April 2020, we heard reports of the spread of COVID-19 infection in Japan and the first COVID-19 patient arrived at the Nagao Clinic in Amagasaki, Hyogo Prefecture, adjacent to Osaka, for a checkup.

During the lunch break that day, we held an in-hospital meeting, "Let's start the outpatient fever clinic today! "

After the in-hospital meeting, the first fever patient who had an appointment was examined outside the back entrance of the clinic. At first glance of the CT image of the lungs, I knew intuitively, "Oh, it's COVID-19". I had always believed infectious diseases should be diagnosed early and treated immediately, but at that time I was unsure for a moment whether to treat the patient on the spot.

At that time (until the fall of 2020), the PCR test was a very complicated testing system in which an appointment was made through the public health center and the patient was called to some testing location. All positive patients were supposed to be admitted to a designated hospital under the direction of the public health center, but soon Japan's medical care system collapsed, and more and more patients had to wait at home. It took one to two days from specimen collection to the determination of results. From the patient's point of view, it took more than a week from the time of fever to the positive result. Moreover, there was no treatment. I thought, "If this is the case, high-risk patients will become seriously ill and, in the worst case, lose their lives".

Fortunately, our hospital had a state-of-the-art CT scanner. Using it, COVID-19 pneumonia could be diagnosed in only five minutes. Therefore, from the beginning, we aimed to diagnose COVID-19 early and treat it on the spot, because a PCR test can take up to a week, while a CT scan can provide an answer in only five minutes, allowing for immediate treatment.

24-HOUR MANAGEMENT BY CELL PHONE

From the beginning, all patients with COVID pneumonia on CT scan were given steroid injections on the spot. This was a painful move because Amagasaki's medical care had collapsed since the first wave of cases, and patients whose CT scans showed typical COVID pneumonia were, of course, faxed to the public health center for PCR testing. Otherwise, patients could not be admitted to the hospital. However, the number of patients was so large that for several days there were many patients from the first wave of COVID-19 in Japan who could not be hospitalized without being contacted by the public health center.

Therefore, once I diagnosed COVID-19 pneumonia, I gave all patients my cell phone number on the spot and managed them 24 hours a day for about 10 days via e-mail and phone calls. This was necessary not only for the early detection of serious illness, but also to dispel the anxiety of the patients. We treated all of our homebound patients the same way. Later, however, I learned that my clinic was the only one in all of Japan doing so. Because COVID-19 was treated as a Class 2 disease (in reality, Class 1 or higher) under the Infectious Diseases Control Law, almost all general practitioners were aware that COVID-19 was a disease that general practitioners were not allowed to treat. I didn't care if the police caught me, so I said, "Anyway, early treatment, immediate treatment. The patients I treat will not die from COVID-19 ." However, I did not only treat COVID-19. Even during COVID-19 pandemic, I spent only 10-20% of my energy dealing with COVID-19, since I had a large number of patients in regular medical care and in regular home care.

The 2020 guidelines for the treatment of COVID-19 included Ivermectin as a therapeutic option. Coincidentally, the Nagao Clinic had prescribed Ivermectin several times a year for scabies patients whom we occasionally treated at home before COVID-19. Therefore, although we were relatively familiar with prescribing Ivermectin, we did not know whether the same dosage of Ivermectin for COVID-19 was appropriate as that for scabies.

During the year until spring 2021, we prescribed Ivermectin to some patients, but mistakenly believed that it was a last resort in the treatment plan. In addition, the amount and number of days of Ivermectin prescriptions were insufficient.

Initially, my clinic administered Ivermectin to patients based on the following criteria.

1. We did not know we should have given them 3 days in a row and only gave them 1 day.

2. They were giving it between meals, not after meals.
3. Did not vary the prescribed dose according to body weight.
4. They administered the drug only to patients with severe illnesses.

In other words, I had no idea that Ivermectin was the drug of choice for the initial treatment of COVID-19. Although it takes time, many severely ill patients are admitted to the hospital and treated there after a few days, and therefore did not feel that Ivermectin was remarkable in terms of its effectiveness.

MEETING WITH DR. OMURA

Since I wanted to know more about Ivermectin, so in the summer of 2021 I requested a meeting in person with Dr. Satoshi Omura of Kitasato University. I thought that it was impossible to meet a Nobel Prize-winning scientist, but I decided to give it a shot. I was determined to save as many patients as possible with Ivermectin. I was so happy to have an interview with Dr. Omura that I went to Tokyo to visit the Kitasato Research Institute.

1. Ivermectin is a drug for initial treatment.
2. Ivermectin is prescribed in proportion to body weight.
3. Ivermectin should be given after meals for three consecutive days.

I learned these things through my meeting with Dr. Omura.

The very next day, I decided to give both Ivermectin and clarithromycin to all of the dozens of infected patients every day, and I also gave steroid injections to patients whose CT scans showed pneumonia. As if I were a textbook myself, I shared information with the approximately 100 doctors, nurses, and staff who worked with me day after day. The hospital's prescribing manual and instructions were revised weekly. In the fifth wave in 2021, even though there were patients with severe cases with sPO2 (oxygen levels in the blood, as read by an oximeter) as low as 60%, the health center could not be reached by phone, and as a result, they could hardly be admitted to the hospital. Even when they requested an ambulance, it did not come. The term "medical collapse" refers to the situation in which there was no doctor other than me to treat patients with severe COVID-19. As a town doctor, I was both the first and the last to be able to treat patients with severe COVID-19.

Doctors and nurses went into the homes of patients with severe pneumonia day after day, and we did everything a hospital would do, including oxygen inhalation and steroid pulse therapy. They were managed 24 hours a day by cell phone and e-mail. We collaborated with the health center, always triaging the patients.

THANKS TO IVERMECTIN, ZERO DEATHS

The fifth wave in August 2021 had the most severely ill patients. But after administering Ivermectin and clarithromycin to patients we were able to save everyone. Fortunately, we have not experienced a single death case to date, including a patient who was able to be hospitalized a few days later.

In three and a half years, I have treated about 10,000 fever patients and more than 3,000 COVID-19 patients, and there were no deaths. The details are described in my book, "Hitori mo, shinase hen" (I will not let anyone die, Bookman, Inc.).

In total, we have treated more than 300 COVID-19 patients with Ivermectin for 3 days, and all of them have responded effectively and without any significant side effect. Many of the cases were also treated with a combination of Ivermectin, clarithromycin and steroid injections. We had only a few cases were treated with Ivermectin alone.

I gave all the patients my cell phone number and managed them during the home care period. As a home health care provider, I was accustomed to 24-hour management. The advantage of this was that I could get real-time information about the effect of Ivermectin from the patients. The improvement rate at 1 day after Ivermectin administration was almost 100%. For patients with mild infection, their symptoms disappeared in one or two days. Even in patients with persistent or moderate infection, their symptoms disappeared in two one or two days. Even in patients with persistent or moderate infection, their symptoms were almost completely resolved in 7 to 10 days.

SUDDEN BAN ON USE

With Ivermectin, I was not afraid of COVID-19. Convinced of this, I went on national TV and You Tube to talk about the effectiveness of Ivermectin. I appealed, "The prime minister should distribute Ivermectin to all the people". I was later told that many people were very surprised when they saw it.

Ivermectin was prescribed to patients in the 6th, 7th, and 8th waves as an initial treatment, and it was successful. However, the use of Ivermectin was suddenly "banned" from September 2022. Although there was no specific notification from the government, the receipt insurer began to send back the requests and said that the use of Ivermectin was not allowed. The sudden flip-flop left us in a panic, as prescriptions for COVID-19 had been allowed from 2020 to September 2022. In Japan, with its universal health insurance system, the Ministry of Health, Labor, and Welfare (MHLW) is absolutely obedient to its directives. We had no choice but to comply because we would be punished if we did not. Fortunately, there were a few patients who had imported Ivermectin over the Internet and stockpiled it, so we advised them on how to take it.

THE EFFICACY RATE FOR POST-VACCINE SEQUELAE IS 60-70%

On the other hand, since the fall of 2021, a series of patients with poor health after COVID-19 prophylactic vaccination began to visit our clinic. People complaining of a wide variety of symptoms known as vaccine aftereffects, such as chronic fatigue syndrome and brain fog, began to visit our clinic every day. Of course, people with COVID-19 sequelae (Long COVID) also came to see us, but most of them had milder symptoms than those with vaccine sequelae.

The causal relationship between the COVID-19 mRNA vaccine and the symptoms is undeniable. These vaccinated patients find it difficult to lead their previous social lives at school, work, and other places. Their symptoms are called "post-vaccine sequelae," and as of the end of December 2022, their number exceeded 200 in our clinic alone. Almost all of them had consulted several medical institutions and were told that the cause was unknown until I saw them. I recommended that these patients try Ivermectin. However, insurance would not cover it, so I had the patients buy the generic version to save on costs.

The efficacy rate of Ivermectin in post-vaccine patients at our hospital was 60-70%. Coincidentally, I was surprised to find that the efficacy rate was consistent with that reported by the U.S.-based Front Line COVID-19 Critical Care (FLCCC) Alliance.

I asked the patients to take the drug for 1 to 2 weeks in a row and then judged the efficacy of the drug. If there was no effect, I stopped the treatment and combined Chinese herbal medicine, supplements, and acupuncture and moxibustion treatment. Although I was tempted to double or triple the dosage, I did not do so because I was being scrutinized by the health authorities for recommending Ivermectin, I had received death threats from strangers and thus had cause to fear for my safety.

Chapter 7   Encounter and Experience with Ivermectin

EFFECTS OF EARLY IVERMECTIN ADMINISTRATION ON COVID-19 PATIENTS

The results of the early administration of Ivermectin to patients with COVID-19 can be summarized as follows.

- The efficacy rate of Ivermectin administered for 3 consecutive days was almost 100%.
- Half of the patients showed dramatic results, with fever resolving the next day.
- Almost all patients with mild disease were cured within a week.
- Above all, there were no deaths among COVID-19 patients diagnosed at our hospital.
- We have not experienced a single adverse reaction to Ivermectin.

However, we could no longer prescribe Ivermectin since it has been banned from September 2022. The patients had to purchase it voluntarily on their own accord.

On the other hand, the efficacy of Ivermectin administration for post-vaccine sequelae is as follows.

- The efficacy rate of Ivermectin is 60-70%.
- Vaccine sequelae are difficult to treat to begin with.
- Ivermectin is often used in combination with zinc preparations, herbal medicines, and supplements.
- No side effects have been reported with Ivermectin.
- The Ministry of Health, Labour and Welfare (MHLW) has not approved the prescription of Ivermectin for post-vaccine sequelae from the beginning to the present.

Some testimonies of patients with vaccine sequelae after taking

Ivermectin included the following.

- *I felt lighter after a few hours of taking Ivermectin.*
- *Junior high school students who could not understand what their teachers were saying became able to understand.*
- *But the effect lasts only for three days, so I have to take it once every few days.*
- *When I take 12 mg tablet, I cannot sleep because of palpitations, so I reduce the dose to 3 mg.*
- *I take it on demand because my physical condition ebbs and flows.*

Many people say that they adjust the dosage according to their physical condition on a given day.

EFFECTS OTHER THAN COVID-19 INFECTION OR COVID-19 / VACCINE SEQUELAE

I held a symposium on "Vaccine Sequelae" at Grand Cube Osaka on December 25, 2021. The capacity was for 300 people, but to my surprise more than 1,000 people came, so I asked for a photo shoot on short notice.

In early 2022, we made a documentary film titled "Recorded Footage: Vaccine Sequelae". This film, with the consent of the people involved, presents the faces and voices of those affected by the vaccine and asks the world about the reality of the aftereffects of the vaccine. The film was shown in movie theaters nationwide until the spring of 2022. At the same time, independent screenings of the film were actively held in various regions.

As the producer of the film, I gave more than two dozen one-hour greetings on stage. During the question-and-answer session at the end of the film, the audience members had some surprising stories to

Chapter 7 Encounter and Experience with Ivermectin

tell about Ivermectin. They were spontaneous comments made in the presence of a large audience.

The following is a list of what we heard about the effects of Ivermectin other than COVID-19 and vaccine sequelae, listed in order of frequency.

- A person who had been blind regained their sight after taking Ivermectin for a long time.
- Improvement in presbyopia and other vision problems.
- Cancer has regressed or disappeared.
- Cure of hay fever and hives.
- Motivation increased.
- Dementia improved.
- Irregular menstruation improved.
- Hair loss stopped, and hair grew back.
- Male sexual function improved.
- Shedding symptoms disappeared.
- Improved high-pitched voice.
- Improved appearance.
- Improved sleep quality.
- Improved bowel movements.

To what extent are these effects due to Ivermectin? We have not examined the cause-and-effect relationship. This is just a list of personal impressions. The placebo effect should be considered but I was surprised at the wide variety of testimonies, even though I cannot take all of them as they are.

IMPROVEMENT OF EYESIGHT

The most impressive and unexpected testimonies were the

"improvement in eyesight. This is most felt by the person who experienced this effect, so it seems highly credible. However, the details of the original disease and the degree of presbyopia are unknown. These are only the words of many people. Research is needed.

When I first met with Dr. Omura in the summer of 2021, he told me the following. "I know only 10% of what Ivermectin can do. Ivermectin has 90% of the effects that have yet to be elucidated. I hope you will do your best to elucidate the wide range of clinical effects of Ivermectin". I am reminded of these words every time I hear the real voices of Ivermectin users at movie theaters or lectures.

MULTIFACETED EFFECTS OF IVERMECTIN

It should be clear to everyone that Ivermectin's effects are no longer limited to parasites, ticks, and COVID-19. Let me list some of Ivermectin's potential effects.

1. Immunomodulatory or immunostimulatory effects
2. Improvement of blood flow
3. Antiallergic action
4. Activation of autophagy
5. Anti-aging action
6. Anti-dementia action
7. Intestinal environment improvement action
8. Anticancer action
9. Immunity enhancing action
10. Mental stabilizing or uplifting action

Ivermectin does not cross the brain-blood barrier. However, there is no doubt that Ivermectin has a positive effect on brain hormones and neurotransmitters through some mechanism such as the brain-gut connection.

CONCLUSION

Ivermectin played a major role in the COVID-19 disaster and other vaccine-related diseases. In addition, it is effective against influenza and several RNA viruses. Ivermectin has not only antiviral but also immunomodulatory and antitumor activities, which are indeed very diverse and mysterious. It is extremely safe. It is a drug that works extremely well for humans. Moreover, it is inexpensive.

After nearly four years of the COVID-19 disaster, I would like to exclaim: "Thank you, Ivermectin. Thank you, Dr. Omura. Thank you, Japanese people, for believing in me! "

Kazuhiro NAGAO, M.D., former director of the Nagao Clinic.
After graduating from Tokyo Medical University in 1984, he joined the Second Department of Internal Medicine at Osaka University and became chief of internal medicine at Ashiya Municipal Ashiya Hospital in 1991. In 1995, he opened Nagao Clinic in Amagasaki City, Hyogo Prefecture, which provides both outpatient and home care services 24 hours a day, 365 days a year with multiple doctors, focusing on early detection of lifestyle-related diseases and cancer, and medical care for elderly patients including dementia. He retired in 2023 and is currently involved in volunteer activities. He is the vice-chairman of the Japanese Association for Death with Dignity, a specialist of the Japanese Society of Gastroenterology, a specialist and advisor of the Japanese Society of Gastrointestinal Endoscopy, a Japanese Society of Home Medicine Specialist, a certified physician of the Japanese Society of Internal Medicine, a visiting professor at Kansai International University, and a researcher at Kitasato University Center for Infection Control. His book "How to Die Without Pain" became a bestseller and was made into a movie. He has also produced a documentary film "Kettai na Machi-isha" (Quirky Town Doctor), which closely follows Nagao, a specialist in home medical care who has taken care of 2,500 people, as well as a documentary film "Vaccine Sequelae" (Vaccine Sequelae), which he has produced himself. His recent books include "Hitori mo shinasehen" (I won't let anyone die) - Diary of 551 days of a town doctor in Amagasaki fighting the COVID-19 disaster, "Hitori mo shinasehen2, Diary of vaccine conflict of a town doctor in Amagasaki fighting the Covid-19 disaster", "Politics and Vaccine" and "Covid-19 and Dementia".

Chapter

8

Japan

Dr. Katsuhiko FUKUDA

Flash in Japan
Survival Wisdom from a Vaccidemic Superpower

INTRODUCTION

For more than 30 years, I have treated patients in various clinical settings as an internist practicing integrative medicine.

Immediately after the SARS-CoV-2 vaccination began in Japan in February 2021, there were a number of medical professionals who had to take leave or quit their jobs due to physical and mental illness. Clinicians in the U.S. reported to me a sharp increase in deaths after the vaccination, especially among the elderly. I sent the following warning message to the Japanese medical associations before the SARS-CoV-2 vaccination of the elderly began in April: "COVID-19 vaccination physicians should be required to report not only short-term adverse reactions, but also periodic follow-up of adverse reactions on an annual basis."

Thus, I became known as the first doctor to advocate "COVID-19 vaccine-induced sequelae (mRNA PVS: post-vaccine syndrome / LPCVS: Long post-COVID vaccination syndrome)" in Japan, and in May of the same year I started an "outpatient clinic for the treatment of the sequelae."

Since the opening of the Fever Outpatient Clinic in 2020, the clinic has treated more than 2,000 patients each with COVID-19 infections, Long-COVID, and the vaccine-induced sequelae.

In September 2020, I started to prescribe Ivermectin, herbal medicines, and homeopathy to patients against COVID-19 infection who had not improved after receiving antipyretic and analgesic prescriptions from their previous doctors. At the end of the same year, I started to administer Ivermectin to Long-COVID patients who had persistent fatigue and cough even after fever had gone down. In addition, I began administering Ivermectin for the treatment and prevention of adverse reactions immediately after mRNA vaccination and for patients with the vaccination-induced sequelae (Long-Vax).

Chapter 8 Flash in Japan

As of early January 2024, the 9th wave (7th vaccine transmission wave?) of COVID-19 infections in Japan has ended, followed by the beginning of 10th wave, mainly of the JN.1 strain (self-amplifying replicon vaccine shedding wave?) that arrived in Japan.

Most outpatient fever doctors are fully protected with masks, gowns, gloves, and face shields, but would not dare to touch a patient with their bare hands or even observe the throat. These same doctors, after prescribing antipyretics and antivirals, will leave the patient in isolation saying, "COVID-19 is just a cold, you should stay home and rest". And yet, in the same breath, they will recommend that the patient receive an additional booster vaccine.

Even infectious disease experts are unaware that such sloppy initial treatment has led to the massive occurrence of Long-COVID and Long-Vax cases.

CUTTING THROUGH JAPAN'S COVID-19 INFECTION CONTROL AND VACCINE MEDICINE

I have given Ivermectin to a total of 1,800 patients not only to treat and prevent COVID-19 infection in the past four years, but also started providing the drug to Long COVID-19 patients and vaccine related sequelae over the last 3 years.

I have issued more than 8,000 COVID-19 vaccine preventive inadmissibility certificates since 2021, starting with Japanese music students in Germany to enable their participation in orchestras.

The certificates allowed anyone worldwide to continue their education, employment, and international travel. Most of those issued the certificates were Japanese families who worried about the adverse effects of vaccine shots and shedding whose movement of livelihood was restricted by the pandemic.

In the course of this work, I kept in mind the humanitarian efforts

In May 2021, our clinic began offering outpatient Long COVID and mRNA PVS services as well as outpatient, online, and home visits following initial treatment of COVID-19 infection. My clinic has treated over 2,000 patient each with Covid-19 infection, Long-COVID, and Long-Vax.

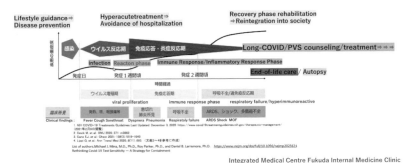

Figure1. From prevention of COVID-19 infection to treatment, rehabilitation, end-of-life care, and autopsy

of Chiune Sugihara, known as the 'Schindler of the East', who issued 'life visas' to Jews persecuted by Nazi Germany during the Second World War.

Figure 1 shows the outpatient services of my clinic for the treatment of the COVID-19 infection.

Currently, the clinic continues to provide guidance in the prevention of COVID-19 infection, therapeutic intervention during the very early stages of infection, home rehabilitation after intensive care management of severe infections, associated treatment of Long-COVID and mRNA PVS, and end-of-life care such as advanced cancer and cardiac/respiratory failure.

SYMPTOMS, DIAGNOSIS AND TREATMENT OF mRNA PVS/ LPCVS

Figure 2 shows the symptoms and diagnosis of adverse effects mainly caused by mRNA PVS in my clinic up to May 2024. Some of the diagnoses include those observed in other medical institutions. As

Chapter 8　Flash in Japan

Adverse symptoms and Diagnosis after mRNA vaccination

Adverse symptoms
Edema, Headache, Eye pain, Lightheadedness, Brain-fog, Dizziness, Fire-burning, Cold sensation, Lymphadenopathy, Othrrhea, Tinnitus, Hearing loss or sensitivity, Rhinorrhea, Posterior rhinorrhea, Pharyngolaryngeal discomfort, Taste/smell disorder, Red/White blood cell abnormalities, Thrombocytopenia, Liver/Renal dysfunction, DIC, Palpitations, Chest pain, Chest agony, Dyspnea, Cough, Difficulty expectorating, Wheezing, Nasal hemorrhage, Hemoptysis, Lethargy,Decreased memory, Difficulty in attending school/work, Fatigue, Deficiency of dexterity, Pain, sensory disturbance, Muscle weakness, Gait disturbance, Anxiety, depression/Mania (symptoms), Emotional instability,anorexia, insomnia, ED, Frigidity, Abdominal pain/discomfort/distention/bloating, Hemorrhoids, Chemical and electromagnetic hypersensitivity

Diagnosios
Anaphylaxis, Herpes zoster (neuralgia), Cellulitis, Palmoplantar pustulosis, Alopecia, Trigeminal neuralgia, Oculomotor/facial/ glossopharyngeal/ nerve palsy, Thyroid dysfunction, Fibromyalgia, Adrenal fatigue, MCAS, Reward Deficiency Syndrome, Chronic nasopharyngitis, Bronchial asthma, COPD, ILD (anti-MDA5), Sleep apnea syndrome, GERD, NUD/FD, IBD/IBS, SIBO, Gastro-duodenal ulcer, Ulcerative colitis, Diverticulitis, Menstrual Abnormalities, Abnormal Pregnancy, Hyperemesis gravidarum, Menopausal disorders/LOH, Cerebral infarction, Subarachnoid hemorrhage, Rectal lacerations, Subdural hematoma, Rheumatoid arthritis, ANCA-associated vasculitis, Systemic lupus erythematosus (SLE), Idiopathic thrombocytopenic purpura, Aplastic Anemia, Acute lymphocytic leukemiam, Multiple myeloma, Adult T-cell leukemia, Lymphoma, Multiple solid tumors, ALS, ME/CSF, Guillain-Barre/Fisher syndrome, Adrenal fatigue, PANS/PANDAS, Lyme disease, Cat scratch disease, Autoimmune encephalitis, ADEM, Creutzfeldt-Jakob disease, Dysmenorrhea, Dysautonomia, Temporal arteritis, Lymphoedema, Varicose veins, Deep vein thrombosis, Malignant neoplasms (various types), Heart failure, Paroxysmal atrial fibrillation, Angina pectoris, Myocardial infarction, Aortic dissection, Schizophrenia, Autism, ADHD, Dementia (MCI), Alcohol/drug dependence, Charcot-Marie-Tooth disease, Falls (bruises, fractures, cerebral contusions), Suicide attempts, Accidental death

Integrated Medical Centre Fukuda Internal Medicine Clinic

Figure2. Adverse (sequelae) symptoms and diagnosis due to mRNA PVS

this table shows, mRNA PVS/LPCVS has a wide range of symptoms and diagnoses.

In Japan, however, there are no established diagnostic criteria for post-vaccination syndrome, and in many cases, no abnormalities are found upon examination and thus no professionally confirmed diagnosis can be made.

It is necessary to persistently and carefully counsel patients about innate vulnerabilities, and latent pathologies of the epidemic before simply confirming a diagnosis of vaccine injury.

Therefore, it is crucial to provide systematic and longitudinal feedback on the mind and body's biological responses to environmental stimuli before and after treatments if the aim is to prevent vaccine injury and/or the onset of COVID-19 infection.

The CHI Fractal System (www.chi-fractal.com) is grounded in sound scientific principles, incorporating Stress Theory (pioneered by

207

the father of stress, Hans Selye); fractal dynamics in human biology; heart rate variability; and proprietary neurodynamic software and algorithms.

This system proves invaluable for examining brain wave patterns, maintaining homeostasis, and regulating higher-order systems affected by environmental changes and pathological processes from a neuro-psycho-endocrinological perspective.

NEW TECHNOLOGIES AND TREATMENTS

CHI-Airnergy/Stream HS employs the photosynthesis principle, utilizing its proprietary photodynamic technology to create activated oxygen from the air. This activated oxygen, a source of essential electric energy, is then seamlessly integrated with water—the magical molecule that sustains life.

Through the gentle act of nasal breathing, a combination of this revitalized water and detoxified fresh air is simultaneously delivered into the body. The inhaled water droplets, charged with stored energy, set in motion a harmonious cascade of detoxification, revitalization, and rejuvenation processes.

DENBA[H] technology (https://denbahealth.com) which is based on preserving food freshness by weak electrolysis, was also effective for sleep disorders, including sleep apnea syndrome, by increasing the activity of the autonomic nervous system in post-vaccine syndrome by creating an electric field space by applying fine vibrations to water molecules. These daily care practices are essential for the rapid reduction of post- vaccine injury and the promotion of holistic recovery.

In the strategy for post-vaccine syndrome, my clinic offers not only prevention and treatment, but also special emphasis on home rehabilitation, which has helped several patients return to social life after being bedridden.

Clinical manifestations of Long-COVID and Post-Vaccine Syndrome(PVS)

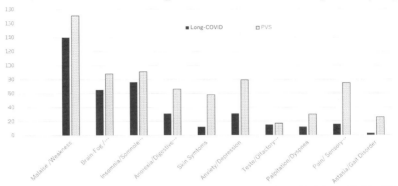

Integrated Medical Centre Fukuda Internal Medicine Clinic

Figure3. Comparison of symptoms lasting more than 2 months at the previous physician between the two groups.

Kidojutsu (http://www.kidojutu.com) 'chi-guiding technique', is a novel wave energy therapy that instantly stimulates the body and mind's natural self-healing powers to quickly relieve stress and pain and revitalize muscles and organs without training or discipline.

The Relive Shirt-related products (https://www.relivewear.net) have also been proven to increase muscle strength and flexibility, improve posture, gait and physical function, and to provide a good night's sleep, thereby reducing the burden on caregivers, rehab professionals and athletes by simply wearing them.

Figure 3 shows the main clinical manifestations of each of the 300 cases of Long-COVID and mRNA PVS in my clinic.

It is generally believed that the symptoms of Long-COVID and PVS, are very similar (due to the spike protein) and, many medical institutions specializing in treatment of COVID-19 sequelae still recommend SARS-CoV-2 vaccination as a prophylactic against the progression of Long-COVID/Long-Vax.

The US-based Front Line COVID-19 Critical Care (FLCCC)

Alliance and others have also proposed a common treatment protocol for Long-COVID/LPCVS.

While many cases of Long-COVID often resolve mildly with various diagnostic treatments, the clinical manifestations of Long-Vax often persist for months or longer, and in some cases may worsen and become more severe. In addition, Long-Vax is more commonly associated with cutaneous and gastrointestinal symptoms, pain and numbness, physical and mental dysfunction such as difficulty standing and walking, and persistent psychiatric and neurological symptoms when compared to Long-COVID.

I usually recommend Ivermectin at about 300 µg/kg orally for minimum 4 consecutive days in the early stages of COVID-19 infection.

However, Ivermectin is rarely used alone in the treatment of Long-COVID and LPCVS as well as in the early stages of infection, but rather in combination with psychological counseling, nutritional

Integrative therapies for Long-COVID/mRNA PVS (LPCVS)

Psychotherapy (Cognitive-behavioral therapy, Hypnotherapy, Meditation, etc.), Kinesiology/Kinesiaroma (HSK)
Chinese Medicine, Acupuncture, Osteopathy, Homeopathy, Aromatherapy, Flower essence, Ayurveda
Rehabilitation/Palliative care (respiratory & circulatory/nerve & motor), Kidojutu, RELIVE shirt, SSS stretch

Dietary/ Nutritional therapy: Medical Rice/ VitaminB/D, Zinc, Magnesium, Silica, Selenium, Iron, Plasmalogen
Sodium Silver Thiosulfate/Molecular Iodine Solution/CBD (CFS), DHA/EPA, Quercetin, CoQ10,Taurine, AHCC
Melatonin,Powerfucoidan, Bromelain, Nattokinase, Curcumin, Berberine, TwendeeX/Mtcontrol, Asaigermanium,
5-ALA, Taxiforin, M-Guard, Fergard B, Lumbrux(V-cure), Milk thistle, Artemisin, Cat' s claw, 5-Deazaflavins,
d-Gs(Selista), NAD, NMN Plus+/Body Vitality/Revive/Easy Sleep/Anoni/TRI-BIOTIC (ENVISIONARY LIFE)

Ivermectin, Nobiletin, Hydroxychloroquine, Mebendazole, Favipiravir, Naltrexone, Resveratrol, Baobab, EGCG
BHRT, Beta-glucans (BRMGs), Autologous formalin-fixed tumor vaccine (Cell-Medicine), IgYAb (Covinax)

Normalization of the internal/external environments:Multi probiotics, Bowel Nosods, Creatine, L-Arginine
Removal of Electromagnetic waves/Pesticides (glyphosate) / Toxic mold, metal (amalgam), and Chemicals
Chelation/Detoxification: DMSA, EDTA, IMD Cleanse (QSS), Augmented NAC, Nicotinell-patches
Vitamin C (IVC, Liposomal), Ozone (MAH)/Biophoto therapy(UVBI), Methylene blue (IVC, PO)
Glutathione (IV, Liposomal), Placenta: Vertebrates/Fishes/Plants(MF+), Cordyceps militaris (Caitac), SHIRAJIT

QUINTON (Inhalation, PO, IV,IM,IC), Nasopharyngeal abrasion and washing (EAT), PDT-PLUS (H4CTC)
The RASHA, Vielight(PBMT), CHI-Airnergy/Stream HS, DENBAᴴ, Hydrogen (Suisonia, Lita Life, H2Elite)
α-Radiorespiro-Rn, Radon/Bicarbonate NO bathing (Medicated HOT TAB), Exosome(CellSource)
Stem cell therapy(PSC/MO/NOP):PlaqX, Pandemic Booster, HGH,HFR, GcMAF, STF, ASI (European Wellness)

Integrated Medical Centre Fukuda Internal Medicine Clinic

Figure4. Integrative medicine by Fukuda Internal Medicine Clinic in Long-COVID/LPCVS

and detoxification including diet. And as individualized treatment, it is combined with digestive enzymes and multibiotics to correct the intestinal microbiota and the gut-lung axis, and also traditional Japanese and Indian medicine such as Chinese herbal medicine and Ayurveda, some wave/energy therapy such as homeopathy, and stem cell therapy (Figure 4).

The SARS-CoV-2 spike protein (SP) binds to the ACE2 receptor on a cell's vascular endothelium during infection and is thought to be involved in angiogenesis and thrombus formation. Since Ivermectin has binding affinity for the fibrinogen peptide portion of SARS-CoV-2 SP, it has been suggested that Ivermectin may interfere with the binding of SP and fibrinogen, thereby reducing fibrin clot formation and microthrombus formation.[1]

Pentosidine, a marker of renal dysfunction and end product of protein glycation (AGEs); D-dimer, a marker of bone matrix, coagulation/fibrinolytic system, vascular endothelial damage and deep vein thrombosis; and homocysteine involved in methionine

Changes in Thrombosis and AGEs Indices with treatment

	Unvaccinated Long-COVID(-) n= 29	Unvaccinated Long-COVID n=188	Vaccinated Long-COVID(-) n=60	PVS Uninfected n=48	PVS COVID-19Infected n=17
Homocystein Untreated (5.1-11.7 nmol/mL)	6.9	14.6	15.1	18.7	20.1
Homocystein Treated		9.4		13.3	14.9
Pentosidine Untreated (0.00915-0.0431µg/Ml)	0.541	0. 703	0.775	0.891	0.704
Pentosidine Treated		0.640		0.773	0.652
D-dimer Untreated (1.00µg/mL>)	0.77	2.06	1.29	1.70	1.88
D-dimer Treated		1.40		1.59	1.76

Survey by Integrated Medical Center Fukuda Internal Medicine Clinic

Figure5. Changes in diagnostic markers at initial visit and after treatment in Long-COVID/ LPCVS

metabolism and is an indicator of atherosclerosis, are considered as biomarkers that can predict the severity of COVID-19 infection as well as the improvement of symptoms such as dementia.

In addition, homocysteine and pentosidine levels were higher in the Long-COVID/LPCVS group regardless of infection or vaccination history, and these indices improved with various treatments such as Ivermectin.[2]

In this research of the Long-COVID and mRNA PVS/LPCVS groups, these biomarkers were expected to predict the severity of COVID-19 infection in the post-vaccine group with a history of COVID-19 infection versus the unvaccinated group or the group without post-vaccine sequelae (Figure 5).

My clinic had been providing nutrition/detoxification instruction to outpatients before the COVID-19 pandemic. In my survey, I reported that the Long-COVID/LPCVS group may have more anemia, endocrine dysfunction such as thyroid, adrenal cortical function, and sex hormones, and various vitamin and mineral deficiencies versus the unaffected group.[3]

Zinc has antioxidant, anti-inflammatory, immunomodulatory, and antiviral effects mediated by RNA-dependent suppression of RdRp.[4]

Vitamin D supplementation has also been reported to have the potential to reduce Long-COVID and vaccine adverse events, as well as prevent severe COVID-19 infection and reduce the risk of hospitalization, treatment, and death.[5]

In my research, blood levels of serum vitamin D and zinc were higher in the group with no post-vaccine sequelae after COVID-19 vaccination compared to the group with initial COVID-19 infection and the group with post-corona/post-vaccine sequelae at the initial visit.

Serum Zinc and 25(OH)Vitamin D levels

Unvaccinated	Before supplementation	After 3 months of intake		COVID-19 initial infection	Long-COVID	Vaccinated PVS(+)	Vaccinted PVS(-)
Serum Zinc (μg/dL)	68.2	98.2	Serum Zinc (μg/dL)	60.5	68.4	63.8	71.0
Serum 25OH-VD (ng/ml)	21.7	47.3	Serum 25OH-VD (ng/ml)	12.9	16.6	14.4	23.1

Zinc: 50 mg/day and VitaminD3: 5000 IU/day preadministration in the unvaccinated group

➡

COVID-19 infection: 32% reduction compared to non-treated group
Long-COVID: 26% reduction compared to the non-treated group

Survey by Integrated Medical Centre Fukuda Internal Medicine Clinic

Figure6. Relationship between serum zinc/vitamin D and COVID-19 infection/Long-COVID/LPCVS

Furthermore, when vitamin D and zinc supplements were taken for more than 6 months in the unvaccinated group with zinc and vitamin D concentrations below reference levels and who were not infected with COVID-19, the rate of new cases of COVID-19 infection and vaccine sequelae was lower than in the untreated group (Figure 6).

For COVID-19 infection, it has been reported that combination therapy with Ivermectin, zinc, nitazoxanide and ribavirin resulted in negative SARS-CoV-2 RT PCR in a shorter time than symptomatic therapy.[6, 7]

Similarly, I found that the prophylactic use of Ivermectin on a weekly basis in addition to vitamin D and zinc further reduced the incidence of new COVID-19 infections and Long-COVID and LPCVS than in the group receiving only two supplemental drugs.

IS IVERMECTIN EFFECTIVE IN PREVENTING POST-VACCINE ADVERSE REACTIONS AND VACCINE SEQUELAE?

Ivermectin is recommended as a first-line treatment protocol following intermittent fasting for the prevention and early transient treatment of FLCCC-recommended protocols and as a protocol for long-term COVID and post-vaccine injury. Ivermectin may interfere with the adhesion of spike proteins to human cell membranes at the docking site between the SARS-CoV-2 viral spike and the ACE2 receptor. Ivermectin has also been reported to have high binding affinity not only for the viral S protein, but also for the human cell surface receptor ACE-2 and the expressing cell TMPRSS2, which may inhibit viral entry into the host cell.[8, 9]

However, genetic-based immunohistochemical studies of SARS-CoV-2 antigens have shown that Ivermectin not only blocks the nucleocapsid protein of SARS-CoV-2 infection, but also inhibits the entry of the mRNA vaccine-derived spike protein into the host cell, preventing so-called "vaccine infection".

Recently, spike protein (SP)-induced erythrocyte aggregation induced by SARS-CoV-2 and virus adhesion to other blood cells and endothelial cells have been reported as a possible key factor in COVID-19 susceptibility. Inhibition of the spike protein-induced erythrocyte aggregation reaction (HA) binds strongly to SARS-CoV-2 SP glycan sites. The macrocyclic lactone Ivermectin, which binds strongly to multiple glycan sites on this spike protein, blocks the erythrocyte aggregation reaction (HA) when added to RBCs before the spike protein and later, also reverses HA when added. It has been suggested that Ivermectin or other competitive glycoconjugates may be a COVID-19 therapeutic strategy and may help elucidate the rare serious adverse effects (AEs) associated with COVID-19 mRNA vaccines that use spike protein as the producing antigen.[10]

In a COVID-19 infection, it has been reported that as the number of mutations in the S-1 site increases, the + charge on the surface of the spike protein increases, attracting the + charge on the surface of red blood cells, resulting in red blood cell aggregation. This report suggests that microthrombi may occur in the body via spike proteins.

Professor Hideaki Hanaki, representative of the Kitasato Project for COVID-19 Countermeasures at Kitasato Institute, Kitasato University, speculates: *"If the binding of spike protein to Ivermectin electrically inhibits the binding of red blood cells and also to spike protein by coronavirus vaccine, microthrombi can be prevented. If Ivermectin can bind to the spike protein of the COVID-19 vaccine and prevent microthrombosis, it may contribute to the treatment of mRNA PVS/LPCVS as well as Long-COVID."*

Ivermectin is believed to be able to block the progression of COVID-19 infection in its early stages, and it has been reported that a single dose of Ivermectin can reduce symptoms of infection in COVID-19 patients undergoing outpatient treatment.[11]

Therefore, I recommend Ivermectin for prevention of COVID-19 infection and early onset of the disease. In cases where mandatory vaccination is required for nursing student practice or workplace conditions, Ivermectin prophylaxis prior to vaccination has been shown to reduce the incidence of adverse reactions to booster vaccination, such as fever, redness and pain at the injection site, fatigue, and anaphylaxis (shock).

Ivermectin has also shown to be effective in treating not only Long-COVID, but also vaccine sequelae. The administration of Ivermectin at the time of initial infection suppresses the onset of these sequelae.

Cases have been reported in my clinic where Ivermectin administration reduced various sequelae such as depression, insomnia, fatigue, lethargy, brain fog, MCI, various skin symptoms including hair loss, visual disturbances such as photophobia and double vision, hearing, smell and taste disturbances such as hypersensitivity and dullness, numbness in extremities, pain in various parts of the body, palpitations and dyspnea.

In some cases, the homeopathic remedy "Grus Japonensis: TANCHO" has been effective in combination with Ivermectin for post-vaccination nasopharyngitis, brain fog, photophobia, hearing and olfactory sensitivity, and peripheral neuropathy.

B-spot therapy (B for Biinku = nasopharynx) is a treatment invented by Dr. Shinsaku Horiguchi, M.D., in which the nasopharynx is washed with zinc chloride, which has bactericidal and anti-inflammatory effects. Recently, this treatment is called EAT (Epipharyngeal Abrasive Therapy).

In my clinic, I have found that the addition of Ivermectin and Augmented NAC to the zinc chloride nasopharyngeal lavage solution cures suppresses various focal infection symptoms, including upper respiratory tract symptoms caused by Long-COVID and Long Vax, more effectively than the zinc chloride solution treatment alone.

In addition, rapid improvement of nasopharyngitis-related focal infection symptoms has been observed with these combination of EAT, photobiomodulation therapy and Methylene blue administration.

The duration of symptoms such as fever, generalized sore throat, and cough was shorter in patients treated with Ivermectin alone for very early COVID-19 infections (within 24 hours of symptom onset) than in those treated with antipyretics/analgesics, Chinese herbal extracts, or azithromycin/clarithromycin alone in my clinic.

During the 18-month period from June 2021 to the end of 2022 in our hospital, the combination of Ivermectin and antibiotics (AZM or CAM) in the initial treatment of COVID-19 infection showed a significant reduction in the duration of various symptoms, such as fever, generalized/pharyngeal pain, and cough when compared to the no treatment rest group, antipyretic/analgesic group, Chinese medicine group, antibiotics alone group, and the antiviral drug(Molnupiravir) group. This combination also, significantly reduced the incidence of

Long-COVID and vaccine sequelae (Long-COVID/LPCVS) within 3 months of infection compared to the no treatment rest group, antipyretic/analgesic group, herbal medicine group, antibiotics alone group, and antiviral drug (Molnupiravir) group (Figure 7).

Incidence of Long-COVID
- 3 of 27 patients (11.1%) in the IVM + AZM/CAM
- 4 of 30 (13.3%) in patients treated with Lagevrio® (Molnupiravir) alone
- 31 of 218 (14.2%) in the no treatment group with rest and isolation only
- 28 of 189 patients (14.8%) in the various herbal extracts alone
- 7 of 59(11.8%) patients in the Ivermectin (IVM) alone
- 71 of 390 patients (18.2%) in the group receiving antipyretic/ analgesic drugs alone
- 29 of 177 patients (16.4%) in the no treatment (rest and isolation only)

Incidence of mRNA PVS
- 2 of 19 (10.5%) patients in the IVM + AZM/CAM
- 4 of 29 (13.8%) in patients treated with Molnupiravir alone
- 5of 31(16.1%) patients in the AZM/CAM
- 29 of 175 (16.6%) patients in the various herbal extracts alone
- 13 of 94 (13.8%) patients in the Ivermectin (IVM) alone
- 65 of 286(22.7%) patients in the antipyretic/analgesic drugs alone (Figure 7)

Prescriptions by previous physicians for early COVID-19 infection tended to include no treatment/rest and isolation, and prescriptions for antipyretic/analgesic or antitussive/expectorant drugs. On the

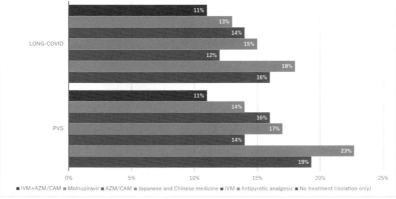

Figure7. Incidence of Long-COVID and PVS by initial treatment of COVID-19 infection

other hand, treatment was individualized according to the progression and improvement of various symptoms and was mainly based on Ivermectin in combination with AZM/CAM, Chinese herbs (extracts or decoctions), homeopathic remedies, antiviral agents such as Molnupiravir, and steroids (oral, injectable, or inhaled), depending on the patient's condition and symptoms in my clinic.

Lagevrio® (Molnupiravir), which is not as effective as Ivermectin, has been administered early in the course of infection to shorten the duration of onset of symptoms such as fever, sore throat, and wet cough, and to reduce the incidence of long-lasting COVID/LPCVS. Between the two, Ivermectin has fewer side effects in pediatric patients, but Molnupiravir has age and severity as risk factor limitations for indication.

In addition, precautions must be taken when administering Molnupiravir, because of gastrointestinal symptoms (including vomiting and diarrhea, urticaria, and anaphylaxis) among patients. This is why I have decided to discontinue the administration of antiviral drugs.

Although Molnupiravir still remains the most commonly administered antiviral drug in Japan during the 11th rippling wave of infection began in May 2024, its efficacy is declining and there is concern that this drug may increase the amplification of mutant strains by mRNA replicon vaccines against SARS-CoV-2 virus.

Clinical data before the patient came to my clinic suggest that inadequate home rehabilitation after intensive care treatment of severe infections and initial treatment of mild/moderate infections with antipyretics and analgesics in addition to home isolation may have contributed to the development of Long-COVID and LPCVS.

THE NEED FOR NEW CRITERIA FOR "POSTVACCINAL SHINGLES"

Herpes zoster is a disease characterized by the appearance of erythema and vesicles and pain along the ganglia in immunocompromised adults infected with varicella-zoster virus (VZV).

Eiki Sano et al. found COVID-19 spike proteins (SP) at the site of rash lesions caused by persistent varicella-zoster virus infection after vaccination in a case of adult varicella that developed 2 weeks after the first dose of mRNA COVID-19 vaccine (Pfizer Inc.: BNT162b), worsened after the second dose, and persisted for 3 months. This report suggests that mRNA-encoded SP may be involved in skin pathology as a side effect of the vaccine.[12]

Whether mRNA COVID-19 vaccination can induce persistent VZV reactivation by disrupting the immune system or whether the expressed spike protein plays a pathogenic role is unknown, but it is usually rare for herpes zoster varicella-zoster infection with blistering and painful cutaneous vasculitis to persist for many months, as in the case of herpes zoster following mRNA COVID-19 vaccination.

In my clinic, I have seen several cases of herpes zoster after COVID-19 vaccination. The refractory symptoms improved promptly after several months of care with antiviral drugs in a specialized medical institution, thanks to integrated medical treatment mainly with Ivermectin (Figure 8).

Herpes zoster after COVID-19 vaccination tends to become recurrent and refractory as the vaccination is repeated. I have also seen cases of so-called "binary infection" where mPVS/LPCV symptoms suddenly appear in previously vaccinated patients triggered by COVID-19 infections like a binary biological weapon.

The following picture shows a teenage girl who lost almost her entire head of hair and became amenorrheic after COVID-19 infection following two mRNA vaccinations. 2.5 months of treatment by dermatologists did not improve her total hair loss and she tended to miss school (Figure 9: left)

After one month of treatment with Ivermectin at a dosage of 6 mg/day, antioxidant (Twendee Mtcontrol®) and stem cell therapy (MF Plus™ Hair Follicle Regenerator), her hair grew back dramatically (middle photo) and by the third month her hair had almost grown back (right photo). Her menstruation resumed after 6 months of treatment, and she now attends school regularly without a wig.

ANNUAL TRENDS IN PHYSIOLOGY AND DEVELOPMENT OF HIGH SCHOOL GIRLS WITH AND WITHOUT VACCINATION

For the past six years, since before the COVID-19 pandemic, we have conducted questionnaires and interviews during medical examinations on menstrual abnormalities and eating disorders among healthy female high school students in and outside the prefecture.

The results showed that the group vaccinated twice or more had

Refractory shingles after COVID-19 mRNA vaccination

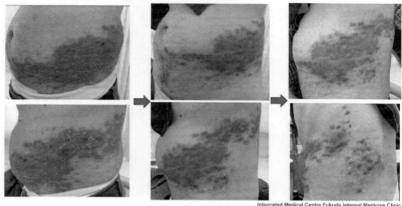

Figure 8. A case of refractory herpes zoster after COVID-19 vaccination relieved by IVM.

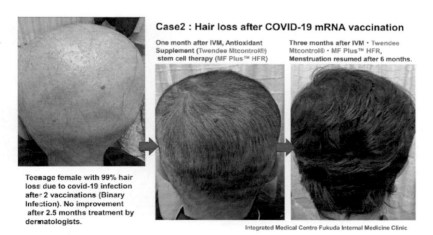

Figure 9. A case of total hair loss after COVID-19 vaccination relieved by IVM.

Refractory shingles after COVID-19 mRNA vaccination

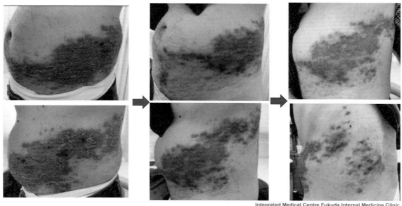

Figure8. A case of refractory herpes zoster after COVID-19 vaccination relieved by IVM.

Refractory shingles after COVID-19 mRNA vaccination: Case 2

Figure9. A case of refractory herpes zoster after COVID-19 vaccination relieved by IVM

significantly more menstrual abnormalities, menstrual cramps, PMS (premenstrual syndrome), persistent headaches and dizziness, and weight loss (rarely weight gain) due to eating disorders when compared to the unvaccinated group (Figure 10).

Annual trends in menstrual abnormalities and eating disorders among high school girls

	Menstrual abnormality	Menstrual pain	PMS	Headace/ Dizziness	Eating Disorder
Unvaccinaed group N=66 (17.1%)	Menstrual irregularity 12.1%→13.6% Irregular M bleeding 3.0% → 4.5% Decreased flow 4.5% Increased flow 6.1%	15.1%→ 16.7%	7.5% → 6.1%	Headache 10.6%→13.6% Dizziness 3.0%→4.5%	Overeating 10.6%→9.1% Anorexia 3.0%→4.5%
Vaccinated group N=321 (82.9%) 2vaccinations 59人 18.4% 3vaccinations 262 81.6%	Mens Irregularity 10.9% → 15.9% Irregular M bleeding 1.9% → 6.9% Decreased flow 8.1% Increased flow 5.0%	17.1%→ 23.9%	6.9%→10.9%	Headache 12.1%→18.1% Dizziness 3.1%→6.9%	Overeating 8.1%→10.9% Anorexia 4.0%→6.9%
N=387 (Total)	※The group that stopped after 3 doses of vaccination had a higher recovery rate of menstrual abnormalities than the group that proceeded to 4 doses of vaccination.				

Survey by Integrated Medical Centre Fukuda Internal Medicine Clinic

Figure10. COVID-19 Vaccination and Annual Trends in Menstrual Abnormalities and Eating Disorders Among High School Girls *Excludes female students who have only been vaccinated once, as symptoms such as menstrual abnormalities are unlikely to be noticed immediately after vaccination.

The increase in menstrual abnormalities with each passing year in the unvaccinated group may be related to the stress of promotion to the next grade or to vaccine shedding. In addition, among female students who complained of menstrual abnormalities, the group that voluntarily proceeded to participate in the 4-dose vaccination program showed less improvement in menstrual abnormalities than the group that discontinued the vaccination program, according to the questionnaire survey and interview in 2023.

In fact, we observed an improvement of 53.8% (7 out of 13) in menstrual abnormalities in those that remained unvaccinated for 1 year after 3 vaccinations.

I also found out from interviews, that students who consulted a gynecologist or health care provider (without consulting their parents or teachers) about their menstrual abnormalities and other physical/ or mental disorders (before and during the COVID-19) may have been caused by vaccination. Most health care providers automatically prescribed low-dose pills and/or painkillers without asking about their vaccination history.

As in this study, it has proven difficult to conduct large-scale investigation on the annual trends in menstrual abnormalities by number of vaccinations, especially when going back to the period before mass vaccination began. With Japan holding the world record for the number of mRNA vaccinations (up to 7doses), it would be ideal track annual trends in tests, higher education, employment, pregnancy, even childbirth and cancer incidence status over a long period.

CAUTION AGAINST ASYMPTOMATIC RENAL DYSFUNCTION AFTER mRNA VACCINATION

Many acute kidney diseases, such as MCD (minimal change disease, which causes nephrotic syndrome), IgA nephropathy, where the immunoglobulin protein IgA is deposited in the glomeruli of the kidney, thrombotic thrombocytopenic purpura (TTP), and autoantibody ANCA-associated vasculitis have been reported to occur within 2 weeks of mRNA vaccination with a higher risk of AKI-related mortality compared to the unvaccinated group.[13, 14]

When podocytes (the foot processes of glomerular epithelial cells from which the protein, dendrin, is expressed), are injured, dendrin is said to translocate to the nucleus and promote kidney damage such as increased proteinuria.[15]

Other reports indicate that Ivermectin treatment of mice with chronic kidney disease, suppressed the translocation of dendrin expressed in glomerular foot cells to the nucleus, thereby reducing proteinuric kidney damage and prolonging survival.[16, 17]

I have been routinely tracking renal function prior to the mRNA vaccination in 2021. The mRNA PVS/LPCVS group showed

The 5 stages of chronic kidney disease

Managing Chronic Kidney Disease in Type 2 Diabetes (ckdandt2d.com)

Stage of CKD	STAGE 1	STAGE 2	STAGE 3A	STAGE 3B	STAGE 4	STAGE 5
eGFR	90 or greater	Between 60 and 89	Between 45 and 59	Between 30 and 44	Between 15 and 29	Less than 15
Level of kidney damage	Mild kidney damage	Mild kidney damage	Mild to moderate kidney damage	Mild to moderate kidney damage	Moderate to severe kidney damage	End-stage kidney disease. Kidneys are close to failure or have completely failed. You will need to start dialysis or have a kidney transplant.

PVS	STAGE1	STAGE2	STAGE3A	STAGE3B	STAGE4	STAGE5
Type2 Diabetes(+)	6	23(11)	14 (6)	7(5)	5(4)	2(1)
Type2 Diabetes(−)	11	29(8)	19(7)	5(3)	2(2)	1(1)

Evaluation of renal function after COVID-19 mRNA vaccination
※( ) Number of patients with stage progression / reduced eGFR

Survey by Integrated Medical Centre Fukuda Internal Medicine Clinic

Figure11. Changes in renal function after mRNA vaccination (from acute to chronic phase)

a progressive decline in eGFR level, pentosidine and other renal function indices with each booster vaccination, even in the absence of underlying diseases such as diabetes and hypertension, compared to the unvaccinated group. Pentosidine progressively declined with each booster vaccination, even in the absence of underlying diseases like diabetes or hypertension (Figure 11).

In my clinic, renal dysfunction cases which progressed due to mRNA PVS/LPCVS, receiving a combined treatment of Ivermectin and low-protein brown rice: Medical Rice developed by Dr. Shaw Watanabe et al resulted in downstaging and improvement of renal function in one case of stage 5 chronic kidney disease (CKD) and three cases of stage 4 CKD. And two cases of stage 4 CKD and one case of stage 5 CKD have shown benefit from anti-aging therapy with 5-deazaflavin (TND1128).[19, 20]

In Japan and Russia, hydrogen inhalation therapy with AfH:H

(H2O) m (Suisonia Gas) has been demonstrated to improve respiratory and renal function in the rehabilitation of Long-COVID and is useful in my clinic as Long-Vax-related interstitial pneumonia, heart failure, and turbo cancer.

My clinic has also reported that silver sodium thiosulfate and sodium thiosulfate hydrate are effective against renal damage and interstitial pneumonia, and molecular iodine solution was effective in relieving thyroid cancer pain after mRNA vaccination. (Cancer-Free Co., Ltd.)

Dr. Farokh Master of Homeopathic Health Center documents effective cases of homeopathic medicine for allopathic treatment-resistant kidney disorders at hospitals in Mumbai. (https://drfarokhmaster.com)

Regenerative medicine using xenogeneic progenitor stem cell transplantation for renal failure has been reported.[21]

My clinic will continue to support the treatment system (European Wellness Centers) for renal failure based on stem cell transplantation for patients who wish to avoid dialysis or kidney transplantation.

IS IVERMECTIN EFFECTIVE FOR TURBO CANCER AFTER mRNA VACCINATION?

Ivermectin has been implicated in the regulation of signaling pathways via PAK1 kinase (a general term for enzymes that transfer phosphate groups from molecules with high-energy phosphate bonds to substrates or target molecules) and thus has anti-tumor effects in cancer cells, including inhibition of proliferation. It is believed to have anti-tumor effects such as inhibiting proliferation, metastasis, and angiogenesis in cancer cells, inducing apoptosis to promote programmed death of cancer cells, inhibiting angiogenesis of tumor stem cells, and reversing multidrug resistance in chemotherapy.[22]

Patients with high levels of PAK1, which is highly expressed in lung adenocarcinoma (LUAD) tissue, are reported to have shorter overall survival. Ivermectin-induced non-proteolytic autophagy mechanism was also found to inhibit PAK1 protein expression in LUAD cells and promote apoptosis (a form of cell death), as well as inhibit colony formation, cell survival and cell proliferation. In addition, IVM has been reported to efficiently inhibit LUAD cell proliferation in nude mice.[23]

It has also been reported that Ivermectin selectively induces apoptosis in chronic myeloid leukemia by inducing mitochondrial dysfunction and oxidative stress.[24]

The spike protein of the COVID-19 mRNA vaccine binds to estrogen receptor alpha and activates transcription, and the addition of S protein is observed to increase the proliferation of breast cancer cell lines.[25] And that Ivermectin inhibits tumor growth and metastasis by degrading PAK1 in esophageal squamous cell carcinoma, and as a target of Ivermectin in prostate cancer, the anticancer effect of Ivermectin by binding to two proteins, FOXA1 and heterodimer (formation Ku70/Ku80), which are important for chromatin opening and transcriptional activation of estrogen receptor (Erα) responsive genes in breast cancer cells, has been reported.[26]

There is a possible risk of accelerated progression of breast cancer when the vaccine spike proteins are produced in the body. It has been reported that cell proliferation is observed when ERα is activated in breast cancer, uterine cancer, ovarian cancer, and acute myeloid leukemia, which have ERα.

In Japan, the incidence of these ERα-positive cancers and deaths increased in the two years following vaccination.

In my clinic, the number of new-onset advanced cancers and simultaneous multiple cancers, called "turbo cancers," has increased rapidly in the last two years after the start of vaccination, and the types of cancers include lung cancer, breast cancer, esophageal cancer, gastric cancer, pancreatic cancer, rectal cancer, ovarian cancer, and malignant lymphoma. In most core oncology hospitals, the combination of chemotherapy and booster vaccination is repeated without considering the immune abnormality caused by vaccination. In my clinic, I have experienced a case in which lung metastasis of uterine cancer disappeared by autologous cancer vaccine therapy alone after chemotherapy was avoided.[27]

Also in my clinic, there have been cases in which tumor lesions partially shrank and various tumor markers improved after Ivermectin administration, but it is currently unclear whether Ivermectin alone or in combination with other anticancer therapies can inhibit the progression, improve the prognosis of turbo-cancer with or without vaccination and shedding.

Photodynamic Therapy (PDT) is a more direct application of low-level laser light based on sonophotodynamic therapy. PDT-Pulsed Laser Watch combines acupuncture, local pain treatment and external blood irradiation in four frequency spectra to provide supportive effects such as cancer treatment. (hope4cancer.com),

Methylene blue combined with the PDT/PBM (vielight.com) is more effective in further enhancing therapeutic efficacy against 'Vaccine Jacob', turbo-cancer and chemotherapy-induced nephrotoxicity.

In patients with "multiple concurrent turbo-cancers" after mRNA vaccinations, the sensitivity of Ivermectin (e.g. cytotoxic agents, immunostimulants/immunomodulators, PK inhibitors) to CTCs/CSTs in circulating tumor stem cells (R.G.C.C. International GmbH) is informative, but there are some cases of Ivermectin's significant response without sensitivity to these CTC assay.

THE ASSOCIATION OF mRNA VACCINE AND PRION DISEASE

Conventional Jacob's disease, caused by dural grafting or other means, was a fatal human prion disease that progressed for decades. Luc Montagnier et al. reported 26 cases of Jacob's disease that progressed rapidly and died suddenly after vaccination, out of 50 cases of Jacob's disease that developed after mRNA vaccination, mostly in Europe. The number of sudden death cases was reported as 26. The spike sequences of the Wuhan strain SARS-CoV-2 mRNA vaccine from each vaccinated company were reported to contain identical prion regions.[28]

The number of cases of Jacob's disease in Japan after the start of mRNA vaccination was reported by the MHLW to be 179 (in 2021) and 166 (in 2022). Although there has been no increase in the number of new cases over the past three years, it is not clear how many of these patients developed the disease after vaccination and whether the vaccine is suspected, as the cause of death, even in autopsy cases.

I have been treating a patient who developed prion disease after mRNA vaccination at home for almost 3 years now. After administration of Ivermectin, the myoclonic seizures disappeared, and after discontinuation of antiepileptic drugs, the patient's liver and kidney function improved. Unfortunately, there was no improvement in her comatose level of consciousness (Japan Coma Scale: 200), however, she could barely communicate through "yubidan", an original Japanese finger language.

A case of suspected adverse reaction of multiple malignant neoplasms such as neuritis, encephalitis and pancreatic cancer was reported to the MHLW after this patient received the same dose of mRNA vaccine derived from the Wuhan strain. Another prion patient, given the same dose of vaccine, developed a similar adverse reaction and died a few months later.

The market for therapeutic research into prion diseases is still growing, but no effective treatment has yet been found for 'vaccine-associated Jacob'.

Augmented NAC uses quantum technology to magnify ("augment") the key beneficial properties of the molecule N-acetylcysteine (NAC). These include potent antioxidant capabilities and the denaturation of up to 99.8% of the toxic spike protein, as well as its detachment from ACE2 receptors, as demonstrated in vitro and with strong empirical evidence attested many times.

- https://zerospike.org

In my clinic, I have seen cases of significant efficacy of augmented NAC as well as Ivermectin in AKI/CKD, turbo-cancer, heart failure and arrhythmias, (rheumatic) interstitial pneumonia (lung fibrosis), neuralgia brain fog, MCL Parkinson's syndrome, stroke encephalitis including ME/CFS, Creutzfeldt-Jakob disease due to mRNA vaccine injury, and various symptoms caused by "shedding".

CONCLUSION

In Japan, the total number of excess deaths in the last three years after the start of COVID-19 vaccination has increased to over 450,000 compared to the previous year before vaccination.

This death toll is said to be more than twice the number of people killed by the World War II bombings of Hiroshima and Nagasaki.

In addition, the number of births recorded in official statistics since 1899 was the lowest since 2022, and the stillbirth rate began to rise a year earlier.

These phenomena are at a rate of 2 deaths per 1 birth. Is the nation of Japan now on the verge of extinction?

Booster vaccination with the mRNA vaccine significantly increases IgG4 levels[29], and these same levels are shown to correlate with mortality in COVID-19 infections[30], in cases where anti spike antibodies are converted to IgG4, the IgG4 antibody level increased with each exposure to the virus due to SARS-CoV-2 reinfection. It has been reported that IgG4 antibodies increased with each exposure to the virus due to SARS-CoV-2 reinfection.

But it still remains to be seen whether IgG4 antibodies are useful as a predictive markers for the development and prognosis of mRNA PVS/LPCVS such as turbo-cancer and prion diseases, or whether Ivermectin can prevent the suppression of IgG4 anti-spike protein antibody production that binds mRNA vaccine-derived RBD.

- Clinical trials, developed by Dr. Yasufumi Murakami et al, are underway to determine whether administration of IgY antibodies derived from the Omicron mutants will inactivate the emerging mutant infections, suppress S protein IgG4 antibody production after several months, and reduce the number of patients with IgG4-related disease and mRNA vaccine sequelae in Japan.

In September 2023, a monovalent vaccine against Omicron strain XBB.1.5 was approved by the pharmaceutical affairs bodies, ahead of the rest of the world, with only antibody induction experiments in mice, and human gene manipulation experiments using mRNA vaccination were conducted as the seventh vaccine, which in turn led to the 9th(vaccine) wave in Japan.

It is predicted that this vaccine is not only ineffective in producing Omicron-type antibodies but will also produce harmful IgG4 antibodies that cannot neutralize the pathogen.

Despite reports of severe cases of anti-MDA5-positive DM-RPILD after vaccination with mRNA vaccine and pneumococcal vaccine, as well as increased cases of "double vaccine sequelae" by COVID-19

Chapter 8 Flash in Japan

and influenza vaccine. Rapidly progressive interstitial lung disease (anti-MDA5-positive DM-RPILD), occurring after COVID-19 and pneumococcal vaccines, self-amplifying mRNA vaccine trials are already underway, and clinical trials of an mRNA-based influenza vaccine, as well as the Replicon vaccine, are already planned to begin before the next planned pandemic season, whether there will be a bird flu outbreak.

This type of vaccine not only expresses the mRNA of the spike gene, but also continues to produce epitope-containing proteins by adding other antigen T-cell receptors, and eventually, genomic modification in the body can easily spread the mutant strain to unvaccinated individuals, as mRNA replication and antigen gene production continue in cells for a long time after induction of antibody and cellular immunity, thus resulting in high IgG4 antibody induction and suppression of immunity against infection and tumor immunity, rising concern that this could become a human experiment in acquiring functionality that is passed on to offspring.[31]

It is unfortunate that we Japanese, seem to be living in the world's largest genetic human experimentation country by bioterrorism. We are being treated like yellow monkeys and cattle in a lab! I fear we may be the first humans to wander into the "Planet of the Apes" and be trapped in a cage of our making.

We have gone from pandemic to infodemic to "vaccidemic", and from national territorial domination to national brain domination in cognitive warfare. The One World, One Health policy of the world's supranational powers has ensured that the non-kinetic occupation of cognitive space is underway.

Now is the time for us Japanese to write our own destiny: to create a future-proof social health care system, free from awe and coercion!

Flash in Japan, or is it just another flash in Japan…The flash of the

231

two atomic bombs were perceived as a tremendous deadly weapon in the next moment 80 years ago, but most Japanese are still unaware of the after-effects of the mRNA vaccination reflash. As is the fate of doctors, we will have to hold science in both awe and fear for the rest of our lives.

I wish that Ivermectin will be the detonating key drug for the eternal health of the human being, the free choice of the natural right and the enlightenment of natural healing.

CONTRIBUTION FROM DR. MINORI SASAKI

I would like to introduce a contribution from Dr. Minori Sasaki, Deputy Director of Osaka Anorectal Clinic, she has experienced many cases of Ivermectin administration for prevention of COVID-19 infection, treatment of early infection, mRNA PVS (Post Vaccine Syndrome) and shedding cases.

Ivermectin is the medicine that led Dr. Satoshi Omura of Kitasato University to win the Nobel Prize. Onchocerciasis, an infection caused by nematodes, is called river blindness because it often leads to blindness and has been a major cause of blindness in developing countries.

Since the introduction of Ivermectin as a treatment for this disease, the number of people going blind has decreased dramatically, and this medicine is still distributed to free of charge. In Japan, Ivermectin is a safe medicine that is also administered to very elderly people as a treatment for scabies. It is probably fresh in your mind that Ivermectin was found to be effective against COVID-19 and it was used in India and all over the world.

Ivermectin has been found to have the following effects:

- Inhibits binding of spike protein to ACE2 receptors (inhibits invasion)

- Inhibits intracellular replication
- Anti-inflammatory
- Immune modulatory
- Enhancement of neutralizing antibodies
- Inhibits cytokine storm
- Inhibits progression of chronic kidney disease (Chiba University)
- Inhibits red blood cell aggregation
- Thromboprophylaxis
-

In our hospital, 293 patients (male: 41, female: 252, average age: 53.9 years) were treated with Ivermectin from January 2022 to August 2023. The total number of prescription tablets was 11,373.

A questionnaire survey on Ivermectin was conducted in 2023. As of August 21, number of responses reached 206 out of 293 (with a response rate of 70.3%). The breakdown is as follows:

- Prophylactic oral medication 107 cases
- COVID-19 treatment 106 cases
- PVS sequelae treatment 54 cases
- Shedding treatment 26 cases
- Ivermectin not used 35 cases

The results are shown below:

- Prophylactic oral medication
  Ivermectin was taken 12 mg once a day, twice a week. 71% of patients were able to prevent COVID-19 infection by taking it.
  As stated by Professor Hideaki Hanaki of Kitasato University, *"Ivermectin works best only when used for prophylactic purposes."*, It would have been extremely effective.

- COVID-19 treatment
The results showed that it was effective in 83% of the patients.
- PVS Sequelae treatment
58% showed efficacy, when administered for COVID-19 sequelae and PVS sequelae.
- Shedding treatment
76% showed efficacy.

Based on these results, it appears that the pandemic was contained more quickly with the use of Ivermectin, which has an established safety profile and is inexpensive, than with a vaccine whose safety is unknown.

I am going to end with the words of the patient who was saved by Ivermectin.

"I hope Ivermectin will be widely available. Why not deploy emergency Ivermectin, which is guaranteed to be safe, nevertheless emergency approval of an incomplete vaccine?

There must have been many lives that could have been saved. Also, it would have been effective for a significant number of those suffering from PVS aftereffects."

Experience with Ivermectin in the clinic

January 2022 to August 2023
Number of patients: 293
41 men
252 women
Average age: 53.9 years old

Total number of prescription tablets: 11,373 tablets

Figure12. Experience with Ivermectin in the clinic

Chapter 8　Flash in Japan

Results of Ivermectin dose questionnaire

• Survey on ivermectin
206/293 responses (70.3% response rate) as of August 21, 2023

Scheduled oral medication 107: cases
COVID-19 treatment 106: cases
Seauelae treatment: 54 cases
Shedding treatment: 26 cases
Ivermectin-free 35: cases

Figure13. Results of Ivermectin dose questionnaire

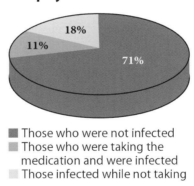

Figure14. Prophylactic internal use

COVID-19 Treatment

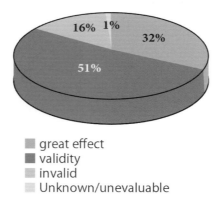

- great effect
- validity
- invalid
- Unknown/unevaluable

Figure15. COVID-19 Treatment

Treatment of sequelae

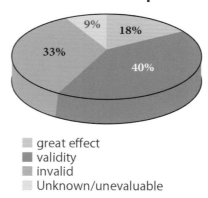

- great effect
- validity
- invalid
- Unknown/unevaluable

Figure16. Treatment of sequelae

CONTRIBUTION FROM DR. TAKAO IKEZAWA

A report by Dr. Takao Ikezawa, an obstetrician/gynecologist from Ikezawa Ladies Clinic, of an mRNA PVS case that was successfully treated with Ivermectin. He has reported his own guidelines in the therapeutic diagnosis of many mRNA PVS and shedding cases, particularly in the field of obstetrics and gynecology.

TWO CASES OF MASSIVE GENITAL BLEEDING AFTER TWO DOSES OF mRNA VACCINE

1. 51-year-old woman with a history of adenomyosis and confirmed menopause. On the 60th day after vaccination, she had massive genital bleeding and severe abdominal pain. But the bleeding stopped after only 2 doses of Ivermectin (IVM) 12 mg. It was speculated that the spike protein produced in the remaining oocytes caused an increase in E2, which in turn caused heavy bleeding and abdominal pain due to uterine adenomyosis, but the competitive inhibitory effect of IVM reduced E2, which may have been effective.

2. 21-year-old woman, with a regular menstrual cycle experienced massive hemorrhage, about 90 days after vaccination. EP combination drug reduced the amount of bleeding but did not completely stop the bleeding. Therefore, Ivermectin 12 mg twice and EP combination drug were used to completely stop bleeding. However, this time, after discontinuation of the EP combination drug, the patient did not bleed out. The suspected cause was the spike proteins, as in the above case, since endogenous E2 was being secreted in large amounts.

After the third and subsequent vaccinations, there are fewer cases of spike protein causing the ovaries to increase E2 production, and more cases of ER-mediated menstrual abnormalities, as described below.

IVERMECTIN THERAPY FOR ANOVULATORY CASES AFTER mRNA VACCINATION

There are cases in which ovulation is restored when Ivermectin 12 mg each is administered at D1 and D3 after menstruation has started. In such cases, it is possible that the spike protein binds to the ER, and the hypothalamus/pituitary system is no longer working properly due to incorrect estrogen signaling. Ivermectin probably has a competitive inhibitory effect with spike protein on the ER as well.

IVERMECTIN ALSO STOPS HEAVY BLEEDING AFTER VACCINATION DURING MIRENA INSERTION

There is another observed menstrual abnormality where the amount of menstrual blood loss increases after vaccination. There have also been cases of heavy menstrual bleeding after mRNA vaccination, even though the menstrual flow had decreased after insertion of Mirena to reduce menstrual flow. In these cases, two doses of Ivermectin 12 mg reduced the amount of bleeding, but it does not appear to be an abnormal secretion of E2 due to spiked protein. The mechanism suggests that the normal function of the endometrial vessels may have been more easily disrupted by the spike protein.

Special thanks to Dr. Hideo Ikezawa and Dr. Minori Sasaki for their contributions.

References

1. Computational Prediction of the Interaction of Ivermectin with Fibrinogen / Int J Mol Sci. 2023 Jul; 24(14)
2. Homocysteine in coronavirus disease (COVID-19): a systematic literature review/ Diagnosis (Berl). 2022 Jun 16
3. Coming of a Post-Vaccine Society -Wisdom to Survive the Vaccidemic- " (Japanese edition)
4. Zinc role in Covid-19 disease and preventionPapel del zinc en la prevención y la enfermedad de COVID-19/ Vacunas Volume 23, Issue 2, May- August 2022
5. Protective Effect of Vitamin D Supplementation on COVID-19-Related Intensive Care Hospitalization and Mortality: Definitive Evidence from Meta- Analysis and Trial Sequential Analysis/ Pharmaceuticals (Basel)2023 Jan 16
6. Effect of a combination of nitazoxanide, ribavirin, and ivermectin plus zinc supplement (MANS.NRIZ study) on the clearance of mild COVID-19/ Journal of Medical Virology Volume 93, Issue 2 Journal of Medical Virology Volume 93, Issue 5
7. Ivermectin-Induced Clinical Improvement and Alleviation of Significant Symptoms of COVID-19 Outpatients: A Cross-Sectional Study: Iran J Sci Technol Trans A Sci 2022;46(5)
8. Ivermectin Docks to the SARS-CoV-2 Spike Receptor-binding Domain Attached to ACE2 / in vivo 34: 3023-3026 (2020) The binding mechanism of ivermectin and levosalbutamol with spikeprotein of SARS-CoV-2 /Structural Chemistry (2021) 32:1985-1992
9. Molecular Docking Reveals Ivermectin and Remdesivir as Potential Repurposed Drugs Against SARS-CoV-2/J Front.
10. SARS-CoV-2 Spike Protein Induces Hemagglutination: Implications for COVID-19 Morbidities and Therapeutics and for Vaccine Adverse Effects / Int. J. Mol. Sci. 2022, 23(24), 15480
11. Ivermectin-Induced Clinical Improvement and Alleviation of Significant Symptoms of COVID-19 in Outpatients: A Cross-Sectional Study: Iran J Sci. Technol Trans A Sci 2022;46(5)
12. Persistent varicella zoster virus infection following mRNA COVID-19 vaccination was associated with the presence of encoded spike protein in the lesion Persistent varicella zoster virus infection following mRNA COVID-19 vaccination was associated with the presence of encoded spike protein in the lesion/ The Japanese Society for Cutaneous Immunology and Allergy/Case Study
13. New-Onset Acute Kidney Disease Post COVID-19 Vaccination/ Vaccines (Basel). 2022 May 9;10(5)
14. Acute kidney injury after COVID-19 vaccines: a real-world study / Ren Fail. 2022 Dec;44(1):
15. Inhibition of importin-α-mediated nuclear localization of dendrin attenuate podocyte loss and glomerulosclerosis / J Am Soc Nephrol. 2023 Jul 1;34(7)
16 . Nuclear relocation of the nephrin and CD2AP-binding protein dendrin promotes apoptosis of podocytes Asanuma et. al. Proc Natl Acad Sci USA. 104. 2007
17. Inhibition of importin-α-mediated nuclear localization of dendrin attenuate podocyte

loss and glomerulosclerosis / J Am Soc Nephrol. 2023 Jul 1;34 (7)

18. Dietary therapy with low protein genmai (brown rice) to improve the gut-kidney axis and reduce CKD progression / Asia Pac J Clin Nutr 2022;31(3)

19. Effects of TND1128 (a 5-deazaflavin derivative), with self-redox ability, as a mitochondria activator on mouse brain slice and its comparison 2023;151(2)

20. The novel mitochondria activator, 10-ethyl-3-methylpyrimido[4,5-b] quinoline-2,4(3H,10H)-dione (TND1128), promotes the development of Biochem Biophys Res Commun. 2021 Jun 30;560

21. Efficacy of Renal Precursor Stem Cells in Management of Chronic Kidney Disease: A cohort study/Journal of Scientific Research and Studies Vol. 3(6) June 2016

22. Ivermectin, a potential anticancer drug derived from an antiparasitic drug: Pharmacol Res. 2021 Jan

23. Ivermectin induces nonprotective autophagy by downregulating PAK1 and apoptosis in lung adenocarcinoma cells / Cancer Chemother Pharmacol. Cancer Chemother Pharmacol. 2023 Sep 23

22. Antibiotic ivermectin selectively induces apoptosis in chronic myeloid leukemia through inducing mitochondrial dysfunction and oxidative stress: Volume 497, Issue 1, 26 February 2018

23. The SARS-Co-2 spile protein binds and modulates estrogen receptors: Sci.Adv. November 30 2022,

24. Ivermectin suppresses tumour growth and metastasis through degradation of PAK1 in oesophageal squamous cell carcinoma:Journal of Cellular and Molecular Medicine 31 March 2020

25. Integrated analysis reveals FOXA1 and Ku70/Ku80 as targets of ivermectin in prostate cancer: Cell Death Dis. Cell Death Dis. Cell Death Dis. 2022 Sep1

26. Estrogen Receptor Alpha and Beta in Acute Myeloid Leukemia: Cancers 2020,12,907

27. Successful monotherapy with autologous formalin-fixed tumor vaccine for a Stage IV uterine cancer patient who rejected rational chemotherapy and immune checkpoint inhibitor treatment / Clin Case Rep.2023 Jun 8;11(6)

28. Emergence of a New Creutzfeldt-Jakob Disease: 26 Cases of the Human Version of Mad-Cow Disease, Days After a COVID-19 Injection / International Journal of Vaccine Theory, Practice, and Research, January 16, 2023

29. Class switch toward noninflammatory, spike-specific IgG4 antibodies after repeated SARS-CoV-2 mRNA vaccination /SCIENCE IMMUNOLOGY 22 Dec 2022

30. Serum IgG4 level predicts COVID-19 related mortality / Eur J Intern Med. 2021 Nov; 93

31. Self-amplifying RNA vaccines for infectious diseases / Gene Therapy (2021) 28 GRT-R910: a self-amplifying mRNA SARS-CoV-2 vaccine boosts immunity for ≥6 months in previously-vaccinated older adults/ Nature Communications volume 14, Article number: 3274 (2023)

Chapter 8   Flash in Japan

Katsuhiko FUKUDA, M.D. PhD.

Vice President of Integrated Medical Centre Fukuda Internal Medicine Clinic
After graduating from the Faculty of Medicine at Tottori University in 1991 and completing his doctoral studies at the university's Graduate School of Medicine, worked as the head of respiratory medicine at major hospitals in San-in region.
He developed ancient food culture and traditional medicine in Izumo region.
He has been practicing respiratory and allergy medicine, psyconeuroendocrinology, fractalbiology, home palliative rehabilitation, integrative cancer medicine, quantum regenerative medicine, and he has established a new concept of "plasticity medicine".
In April 2021, he was the first Japanese to warn and advocate "COVID-19 vaccine sequelae" (mRNA PVS/LPCVS) and established a "Vaccine Sequelae Outpatient Clinic" and examined more than 1,500 LPCVS patients.
He has issued more than 7,000 vaccine exemption certificates in over 50 countries.
 Author; The Coming of the Post-Vaccine Society - Wisdom of Surviving the Vaccidemic-etc.

Takao IKEZAWA, M.D.

Director of the Ikezawa Lady Clinic
After graduating from Osaka University School of Medicine in 1977, Dr. Ikezawa worked at a major hospital in the Kansai region before opening his own clinic in 1995. He is a board-certified obstetrician and gynecologist in Japan. Since the beginning of the corona disaster, he has continued to disseminate information on Facebook and X (formerly Twitter). He advocates and treats "delayed post-vaccination syndrome," a menstrual abnormality that mainly develops several months late after corona vaccination. He also treats various cases caused by mRNA vaccine shedding and works to disseminate countermeasures and treatment methods for these cases.

Minori SASAKI, M.D.

Deputy Director, Osaka Proctology Clinic
After graduating from Osaka Medical College in 1994, she worked as a dermatologist at a university hospital before becoming a proctologist and opening Japan's first proctology outpatient clinic for women in 1998, making her a pioneer among female proctologists. She is a specialist in Japanese colorectal disease, an instructor of Japanese colorectal disease, and a specialist and instructor in proctology. Author of "If you suffer from pain, itching, or constipation, stop washing your bottom."
She started treatment of post-vaccine syndrome in 2021, and the number of cases has exceeded 100. She has the highest number of Ivermectin prescriptions in Japan.

Southeast Asia

Chapter
9

Philippines
Dr. Allan A. Landrito

The Philippine Experience on Ivermectin During and After the Pandemic

At the onset of the pandemic, people in the Philippines were panic-stricken as every channel and program in the media were showing nothing but gruesome pictures on how the pandemic was occurring in other countries. As of March 6, 2020, there were only 5 confirmed cases of SARS-CoV-2 infection in the Philippines. But by March 26, there were already 709 cases, of which 45 were reported to have died. On that particular day, the big headline was the shocking news about the death of 9 doctors, all of them died from COVID-19.

They were all frontliners, treating COVID-19 patients in different hospitals. That was a ratio of 1 doctor out of 5 people dying from COVID-19. Within the next five days, by March 31, 2020, 8 more doctors were added to the list, making it 17 out of the total 88 deaths. The total number of cases was already 2,083 by then. Still, this ratio showed that 1 out of 5 people dying from COVID-19 were doctors. Such grim reality terrified the doctors, causing a great number of them abstain from their duties and hide from this seemingly dreadful killer, the novel coronavirus SARS-CoV-2. In an instant, the hospitals and clinics faced shortages of doctors amidst an overflowing number of patients who have developed various types of COVID-19 syndromes.

Government protocols on lockdowns and quarantines were soon implemented. Most hospitals imposed zero visitations for relatives of patients, and this kind of policy deprived the patients their customary rights of having the presence of a loved one at their bedside. It soon became apparent that the rich and the poor alike were facing the same predicament and suffering the same fate. A common scenario in the hospitals was an overpacked emergency room with more patients waiting outside, while all the hospital beds in the wards were filled beyond capacity. Once a patient is admitted in a hospital, their love ones have no way of knowing what is happening to their patient on a day-to-day basis. And there was no certainty as treatment outcome was concerned.

They could only hope that somehow their patients would survive, and that they would not be coming back in urns, as had been the fate of many. This situation was compounded with the government's imposition of mandatory immediate cremation for all patients dying from COVID-19. Many symptomatic patients were taken by ambulances from their residences but bringing them nowhere since all hospitals were already full. Not having received any medical treatment, they were eventually brought back to their residences, then their houses were barricaded. Those who were fortunate enough to have been admitted in the hospitals were most likely given the expensive and toxic drug Remdesivir. And as soon as their conditions got worse, they were subjected to early intubation as this was then the standard treatment protocol.

These kinds of circumstances were the common sad reality during the years 2020 and 2021 in the big cities in the Philippines. While many patients were dying from the viral scourge, a great many patients could be dying also from the very treatment that were given for their viral affliction. Becoming aware of these situations, a large portion of the population who developed symptoms opted not to report their ill conditions to the health authorities, and instead sought treatment from on-line consultations wherever they can be found. They were therefore confined in their own homes where they received their minimum required treatment.

Nevertheless, in the outskirts of the cities, such as the poor slums and depressed areas, the marginalized poor people were not strictly observing the government-imposed physical distancing and other lockdown measures. Commonly, they clamor during food distribution whenever there is an amelioration program by the government or from the non-governmental organizations. They would gather only during food distribution. In a similar way, people in the rural areas and provinces continued with their agricultural occupations while they avoid the use of public roads as these were blockaded and also to avoid being apprehended by the authorities for violating rules on lockdowns. Both the poor people in the cities and those in the provinces were more concerned about their hungry stomachs than they were with the governmental impositions during the height of the pandemic. For them, the problem of hunger caused by the stagnated economy was the greater reality and the more serious problem than the pandemic itself. Noticeably however, these segments of the population were not significantly affected by the contagion despite their violations of the so-called governmental health protocols such as face masking, frequent hand sanitation, physical distancing, staying at home, quarantining, lockdowns, and the like. They turned out to be more resilient as they have relatively lower number of cases and with less severities than those of the middle and upper rich classes.

DOH PROHIBITS IVERMECTIN

As early as August 2020, the Department of Health (DOH) already made an announcement and issued a Health Advisory ordering that doctors should NOT prescribe Ivermectin for the reason that, as they say, 'there is no clinical trial' on the said drug. They were also indifferent and non-supportive in any way on the use of Hydroxychloroquine or any other medicine or herbs or Virgin Coconut Oil (VCO) for the treatment of COVID-19 patients. Later, the Department of Science and Technology (DOST) completed a study and came out with the conclusion that the use of VCO has substantial benefits in the treatment of COVID-19. And yet, the DOH was not optimistic about it, did not support it, and never implemented VCO as part of their treatment protocol.

Amidst all this, I was working in a government emergency clinic in the City of Muntinlupa in Metropolitan Manila where I saw about a hundred patients each day during my days of duty. I was seeing so many patients with common complaints of fever, cough, loss of taste, and loss of smell. These are the pathognomonic signs and symptoms of COVID-19 about which I was fully aware. To protect myself however, I was taking Hydroxychloroquine daily for one week, then repeating this cycle every three weeks. I was also infusing myself with IV Vitamin C (Sodium Ascorbate) 25,000 mg initially, then 50,000 mg every 3 weeks. I realized that I was adequately protected as I was examining and treating the patients the same way as I was doing before the pandemic; continuing with "Facebook–to-face" interaction, physical examination and palpation when necessary. Yet I was not becoming sick. In June 2020, I began searching for Ivermectin sources after I chanced upon the in-vitro study of Ivermectin against SARS-CoV-2 done at Monash University in Australia.

But I could not find any Ivermectin preparation in the many pharmacies I went looking into. Then in the veterinary stores, I found a preparation of a sachet containing 15 mg of Ivermectin in granules. This was of course intended to be given as anthelmintics for pets and farm animals. But after due analysis, I found that it is safe for human consumption, so I started using this for myself, then for my family. I determined that it was working like an 'internal protection', so I then recommended it to my friends and private patients as a form of prevention.

I started using Ivermectin for treatment as early as July 2020. Mild to moderate COVID-19 cases were showing improvement when Ivermectin was added to their Vitamin C, antibiotics, and other medications.

During this time, I encountered a severe case of COVID-19 in a

67-year-old lady who called me to visit her in her house. For one week she had been having cough and low-grade fever. She lost her appetite and become so weak after 3 days with very meager food intake. Her chest x-ray indicated impression of pneumonia. She was very depressed and revealed to me that her husband had just died a week prior, due to COVID-19. Her husband however, was not brought to the hospital, and she was the one who took care of him at home until he died. I instructed her to take a sachet of Ivermectin 15 mg (0.25 mg/kg BW) every 2 days and I administered intravenous Vitamin C (Sodium Ascorbate) 50,000 mg that day. On the third day I gave her another intravenous Vitamin C but this time I administered 70,000 mg plus Dimethyl Sulfoxide (DMSO) 10 ml as she had not shown any significant improvement yet. During the week that followed I became so busy that I entirely forgot about her, only to call her a week later to inquire about her condition. To my surprise, she told me that she has fully recovered. I inquired what she did during that week, and she said she only took Ivermectin 15 mg every 2 days along with my advice to consume a whole fresh young coconut every day.

Then I searched where I could procure pure Ivermectin powder, and I found a source who imports it from China. In early August 2020, I started producing Ivermectin 15 mg in capsule form. Soon, I was providing this to my private patients.

However, I could not do this in my capacity as a government physician in the clinic where I was working, as I was not allowed by the City Mayor and the Chief of the City Health Department. In the later part of 2020, the DOH issued a second Health Advisory against Ivermectin, misinforming the people that Ivermectin is an animal medicine and should not be used for human consumption. Despite this, I persisted in making Ivermectin popular as I claimed that it is the solution to the pandemic and continued distributing it widely. From

Chapter 9 The Philippine Experience on Ivermectin During and After the Pandemic

July to December 2020, I was proactively recommending Ivermectin as prophylaxis for everyone I met in person and even on the social media, advising them to take one 15 mg capsule every 3 weeks.

During this time, 99% of my patients did not acquire COVID-19. Later on, I published a written study report based on the data I gathered from a total of 1,273 subjects from all regions in the Philippines who were taking Ivermectin for prevention during the period from October 2020 to March 2021. The result of this study substantiates the prophylactic efficacy rating of Ivermectin against COVID-19 at 95%.

During those months in 2020, I was recommending my Ivermectin 15 mg (0.25 mg/kg BW) capsule to be taken one capsule (for an average 60-kg adult) every 3 weeks for prevention. In January 2021, I revised my recommendation to increase the intake of Ivermectin to one capsule every 2 weeks; then from May 2021 to increase frequency to once a week; and then from October 2021 to twice a week or every 3 days.

These adjustments were made as I followed the recommendations from the FLCCC (Frontline COVID-19 Critical Care) Alliance in the US. It was in February 2021 when I was prompted to take an indefinite leave of absence from work as I became unimaginably busy engaged in unending demands for consultations on-line and over my cellphone.

Meanwhile, the Concerned Doctors and Citizens of the Philippines (CDC PH) comprised of about 5,000 members or supporters who have been seeking a round-table discussion or a dialogue with the DOH since August 2020 but was being ignored. The CDC PH wanted to propose Hydroxychloroquine and later Ivermectin. On March 30, 2021, doctors from CDC PH were given the chance to be heard by Congress. There were representatives from the DOH, Philippine Food and Drug Administration (FDA) and Philippine Society of Microbiology and Infectious Diseases (PSMID) who were totally opposing all that the

251

CDC PH was proposing. I remember answering them: "I am getting the feeling that we are living in two different planets, because as far as we know there are already a substantial number of clinical studies on Ivermectin in many countries along with a handful of meta analysis, And yet you are citing only this one study which is showing a negative result." And after I presented Ivermectin for about 30 minutes, I proposed that every adult Filipinos be given Ivermectin 1 capsule (15 mg) every week, open the economy and resume the usual social lives (let everyone be exposed to the virus but be 'internally protected' with Ivermectin) and the pandemic will be over in 4 months. Of course they did not listen, and they did not believe, nor did they adapt any of our proposals. But the whole event was aired on the television and people nationwide gained hope and started looking for Ivermectin.

Yet the government suppressed it even more and threatened to cancel the licenses of doctors who will be using Ivermectin. The opposite happened. Ivermectin coming from India and other countries started pouring in and were sold in the black market.

And in October 2021, what I was claiming in the Congress literally happened in Uttar Pradesh in India. During the height of the Delta variant contagion, when their daily new cases numbers were soaring high (to as many as 30,000 a day), then everyone was given Ivermectin. This resulted in drastic drop of the numbers to near zero in just 2 weeks.

Meanwhile, on June 15, 2021, the Secretary of the DOH agreed to hear us in a one-hour Zoom meeting. After we presented the science and the studies on Ivermectin in many countries, we asked him of the possibility of DOH adapting Ivermectin as part of the government's COVID treatment protocol. He answered that it is possible but only after the results of a local clinical trial that the DOH would undertake.

HIGH ENOUGH DOSES IS THE KEY

With regards to the use of Ivermectin as treatment for COVID-19 syndromes, I came to understand its full therapeutic potential during the second half of 2021 as I observed that COVID-19 patients respond in a dose-dependent manner. The doses needed to be increased higher and higher according to the extent of severity of the conditions of the individual patients. When we realized this, we started getting more successful results.

There was this 62-year-old farm neighbor of mine in Quezon province of Luzon Island who got severe COVID-19 and was brought to the hospital. On admission his oxygen saturation went down already to 51%. They wanted him to be transferred to the Provincial Hospital as they did not have access to Remdesivir and were not equipped to do an intubation. We convinced the patient to take Ivermectin and we gave him 6 capsules equivalent to 90 mg (1.5 mg/kg BW). Within 6 hours his oxygen saturation went up to 92%. So, he was no longer transferred to the bigger hospital and his treatment was continued using Ivermectin, off the charts, until he fully recovered and was discharged after a few days.

Many similar situations happened. Locked up in their homes, many COVID-19 patients took higher doses of Ivermectin on their own. They would rather take the chance of getting an overdose than to die from COVID-19. So far, there has not been reported any single case of a real overdose that caused injury. Meanwhile, I appointed about 300 persons as my delivery channels so I can systematically distribute my Ivermectin nationwide. We were meeting by Zoom and they heard me relate my story about how I consumed 10 capsules of my Ivermectin 15 mg capsule, totaling 150 mg, (2.5 mg/kg BW) in a single intake as I was experimenting on the safety of this medicine. I did not intend that they would take my statement as an instruction. And they started recommending the same high doses to severe COVID-19 patients. And we were all amazed how the patients were recovering, even the severe cases.

After the original Wuhan coronavirus there came the alpha, then the beta, then the gamma, and then the delta variants in a progressively increasing degree of virulence. And my dosing went up from 10 capsules (2.5 mg/kg BW), to 12 capsules (3 mg/kg BW), to 14 capsules (3.5 mg/kg BW), and even to 16 capsules (4 mg/kg BW) daily on those with very severe COVID-19. In several cases, the patients themselves were taking even higher doses. When given these high daily doses, the patients are experiencing the side effects like visual disturbances (glaring, dimming, tunnel vision, patterned vision, and floating blue bubbles), disequilibrium, disorientation, and hallucinations in ascending order according to doses. But despite these, we have been seeing a reversal of their COVID-19 conditions and many were achieving cures.

I started doing Zoom consultations to groups of people starting in my city, then to the neighboring cities, then later on to almost every province of country. The maximum number of Zoom participants of 1,000 was soon exceeded. I was doing it 3 times in a week from 1pm to 10pm and sometimes extending to 12 midnight and even beyond. Through this program, I treated thousands of patients remotely, online or by phone. I could no longer administer intravenous Vitamin C. I was mainly dispensing Ivermectin capsules along with other oral medicines which they can easily source in their localities such as Vitamin C, Vitamin D, N-acetylcysteine, Colchicine, Doxycycline, Methylprednisolone, VCO and some herbs. Those days were very tiring, but we were always refreshed by the success stories.

Here are some of them.

There was this big family in Quezon Province of Luzon Island with grandparents, uncles, aunts, nephews, nieces, and grandchildren who were regularly taking Ivermectin capsules for prevention except for an 8-year-old granddaughter. They were thinking of not giving her Ivermectin because she has a profound autistic disorder, and they were afraid that this may not be good for her.

It was about this time that the DOH issued its third Health Advisory against Ivermectin saying that it causes brain damage. Then there was a big wave of infection in their town and many people in their community got COVID-19. None in their family manifested a COVID-19 syndrome except for this 8-year-old autistic child. She developed a severe respiratory syndrome, was brought to the hospital, and was admitted to the ICU. An aunt who turned out to be positive on RT-PCR test but was asymptomatic was allowed to stay at the bedside of her niece to help in her care in the hospital. She started secretly giving her niece the contents of one Ivermectin 15mg capsule (0.75 mg/kg BW) everyday as well as Vitamin C syrup through her nasogastric tube. The aunt signed a waiver so as not to let her niece be intubated as I instructed her to do. After one month in the hospital, she completely recovered. Later on, her aunt was relating her observation that during the whole time she was in the ICU all the patients there who were intubated died. But her niece who was not intubated survived.

During my Zoom consultations, a 25-year-old female patient presented with severe respiratory COVID-19 syndrome. Weighing only 45 kg and living alone in her condominium in Mandaluyong City, she consulted me online once or twice a week. In the beginning her condition was worsening even though she has a continuous supply of oxygen. Her oxygen saturation was dwindling from 90% to 78% to 65%. I started her with 4 capsules of Ivermectin 15 mg daily (60 mg) (1.33 mg/kg BW) and increased this to 8 capsules (120 mg) (2.66 mg/kg BW). She showed signs of improvement when she reached the high dose of 8 capsules. This was when we were just realizing that Ivermectin is dose- dependent.

We started seeing improvement, when the high dose was reached. We realized that we have to reach a high enough dose as quickly as possible. So, we started increasing the daily dose by adding 1 capsule each day for women or 2 capsules each day for men. We continued this until we could see signs of improvement, indicating the dose has reached a high enough level.

We gave this high enough dose for three days, and as the patients continued to improve, we tapered the dose by subtracting 1 capsule each day until only 2 capsules remain. Then we continued giving 2 capsules daily until the patient has fully recovered. So, we developed this 3-phase dosing of Ivermectin.

During this time the DOH issued its fourth Health Advisory against Ivermectin stating that it harms the liver and the kidneys. My 25-year-old patient said that at night she could hardly breathe and fear that she would not wake up the next morning.

The high dose Ivermectin put her to sleep and when she was in her highest dose, she started waking up with feelings of improvement in the morning. She fully recovered after 6 weeks and her total consumption of Ivermectin was 230 capsules, equivalent to 3,450 mg.

We then determined her SGPT which was 28 mg%, while her Creatinine was 78 mg%, all turned out normal. A sad ending to my patient's story is three of her office mates had severe COVID-19 at the same time. However, her officemates were brought to different hospitals where they were treated with the usual protocol of Remdesivir and intubation. Unfortunately, her three friends died while she was saved from her home-based treatment.

There was a case of a young family with 2 children in the province of Laguna who got COVID-19. The father got moderate COVID-19 and recovered after one week with a daily intake of 4 capsules of

Ivermectin 15 mg (1 mg/kg BW). The mother got mild COVID-19 and recovered after 4 days with a daily intake of 2 capsules (0.5 mg/kg BW). Their 3-year-old daughter developed symptoms of cough and fever but recovered after one week on one capsule daily (1 mg/kg BW).

Lastly their 5-month-old infant developed profuse diarrhea for 4 days. He had become so weak, and his watery stools became bloody on the fourth day. The mother was terrified that her 6 kg infant lost substantial weight and was so weak, he could no longer cry. She decided to give him a whole capsule of Ivermectin 15 mg (2.5 mg/kg BW) each day by emptying the powder contents of the capsule and mixing this with his milk formula, and feeding him using a dropper. Within 3 days the infant dramatically improved and on the fourth day he had fully recovered.

In the Central Luzon province of Pampanga, there was contagion in a particular village, and many died from COVID-19. In one household, a 50-year-old male and his father got COVID-19 at the same time. The son locked himself in his room and no one knew how many 15 mg Ivermectin capsules he took.

His father and a neighbor both died from COVID-19. His family was alarmed by his silence because he was in seclusion for several days.

They were banging on his door, and he was not responding. So, they decided to force open the door lock and found him completely disoriented and all his things in a topsy-turvy condition. Nonetheless, he has already recovered from his severe COVID-19 but was still deep in his stupor.

After a few days he was back to his senses with complete cognitive functions as if nothing had happened. It was estimated that he could have ingested 20-25 capsules (5 mg/kg BW) in a day for 7 days. We have seen these kinds of situations where people who took very high doses of Ivermectin became disoriented and developed hallucinations.

However, depending on the amount they took, they eventually returned to their normal cognitive functions and become totally free from hallucinations after a few days without Ivermectin.

With the support of my delivery network and the people in my Zoom meetings, I have treated thousands of Filipinos during the pandemic. They were cured with Ivermectin combined with other medicines that are widely available in the Philippines.

I opened a website: www.drlandrito.com, which anyone can visit for information on Ivermectin and COVID-19, which is still active today. Finally, the DOH conducted a clinical trial on Ivermectin in January 2022, but abandoned and discontinued this project just after 3 weeks. They followed the announcement by the World Health Organization (WHO) claiming that Ivermectin is not effective against COVID-19. At this time the DOH then issued its fifth Health Advisory against Ivermectin claiming that it is not at all effective against COVID-19.

I have been applying for approval from the Philippine Food and Drug Administration (FDA) for my Ivermectin 15mg capsule to obtain what is called a Certificate of Product Registration (CPR). My application was classified under a new drug for which I had to provide about 50 different requirements and tests. It should be noted that many years ago Ivermectin was included in the Philippine Drug Formulary. I was struggling to comply with all of these requirements.

One of the tests, the Bioequivalence Test even cost 5 million Philippine pesos (US$100,000), but somehow with the help of some supportive people I was able to comply with all of them. Frustrated with their inaction, I reported them to the Anti-Red Tape Authority, which intervened and ordered the FDA to release my Certificate of Product Registration (CPR) which happened on December 20, 2021.

As early as November 2020, the national government was able to obtain COVID-19 vaccines for a small group, the Presidential Security

Guards. After they were all vaccinated, most of them got the ill effects and became sick. The Department of Health was consulted, and they were at a loss as to what treatment must be given to the elite soldiers. Finally, Ivermectin was suggested, and when they were given this medicine, they all immediately recovered.

Then in March 2021, the national government's COVID-19 vaccine roll out was started. From March to September 2021, the death toll was painfully high. The Philippines Statistics Authority (PSA) reported an overly excessive death rate for the year 2021. The total number of deaths was 879,429 as compared to that of the year 2020 which was only 613,936. The difference of 265,493 is a considerably large number which is something that cannot be attributed to deaths from the COVID-19 malady which only numbered 66,444 during the 3 years of the pandemic (from March 11, 2020, to March 11, 2023). This excess death is indeed so enormous with a staggering rate of 42%. I can surmise no other probable cause except the COVID-19 vaccines. The Philippine FDA has received reports from doctors nationwide on COVID-19 vaccine severe adverse events in the number of 237,871 and deaths in the number of 2,801 as of February 28, 2023. These numbers are underreported because the majority of doctors are incognizant with COVID-19 vaccine injuries. Therefore, I have been recommending to people who were vaccinated to take one capsule of my Ivermectin 15 mg (0.25 mg/kg BW) every day for one month followed by one capsule every 3 days for 5 months in order to neutralize the spike protein that is causing the toxicities from these vaccines.

OTHER USES OF IVERMECTIN

We are now seeing many patients who have developed various kinds of cancers after receiving COVID-19 vaccines. Many of them are in advanced conditions which are very difficult to treat as compared to those who are not vaccinated. For cancer patients, I recommend taking daily Ivermectin at doses from 1mg to 2 mg/kg BW along with high dose intravenous Vitamin C (Sodium Ascorbate) 50,000 mg every other day for 2 months.

Then we determine if there is any improvement. If there is, then we continue treatment while monitoring the progress every month as we adjust the doses according to their development. This recommendation is based on our successful experience with a case of a huge adenocarcinoma of the gallbladder in a 40-year-old female. She had previously failed to achieve any improvement on chemotherapy in 2020 (using Capecitabine, then Oxaliplatin). She was presenting with a tumor with a size of 11.6 cm in diameter. She took a daily dose of 8 capsules of Ivermectin 15 mg (2.4 mg/kg BW) for 6 months plus intravenous Vitamin C (Sodium Ascorbate) 50,000 mg every other day. Every month she was having an ultrasound which was showing that the tumor was gradually decreasing in size. She continued for another 4 months but decreased the Ivermectin to 6 capsules a day (1.8 mg/kg BW) and discontinued the intravenous Vitamin C. And the tumor continued decreasing in size until it was completely gone.

However, she continued taking Ivermectin daily on a reduced dose of 2 capsules (0.6 mg/kg BW). All throughout this time, her SGPT and Creatinine were always on normal levels.

We have also been using Ivermectin in the treatment of tuberculosis. We observed that some pulmonary tuberculosis patients who took Ivermectin as prophylaxis against COVID-19 showed improvements in their general well-being and appetite.

This observation prompted us to discover the many research done before the pandemic on the efficacy of Ivermectin against tuberculosis.

Now, I am giving tuberculosis patients Ivermectin as a monotherapy on a dose of about 0.5 mg/kg BW daily while monitoring their progress for the next 6 to 12 months.

We have also treated a number of patients with Benign Prostatic Hyperplasia with Ivermectin 0.5 mg/kg BW to be taken every night. Most of these patients were so satisfied with the result because they no longer have to get up in the middle of their sleep at night, an effect they have not achieved with the pharmaceutical medicines they have been taking and which we discontinued.

We have seen so many other benefits of Ivermectin and are confident about giving it at high doses. We are no longer afraid and have gained the confidence to give it at high doses. We anticipate the side effects which are usually visual disturbances, but we reassure our patients that these are transient and were off within 24 hours. We complement this with oral Vitamin B complex and the side effects are considerably reduced. We have seen how it can be used in autoimmune disorders like Psoriasis. We have seen how it works with other viral infections like the common flu, herpes, and even dengue hemorrhagic fever which is endemic in the Philippines. We also recommend it to patients with HIV. Most importantly, I recommend Ivermectin for cancer prevention on a one capsule a day dose (0.25 mg/kg BW) every 3 days, as I myself and my whole family have been taking it daily for more than 2 years.

And especially now with the emergence of many post-COVID-19 vaccine diseases, I am using it as a mainstay treatment along with other medications, both oral and intravenous. Ivermectin is indeed a very wonderful drug. And I call it a Jehovah Jireh – a provision that came from God.

Allan A. Landrito, MD

Allan A. Landrito, MD finished his medical degree from De la Salle University in 1991. He was serving as a primary health care physician in the City Health Department of Muntinlupa, Metro Manila when the COVID-19 pandemic suddenly emerged. Some 15 years before this, he has been practicing alternative therapies such as chelation therapy, DMSO therapy, nutrition medicine, orthomolecular medicine, and herbal medicine, espousing an integrative medical approach to prevention and cure that has been the hallmark of his career as a physician. His adept and persistent research in the most fundamental aspects of health and medicine, his application of profound therapies in metabolic syndromes and viral infections, and his compassion for the common people motivated and inspired him to develop a practical, sensible, and efficient way of preventing and treating COVID-19 highlighting Ivermectin as the mainstay therapeutic agent. On December 1, 2020, he published a small book entitled "Freedom from Covid-19 Now! Prevention and Treatment at Hand" where he discussed the different facets of the pandemic and proposed the way to end it. He conducted free consultations nationwide using Zoom and was able to guide the treatment of a hundred thousand patients during the height of the pandemic. Since 2022 he has been treating Covid-19 vaccine injuries and recommends Ivermectin in the prevention of cancers and autoimmune disorders and treatment to a host of diseases.

Oceania

Chapter

10

Australia

Dr. Julian Fidge

Ivermectin in Australia

COVID-19 entered Australia on the 25th of January 2020, when a man who had traveled from Wuhan, China, tested positive for the virus. Two years of chaos followed in Australia, and it will be apparent from my narrative that I am unable to make sense out of what transpired.

The COVID-19 pandemic of 2020-2022 revealed serious failings in Australian health regulation. The most egregious errors were the precipitous approvals of novel COVID-19 vaccines without adequate safety data, resulting in tens of thousands of serious adverse reactions, including myocarditis, thromboses and deaths. But not far behind those stunning errors of judgment was the vilification of Ivermectin, hydroxychloroquine and doctors who were treating patients with COVID-19 in the community. Some doctors were suspended for providing necessary and appropriate treatment for COVID-19 that did no harm and preserved life, while others were suspended for criticizing the government's health policies regarding COVID-19.

The anti-viral activity of Ivermectin had been the subject of on going research since 2012, confirming that it inhibits nuclear import of viral proteins, limiting infection by RNA viruses. This work was applied to COVID-19, and it was established by June 2020 by Caly & colleagues that:

Ivermectin, an FDA-approved anti-parasitic previously shown to have broad-spectrum anti-viral activity in vitro, is an inhibitor of the causative virus (SARS-CoV-2), with a single addition to Vero-hSLAM cells 2 h post infection with SARS-CoV-2 able to effect ~5000-fold reduction in viral RNA at 48 h. Ivermectin therefore warrants further investigation for possible benefits in humans.

Chapter 10   Ivermectin in Australia

... a 99.8% reduction in cell-associated viral RNA (indicative of unreleased and unpackaged virions) was observed with Ivermectin treatment.

. . As we have observed previously (Lundberg et al., 2013; Tay et al., 2013; Wagstaff et al., 2012), no toxicity of Ivermectin was observed at any of the timepoints tested, in either the sample wells or in parallel tested drug alone samples.

The researchers concluded:

Ultimately, development of an effective anti-viral for SARS-CoV-2, if given to patients early in infection, could help to limit the viral load, prevent severe disease progression and limit person-person transmission. Benchmarking testing of Ivermectin against other potential antivirals for SARS-CoV-2 with alternative mechanisms of action (Dong et al., 2020; Elfiky, 2020; Gordon et al., 2020; Li and De Clercq, 2020; Wang et al., 2020) would thus be important as soon as practicable. This Brief Report raises the possibility that Ivermectin could be a useful antiviral to limit SARS-CoV-2, in similar fashion to those already reported (Dong et al., 2020; Elfiky, 2020; Gordon et al., 2020; Li and De Clercq, 2020; Wang et al., 2020); until one of these is proven beneficial in a clinical setting, all should be pursued as rapidly as possible.

Ivermectin has an established safety profile for human use (Gonzalez Canga et al., 2008; Jans et al., 2019; Buonfrate et al., 2019), and is FDA-approved for a number of parasitic infections (Gonzalez Canga et al., 2008; Buonfrate et al., 2019). Importantly, recent reviews and meta-analysis indicate that high dose Ivermectin has comparable safety as the standard low-dose treatment, although there is not enough evidence to make conclusions about the safety profile in pregnancy (Navarro et al., 2020; Nicolas et al., 2020).

Similar work was done for chloroquine by Wang & colleagues by February 2020:

Chloroquine, a widely-used anti-malarial and autoimmune disease drug, has recently been reported as a potential broad-spectrum antiviral drug.8,9 Chloroquine is known to block virus infection by increasing endosomal pH required for virus/cell fusion, as well as interfering with the glycosylation of cellular receptors of SARS-CoV.10 Our time-of-addition assay demonstrated that chloroquine functioned at both entry, and at post-entry stages of the 2019-nCoV infection in Vero E6 cells. Besides its antiviral activity, chloroquine has an immune-modulating activity, which may synergistically enhance its antiviral effect in vivo. Chloroquine is widely distributed in the whole body, including lung, after oral administration. The EC90 value of chloroquine against the 2019-nCoV in Vero E6 cells was 6.90 μM, which can be clinically achievable as demonstrated in the plasma of rheumatoid arthritis patients who received 500 mg administration.11 Chloroquine is a cheap and a safe drug that has been used for more than 70 years and, therefore, it is potentially clinically applicable against the 2019-nCoV.

Our findings reveal that remdesivir and chloroquine are highly effective in the control of 2019-nCoV infection in vitro. Since these compounds have been used in human patients with a safety track record and shown to be effective against various ailments, we suggest that they should be assessed in human patients suffering from the novel coronavirus disease.

In a disappointing demonstration of the capture of the Australian health regulators by the pharmaceutical industry, remdesivir was approved for use in Australia on 10 July 2020 (Victorian Dept of Health), at a cost of about $4,607 per patient, instead of hydroxychloroquine or Ivermectin. An Australian philanthropist, Clive Palmer, purchased 33 million doses of hydroxychloroquine to donate to the Australian government. Some of it was destroyed, and it was reported by The Guardian in October 2023 that 22 million doses remain in storage.

Interestingly, an international study concluded by February 2021 that remdesivir "had little or no effect on hospitalized patients with COVID-19, as indicated by overall mortality, initiation of ventilation, and duration of hospital stay." (WHO Solidarity Trial Results). The approval of remdesivir appears to have been based upon effective marketing to the Australian government, not clinical effectiveness or scientific data.

The use of Ivermectin by Australians increased by a factor of 17 in 2021, presumably for prophylaxis against, and treatment of, COVID-19. This offended the Australian government, and the Australian Therapeutic Goods Agency (TGA) banned the use of Ivermectin for the treatment of COVID-19 on 10 September 2021 in the following terms:

Today, the TGA, acting on the advice of the Advisory Committee for Medicines Scheduling, has placed new restrictions on the prescribing of oral Ivermectin. General practitioners are now only able to prescribe Ivermectin for TGA-approved conditions (indications) - scabies and certain parasitic infections. Certain specialists including infectious disease physicians, dermatologists, gastroenterologists and hepatologists (liver disease specialists) will be permitted to prescribe Ivermectin for other unapproved indications if they believe it is appropriate for a particular patient.

These changes have been introduced because of concerns with the prescribing of oral Ivermectin for the claimed prevention or treatment of COVID-19. Ivermectin is not approved for use in COVID-19 in Australia or in other developed countries, and its use by the general public for COVID-19 is currently strongly discouraged by the National COVID Clinical Evidence Taskforce, the World Health Organization and the US Food and Drug Administration.

Firstly, there are a number of significant public health risks associated with taking Ivermectin in an attempt to prevent COVID-19 infection rather than getting vaccinated. Individuals who believe that they are protected from infection by taking Ivermectin may choose not to get tested or to seek medical care if they experience symptoms. Doing so has the potential to spread the risk of COVID-19 infection throughout the community.

Secondly, the doses of Ivermectin that are being advocated for use in unreliable social media posts and other sources for COVID-19 are significantly higher than those approved and found safe for scabies or parasite treatment. These higher doses can be associated with serious adverse effects, including severe nausea, vomiting, dizziness, neurological effects such as dizziness, seizures and coma.

Finally, there has been a 3-4-fold increased dispensing of Ivermectin prescriptions in recent months, leading to national and local shortages for those who need the medicine for scabies and parasite infections. It is believed that this is due to recent prescribing and dispensing for unapproved uses, such as COVID-19. Such shortages can disproportionately impact vulnerable people, including those in Aboriginal and Torres Strait Islander communities.

There is only one TGA approved oral Ivermectin product, Stromectol Ivermectin 3mg tablet blister pack which is indicated for the treatment of river blindness (onchocerciasis), threadworm of the intestines (intestinal strongyloidiasis) and scabies.

All medical practitioners can continue to prescribe oral Ivermectin *for the approved indications. However, prescribing of oral Ivermectin for indications that are not approved is now limited to certain specialists. (New Restrictions)*

It can be seen from this announcement that the TGA were inconsistent and unable to triage COVID-19 appropriately. The TGA was claiming that COVID-19 was such a serious health threat that emergency approvals of novel vaccines were required, while banning the use of Ivermectin for COVID-19 so that it would remain available for the treatment of scabies and parasites.

The decision was counter-productive, justifying the decision by observing that social media is an unreliable prescriber, while stopping patients from accessing safe doses of Ivermectin being prescribed by a doctor and then dispensed by an independent pharmacist. The ban removed both of these effective, validated safeguards for patients.

Moreover, it was widely known to doctors with an interest in international health that Ivermectin had been widely used in Africa in entire populations of some countries in order to prevent serious parasitic infections. This regular use of Ivermectin in millions of patients for many years proved that Ivermectin was safe to administer to patients.

Furthermore, the large number of deaths that had been predicted in countries which did not use COVID-19 vaccines did not occur in Africa, leading to the possibility that the regular, prophylactic use of Ivermectin was also protecting African people from severe COVID-19 infection.

Accordingly, I made an application to the TGA to delete the ban under a provision of their enabling legislation for this ban to be lifted on the 13th of August 2022. In my defense, the pandemic was a very busy time for me as a country doctor and the preparation of the 33-

page application took me several months. The basis for my application was explained in the following terms:

1. **I request the Appendix D, Item 10 listing for Ivermectin in the Poisons Standard** that was included on 11 September 2021 be deleted in its entirety in order to allow general practitioners to prescribe Ivermectin safely and effectively for patients who wish to use Ivermectin off-label to prevent and treat COVID-19.

2. **The basis for this request is that the Appendix D listing for Ivermectin is clearly irrational**, irresponsible, reckless, negligent and possibly criminal, because it poses a serious threat to public safety and may have caused the unnecessary deaths of thousands of Australians by preventing general practitioners from treating their patients with a safe and effective and cheap medication that may prevent more than 85% of COVID-19 infections and may prevent serious illness and death caused by COVID-19 infections.

3. **The listing forces patients to access Ivermectin on the black market, or to use veterinary** Ivermectin, and to use it without medical or pharmaceutical supervision, while simultaneously preventing the safe prescribing of Ivermectin by doctors and the safe dispensing of Ivermectin by pharmacists, for the prevention and treatment of COVID-19. The listing itself is unsafe and irrational and has the opposite effect to that which was intended.

4. **There was never any rational basis for the Appendix D, Item 10 listing for Ivermectin** in the Poisons Standard. The listing provides for additional controls on possession and supply of poisons included in schedules 4 and 8. There was never, at any time, a specific health risk that could be mitigated by restricting off-label prescribing of Ivermectin to dermatologists and gastroenterologists. There was never any evidence that specialist general practitioners have been

prescribing Ivermectin unsafely, or that the prescribing by general practitioners was undesirable.

5. **The TGA has been aware that Ivermectin is safe in the doses used in the prophylaxis** and treatment of COVID-19 since 2013, when it undertook a rigorous analysis of the safety of Ivermectin which was published in a 2013 AUSPAR.

6. **There is no evidence that Ivermectin is unsafe when prescribed by doctors** and dispensed by pharmacists. There is evidence that Ivermectin is an effective prophylactic and treatment for COVID-10. This application is based on a harm minimization approach to patient care. The listing is causing harm, separate from the question of the efficacy of Ivermectin, in and of itself.

7. **The use of Ivermectin by Australians will be safer if the listing is deleted**, because doctors and pharmacists can then be involved in the use of Ivermectin by patients.

8. **There is a strong possibility, based on published research, that Ivermectin may** help prevent and also treat COVID-19. It is unethical, immoral, and possibly criminal to withhold a safe and effective prophylactic and/or treatment from the Australian public when there is no rational basis for preventing Australians from accessing Ivermectin safely.

9. **The Appendix D, Item 10 listing appears to be a political act that is designed to support** the government and public health authorities, rather than medicine or science or logic.

The application was strongly supported by many thoughtful doctors, who also made submissions in support of my application. But it was strongly opposed by peak bodies in Australia who should have known better. It was, at all times, clear that the ban was motivated by politics, not medicine or science. Prohibition of any substance has never worked, and the ban had the effect of forcing patients to self-medicate with veterinary products. The ban was hysterical, embarrassing and counterproductive. It brought the medical profession and the health regulation authorities into disrepute which continues to reduce trust and confidence in doctors and government.

To their credit, the TGA recognized this and deleted the ban on off-label prescribing on 3 May 2023, and this came into effect on 1st of June 2023. The TGA explained their decision in the following terms:

From 1 June 2023, prescribing of oral Ivermectin for 'off-label' uses will no longer be limited to specialists such as dermatologists, gastroenterologists and infectious diseases specialists.

In its final decision published today, the Therapeutic Goods Administration (TGA) has removed the restriction through its scheduling in the Poisons Standard because there is sufficient evidence that the safety risks to individuals and public health is low when prescribed by a general practitioner in the current health climate.

This considers the evidence and awareness of medical practitioners about the risks and benefits of Ivermectin, and the low potential for any shortages of Ivermectin for its approved uses. Also, given the high rates of vaccination and hybrid immunity against COVID-19 in Australia, use of Ivermectin by some individuals is unlikely to now compromise public health.

However, the TGA does not endorse off-label prescribing of Ivermectin for the treatment or prevention of COVID-19.

A large number of clinical studies have demonstrated that Ivermectin does not improve outcomes in patients with COVID-19. The National Clinical Evidence Taskforce (NCET) and many similar bodies around the world, including the World Health Organization, strongly advise against the use of Ivermectin for the prevention or treatment of

Chapter 10   Ivermectin in Australia

COVID-19.

Ivermectin for oral use is a Prescription Only (Schedule 4) medicine in the Poisons Standard. It is only approved by the TGA for the treatment of river blindness (onchocerciasis), threadworm of the intestines (intestinal strongyloidiasis), and scabies.

The restriction on Ivermectin was introduced in September 2021 because of concerns about the safety of consumers using Ivermectin without health advice to treat COVID-19, widespread use of Ivermectin instead of approved vaccines and treatments for COVID-19, and potential shortages of the medicine for approved uses.

The final decision follows an application to remove the restrictions and has been made according to the process required under the Therapeutic Goods Act 1989. It takes into account advice from the independent Advisory Committee on Medicines Scheduling (ACMS) and two rounds of public consultation.

It can be seen from the change in tone and content that the TGA has become more rational and was finally able to accept my arguments about the safety of Ivermectin. Ivermectin has always been safe when used appropriately. I trust my colleagues have covered this sufficiently and I will not dull this message by dwelling on it here, too.

Another unquestionable virtue of Ivermectin is its affordability. Even packaged as blister packs of four tablets, a 3mg tablet of Ivermectin costs AU$6.00, dispensed and labeled by a pharmacist. I assume this cost drops to 6 cents per tablet in bulk quantities of bottled Ivermectin. I am a scientist. This was forced upon me by my father, a biochemist who spent his entire life performing basic research on cholesterol in humans and teaching me how to construct an experiment while I worked as his unpaid lab assistant. Being a scientist, I know, in my bones, that the Australian health authorities could have easily added

277

Ivermectin to a statistically significant number of patients in most of the treatment regimens they used throughout the COVID-19 pandemic, at different dose regimens, with complete safety. But the health authorities in Australia were completely captured by the pharmaceutical industry, and only implemented therapies promoted by the large pharmaceutical companies. To this day, we don't know how effectively Ivermectin treats COVID-19 because of a paucity of well-designed trials of sufficiently large numbers.

It would also have been completely safe and relatively cheap to provide a statistically significant number of Australians with Ivermectin as a prophylactic. Again, this did not happen, and we are left without a clear answer as to the effectiveness of Ivermectin against COVID-19 infection. I cannot point to the apparent effectiveness of Ivermectin in Africa because it was used in the whole population: there can be no control group, ethically, when the Ivermectin is required for prophylaxis from serious parasitic infections. We could have provided an answer to this question easily and effectively, but again, we still do not know how effectively Ivermectin prevents COVID-19 infections in the Australian setting.

In a telling aside, an Australian university quickly developed the most effective COVID-19 vaccine in the world. It was protein based, and not a genetically modified mRNA vaccine, and had a 99% response rate. Unfortunately, it also caused a false-positive in HIV tests for patients for some time after the vaccination, so it was abandoned. Many informed patients (including myself) would have preferred to have this Australian, protein-based vaccine in order to get better protection and avoid the genetic transfection from the GMO mRNA vaccines. But our choices, like our liberty, were removed during the pandemic.

- Ivermectin became an ethical, moral, and scientific touchstone during the COVID-19 pandemic. The treatment of Ivermectin by the health authorities is an indicator of how immature the Australian health authorities have become, without depth and insight. In an uncomfortable demonstration of the Dunning-Kruger Principle, it was clear from their reaction and attitude toward possible treatment like Ivermectin the health authorities were performing poorly, while thinking they were doing a good job. This was especially frustrating for good doctors and scientists, who were demonized for pointing out the obvious flaws in the health authorities' conduct. A good example of this is my treatment for making an application to the TGA about Ivermectin: one of my colleagues wrote, in the comments section of the news that I had made an application to the TGA, that I required disciplinary action, merely for making the application. The bullying, intimidation and persecution of doctors who questioned the narrative was extraordinary.

One of the things that has become apparent from the way in which the pandemic, generally, and Ivermectin, specifically, was managed by the Australian health authorities is that those authorities are completely hopeless in an emergency. It has long been acknowledged that the less capable doctors and scientists choose bureaucratic careers because they lack the ability to flourish in the private sector and require the structure and support of a government department to be able to function. And for 99 years out of one hundred, this does not matter because these clinicians are supported by a large staff and plenty of resources. It is cumbersome, but the health authorities slowly arrive at reasonable solutions. But when something like COVID-19 comes along, they are immediately intellectually, clinically, and emotionally overwhelmed. The authorities panicked, and it quickly became obvious that there was not a single experienced, calm practitioner anywhere in the public service of Australia. The decisions implemented by the health authorities were usually incorrect and usually worsened the health of Australia.

If we are ever faced with a severe infectious disease, many millions of Australians will die. We do not have sufficient intellectual or ethical health leadership to preserve our health in an emergency, and our health leadership holds all other health providers in contempt. Ivermectin became a pointed example of how poorly equipped the Australian health authorities are for dealing with a widespread health emergency.

Chapter 10   Ivermectin in Australia

References

1. Caly, L., Druce, J. D., Catton, M. G., Jans, D. A., & Wagstaff, K. M. (2020). The FDA-approved drug ivermectin inhibits the replication of SARS-CoV-2 in vitro. Antiviral research, 178, 104787.

2. New restrictions on prescribing ivermectin for COVID-19 - https://www.tga.gov.au/news/media-releases/new-restrictions-prescribing-ivermectin-covid-19

3. Victorian Department of Health - https://www.health.vic.gov.au/covid-19/vaccines-and-medications-in-patients-with-covid-19

4. Wang, M., Cao, R., Zhang, L. et al. Remdesivir and chloroquine effectively inhibit the recently emerged novel coronavirus (2019-nCoV) in vitro. Cell Res 30, 269–271 (2020). https://doi.org/10.1038/s41422-020-0282-0

5. WHO Solidarity Trial Consortium. "Repurposed antiviral drugs for Covid-19—interim WHO solidarity trial results." New England Journal of medicine 384.6 (2021): 497-511.

Julian Fidge
BPharm, Grad Dip App Sc (Comp Sc), MBBS, FRACGP, MMed (Pain Mgt)

Dr. Fidge is a rural general practitioner in Australia. He began his working life as a soldier in the Australian Army, leaving the military to finish high school at 22 years old. He then studied pharmacy and worked in community pharmacy from 1987 to 1996. In 1994/95 he worked for CARE Australia in The Congo with Rwandan refugees. On returning to Australia, he decided to study medicine, which he did at the University of Queensland from 1997 to 2000.

After completing medicine, he worked in various hospitals, before starting general practice training and accepting a commission as a Medical Officer in the Australian Army in 2005. He has worked in South Africa at the Chris Hani Baragwaneth Hospital and Swaziland at the Good Shepherd Hospital. He was deployed on peace-keeping operations as the aeromedical evacuation Medical Officer to East Timor in 2006/7.

He now runs a group practice with 8 other doctors in Wangaratta, a large country town in northeast Victoria, and is a part-owner of two pharmacies. He has been awarded the Humanitarian Overseas Service Medal, the Australian Defence Medal and the Australian Service Medal by the Australian Government, and the Timor-Leste Solidarity Medal by the President of East Timor.

He lives on the family beef cattle farm with his wife and two children near Wangaratta.

South Asia

Chapter

11

India

Dr. Kavery Nambisan

The Pandemic and the Rural Doctor

This is the first time in the history of a disease that its course is so anxiously charted, and its possible surge predicted months in advance. In India, the government rushed into an ill-timed lockdown, announced a mere four hours before enforcement. (South Africa gave four days' notice before locking down and Bangladesh gave a week.) It did not even think about the hundreds of millions migrant workers who were stranded in cities and towns all over the country, with no jobs, no shelter, no transport home and no food. It caused a humanitarian, social and economic debacle of huge proportions.

Everywhere across the country of India, ordinary citizens, NGOs, a few celebrities and corporates went out of their way to help these distressed migrant workers. Sadly, the judiciary delayed hearing the many petitions that were filed against the government for causing this tragedy while those in power underplayed the ill effects of the monstrous goof-up.

The original bungling and the refusal to admit it and address the disaster has left millions in poor health due to under-nutrition and malnutrition. Compounding the tragedy are the new labor laws which will further curtail the rights of the labor force, while favoring the employers. The aftermath of the COVID years continues to have adverse effects on the future course of our nation. One can only hope that we have learnt some important lessons from our mistakes.

PEOPLE HAVE THE RIGHT TO KNOW THE FACTS

When I retired from my surgical career a few years ago, I set up a clinic in a rural town in Kodagu district, Karnataka. The COVID-19 pandemic—which is ultimately connected to our careless handling of the environment—happened at a time when I was truly enjoying my job as a general practitioner, seeing a marvelous variety of cases, and also updating my medical knowledge.

By the end of March 2020, new COVID-positive cases were being reported in India every day. The government announced a near-total lockdown, giving the citizens a less than twenty-four-hour notice. At that time, we had one positive case in a district of one hundred thousand people. The average citizen buckled under the resulting mayhem. The lifting of the lockdown, when it came a few months later, resulted in frenetic attempts to return to work and an influx of people coming from bordering districts and states. There was a surge of COVID infections, which quickly reached 6,000. The district hospital in the town of Madikeri admitted proven cases and managed them efficiently. But having a single center for the entire region was inadequate. The distance from my clinic to Madikeri is 70 kilometers. Systematic surveillance and interaction with all the medical staff in the district were not done.

I spoke to the district health officer at the beginning of the lockdown to find out if he had any advice. He advised me to shut my clinic, stay safe and send all suspected cases to Madikeri. Of the three doctors working in our town, one had tested COVID-positive and was therefore staying off work. I shut the clinic during the lockdown, opened the clinic, shut it again and finally decided to stay open. During the lockdown period, I used to see patients, on the narrow porch in my home.

In our health-care system, there is absolutely no connectivity between the city and the rural professionals. Specialist doctors from nearby cities are ever ready to come on flying visits once a week or once a month and offer their specialist services for which we are grateful. But the chasm between the two is as wide as ever. A large number of doctors in rural India had to rely on their own resources to handle the pandemic. Our efforts are an essential part of the rural struggle to cope with a monumental medical crisis which claimed the lives of at least four hundred thousand Indians.

In the early months of the pandemic, people were reluctant to take social distancing or the use of masks seriously. As for the hand sanitizer, everyone loved the idea of 'washing away' the virus with a few drops of alcohol-scented liquid. A cousin told me how she and her husband took the precautionary measures with complete seriousness and geared up before driving to the town to buy provisions: masked, gloved and goggled. They created a minor scene at the shops where everyone stared, unbelieving, at the pair of aliens.

Epidemiologists warned that for each clinically confirmed case, there would be about sixty more who were afflicted but asymptomatic.

I tried to work within the confines of this crucial detail and did my own bit of clinical detective work in tracing persons who were most likely to be affected. I learned about building immunity against the virus naturally, and about preventive medical treatment through online seminars, data and discussion with those who were knowledgeable.

The best help I could get came from a friend in Pune (non-medical, from the armed forces) who sent me a steady supply of the medicines and alerted me to new developments that I might have missed. The other source of help was my brother (also from the armed forces). He provided me with a stack of N95 masks and gloves and offered to buy me PPE (Personal Protective Equipment) clothing. I declined the last, because I was not working in a hospital environment where the risk of infection was higher. I do know that he helped procure protective gear for many doctors who needed them.

The role of these two army guys was far, far more important and genuine than the showy praise for medical fraternity from the Armed Forces with helicopters showering flowers over hospitals, and serenading medical staff with music, thus expending Rs 68 crore. The banging of steel plates and lighting lamps to promote good health (recommended by our Prime Minister) was a ludicrous and empty gestures.

We had enough evidence from several countries in the use of simpler, effective medicines (Hydroxychloroquine and Ivermectin) which can be given to patients quarantined at home. Why, then, were these measures not checked out, and used in our country and in the west? They are inexpensive and can help the majority of COVID patients avoid hospital admission, intravenous medication and endless investigations.

It is because hospitals need money. Their routine work came to a standstill, so how else could they have survived? Even several months after the pandemic struck, the Indian Council of Medical Research (ICMR) endorsed these simple medications but did not give them enough publicity. Perhaps they were being cautious because there had been no extensive peer-reviewed clinical trials in the use of these medicines for COVID infections. But any reasonably experienced practitioner will tell you that we have used Hydroxychloroquine and Ivermectin for years to treat other medical conditions.

Hydroxychloroquine and Ivermectin for years to treat other medical conditions.

In some countries such as in Bangladesh, innovative methods were backed by the government but in many others, including the US, Germany, Australia and Nigeria, doctor-groups took their own decisions.

Based on the above facts, I devised my treatment strategy. Those who presented at my clinic with symptoms and signs of respiratory infection were given routine treatment for three to five days. If they did not recover within three to five days, blood tests were done to rule out bacterial infections, typhoid, dengue, and malaria. If the tests pointed towards a viral infection, the patient was given the choice to either get tested for COVID or to undergo a week's treatment which I would closely supervise, by having the patient or the family member report to me on alternate days. All such patients were counseled about the illness, the need for distancing from family members and isolation, even within their homes.

Those with upper-respiratory–tract infections (of the nasal cavity, sinuses, ear and throat) were treated with Ivermectin, Azithromycin, Vitamin C, Zinc and Vitamin D3. Patients with lower-respiratory-tract infections (the bronchial tubes and lungs) received Ivermectin with Doxycycline and Bromhexine, besides the three supplements. Many of them were hypertensive, diabetic or had other causes of chronic ill health. Since most of them had been in my care for years, it was easier for me to convince them about their role in containing the disease.

Only those who presented with more severe symptoms like fluid lung infections, breathing distress or extreme fatigue were referred to the district hospital.

Of the sixty-odd patients whom I treated thus, three required hospital admission and care for respiratory distress and declining oxygen levels. One among them was a diabetic with advanced renal disease and already on regular dialysis. The family were financially bereft, and he expired within a week after developing the infection but his wife who got infected, recovered, in spite of being a poorly controlled diabetic.

DOCTORS IN UTTAR PRADESH

Another was found to have tuberculosis underlying the COVID infection. His condition improved after starting appropriate treatment for both but he is not yet fully recovered. The third, also a diabetic with heart disease was lost to follow up. By the end of the pandemic, I had treated a little over eight hundred patients.

The controversy over the use of Ivermectin raged for the last three years. These are the facts on which I based my treatment. In 1979, two scientists – Campbell and Omura discovered the drug Ivermectin, which was found to be effective against a number of parasitic infestations. The drug was produced by the pharmaceutical company Merck and in the last 40 years of its use, 3.7 billion tablets have been consumed worldwide. It figures in the WHO list of essential drugs. The two scientists were awarded the Nobel Prize in Physiology or Medicine for their discovery. Ivermectin is safer than commonly used medicines like Ibuprofen, paracetamol, penicillin and aspirin. In India, every medical practitioner is familiar with this drug which is safe also in children. However, parasitic infestations are the bane of economically backward countries in Africa and Asia. For the manufacturer, it is not a profit-making drug, so Merck did not renew its patent after the early years. Ivermectin is now being produced by several companies.

In 2020, during the early months of the pandemic, an Australian scientist experimenting with Ivermectin in vitro found that it killed the COVID-19 virus. He wrote about his findings, and it was noted by a doctor working in a large government hospital in Bangladesh. He used Ivermectin on 60 patients and found that it cured most of them. Moreover, none of them developed any serious complications of the disease. As the news of this simple drug being effective in treating COVID spread, hundreds and then thousands of doctors began to use it all over the world.

The results were extraordinary: When given in the early stage of viral replication (first five days) and along with other supportive vitamins, Ivermectin is far more effective than other more expensive drugs. In the later stages of the disease also it works because of its anti-inflammatory properties which help avoid serious complications.

By August 2020, Ivermectin was being used in Bangladesh, Mexico, South Africa, Israel, Spain, Italy, Slovakia, and Japan, besides in the UK, US, and many other countries in Europe. In December 2020, a group of medical experts formed the International Front-Line Critical COVID Care (FLCCC) Alliance led by Drs. Paul Marik, Umberto Meduri, Jose Iglesias, Pierre Kory and Joseph Varon. In the UK the British Ivermectin Recommendation Development Panel (BIRD) was founded by team led by Dr. Lawrie. To date there have been over 60 clinical trials and 31 Randomized Clinical trials done on 25,000 patients by 549 scientists on Ivermectin use in COVID-19 infections. They firmly endorse the universal use of the drug.

In India, Dr. Chaurasiya in Deoria district of Uttar Pradesh had, by late 2021, treated over 4,000 patients; Dr. Darrell Demello in Kandilivi, Bombay treated 6,000 (most of them from corporate houses) and a professor of ENT working in Mangalore and Kannur treated over 4,000 patients. Dr. Auburn Jacob used Ivermectin to treat patients and medical professionals in a hospital for leprosy patients in Tamil Nadu and thus prevented the disastrous effects of the disease. There are many others who have treated patients in large numbers. I spoke to and learned from many of these doctors and also, particularly from the work of Dr. Shankara Chetty in South Africa.

Ivermectin can also be used as a preventive medicine for those who are at high risk of infection, like family members of COVID-positive individuals and all frontline workers which includes health care professionals, the police, traffic and railway personnel, bus, auto, taxi drivers, bank employees and more. It was very useful in treating post-COVID complications and in treating the Long COVID, although the most dramatic results are seen when it is used early. We believed that this drug should be quickly cleared for use countrywide and also provided to our urban and village health workers in their health kits, with clear instructions for use. In fact, Ivermectin should be given to all those who are not vaccinated or are partially vaccinated. After the initial three tablets given on three consecutive days, a once weekly dose of 12 mg provides enough protection against the virus. When a drug that was safe and cheaply available could work effectively, what was the reason for not using it, at least until a safe vaccine was widely available?

LETTER TO HEALTH MINISTER

Mass prophylaxis is a sure way of stopping transmission. It could have been urgently implemented by the government, because all mechanisms of mutation and spread were not only of national but also international significance.

I reproduce here the letter I wrote to the health minister of our country in early 2021, urging him to consider the proper and large-scale use of Ivermectin as a preventive and treatment strategy against COVID. It went unanswered.

To Dr. Harsh Vardhan,
Union Minister for Health and Family Welfare
New Delhi

Sub: A safe and economical strategy for stopping COVID transmission before the vaccines arrive

Dear Sir,

Please let me place before you some urgent suggestions regarding COVID care. I am a senior doctor from rural Karnataka. All of us working in health care have seen the extent of suffering caused by COVID-19, the ripples of which have reached every household. It is the first such National Medical Emergency in hundred years. India has suffered immensely, with the loss of lakhs(hundreds of thousands of lives) of lives, loss of livelihood for millions, diminishing strength of the working population due to poor nutrition, mental fatigue and depression. Young doctors are exhausted and fearful of the future.

From the early days, the focus has been on how we can safely treat and prevent the spread of this disease in a way that is safe, quick and affordable. Although the one method by which this could be achieved is within our reach, we have not fully utilized it.

India needs to think clearly and act fast. The drug Ivermectin is known to be highly effective against COVID-19, particularly in the early stage of the disease. It is a very safe and has been in use for other conditions by several million people worldwide without any harmful side-effects. Indeed, it is safer than any antibiotic currently in use and it is cheap. More than 20 large clinical, peer-reviewed trials around the world (links given below) have shown that the drug Ivermectin reduces virus multiplication effectively in 74% of patients and prevents the second or inflammatory stage, when complications frequently happen. Even if an Ivermectin user gets COVID, it will be a mild attack and not serious.

In India, ICMR (Indian Council of Medical Research) has endorsed its use and so had AIIMS Delhi (All India Institute of Medical Sciences), but has endorsed its use and so has AIIMS Delhi, but this has not received the attention and follow up it deserved. Its nation- wide use is highly recommended, and every day wasted means that the virus can gallop on to produce dangerous mutant strains leading to a third wave.

Vaccination of an adequate number of people will no doubt fulfill the need to stop the virus, **but only if the vaccination drive is completed rapidly,** with 70 % of the population vaccinated in five to six weeks. In India, in spite of all efforts, it will take at least eight to ten months to do it. *During that time the large, unprotected population will continue to get infected and transmit the disease. The repeated mutations will lead to a cycle of repeated vaccinations and boosters and India will remain in the 'pandemic mode' for many years. The effect of this on the well-being of our people and on the economy can easily be imagined.*

Repeated, even partial lockdowns are of temporary help, and they come with the loss of livelihood for millions of Indians. No amount of subsidies will suffice to ensure good nutrition and that will lead to long-term problems among the workforce.

Recommendation based on the experience and evidence from doctors worldwide:

1. *Ivermectin 12 mg daily for 7 days at the earliest onset of COVID-like symptoms. Ivermectin is given along with the antibiotic, vitamins and other supportive medicines that are now being used in early cases.*
2. *Ivermectin works as a powerful prophylactic in preventing COVID infections. 12 mg for three days should be given to all family members and contacts of those affected, and then followed with one tablet a week until the risk is low.*
3. *The above preventive measure should be used for all frontline workers – that is healthcare workers, police, traffic inspectors, shopkeeper delivery boys, auto, taxi and bus drivers, bank officials and almost anyone who has to go out of their homes to work and will come in contact with others. It is the best and safest protection against the disease in all those who are waiting to be fully vaccinated.*

The use of Ivermectin will reduce COVID infections, transmission, virus mutations and death. It will drastically reduce the need for quarantine outside the home, hospital admissions and oxygen usage.

It is only among the very few who reach the second or inflammatory stage of the disease that we need to do blood tests and give a short course of low-dose steroid and an anticoagulant. Some of them will need admission, oxygen and critical care. **That percentage will be greatly reduced with the use of Ivermectin.**

Doctors around the country and abroad have been using it for several months, with excellent results. Orissa, Goa and parts of UP (Uttar Pradesh) have recommended its use in a big way. Many of us doctors in Karnataka too have been using it for over six months. Doctors in several countries (Israel, parts of US and UK, Belgium, Spain, Italy, Mexico, Bangladesh, Slovakia, South Africa and others) have strongly recommended its use.

Just as it is the duty of a soldier to fight for his country, it is my duty as a doctor to try and save lives. With this humble request I entreat you as the Union Minister for Health to take a decisive step and make the use of Ivermectin mandatory in the early stages of the disease. It could be provided in the Home Kits distributed to COVID patients by ASHA workers who can also ensure that the family members receive it.

I have attached links to vital information regarding the use of Ivermectin in different countries and continents.

Yours sincerely,
Dr. Kavery Nambisan MBBS, FRCS (London)
Kodagu district, Karnataka.

- *https://covid19criticalcare.com/ from FLCCC Alliance*
- *https://bird-group.org/ from UK*
- *https://covid19criticalcare.com/videos-and-press/flccc-releases/joint-statement-may-03-2021-joint-statement-on-widespread-use-of-ivermectin-in-india-for-prevention-and-early-treatment*
- *https://health.economictimes.indiatimes.com/news/industry/immediate-global-ivermectin-use-can-end-pandemic-scientists/82479538*
- *https://www.ncbi.nlm.nih.gov/pmc/articles/PMC8088823/*

- *https://covid.aiims.edu/clinical-guidance-for-management-of-adult-covid-19-patients/*
- *https://www.researchgate.net/publication/345321623_Title_Role_of_ivermectin_in_the_prevention_of_COVID-19_infection_among_healthcare_workers_in_India_A_matched_case-control_study*
- *https://timesofindia.indiatimes.com/city/bhubaneswar/odisha-to-buy-7-2-lakh-ivermectin-tablets-to-cater-to-needs-of-covid-19-patients-in-home-isolation/articleshow/82570387.cms*

The receipt of the letter was acknowledged but he did not deign to reply.

THE MEDIA ONLY SEES ONE SIDE OF THE COIN

The COVID-19 pandemic exposed clearly the errors made by our government, the most fundamental being to entirely rely one set of advisors and then rushing into an ill-timed lockdown.

The plight of migrant workers who bore the triple blow of hunger, joblessness and COVID is unforgettable. Those in power underplayed the ill effects of their goof-ups; they concealed hard truths under a blitzkrieg of self-congratulatory exaggerations of India's success in defeating the virus. That a second COVID-19 surge was likely in April-May in 2021 through India was foretold as early as January by experts in India and abroad. The government chose to be arrogant and ignorant; and we the people stupidly chugged along - traveling, attending parties and weddings, forgetting to wear masks. The reprisal was swift.

The second wave that came in April 2021 was much more severe than the first. I had to shut my clinic again and get back to seeing patients on my porch.

I was learning every day. The disease had two phases. During the first phase that lasted six to seven days, the virus multiplied in the body, and it was the ideal time for simple, effective treatment. The second stage was one of high inflammation caused by a hypersensitivity reaction to the virus and it could be dangerous if not quickly detected and treated. Blood tests to detect inflammation were essential in those who had persistent fever after five days of treatment, severe lung signs, extreme fatigue, or low oxygen levels. They needed a blood thinner and an antihistamine, if medication is given quickly and in the right dosage, hospitalization could be avoided. Those who deteriorated because of delayed or ineffective early treatment required oxygen; few such patients needed admission for critical care.

During the Pandemic, with no public transport, patients who suffered from chronic and acute ailments of all types were unable to seek medical help. (On an average, our outlying villages are five to fifteen kilometers away from any town which might have a chemist's shop, a public health center, a nurse, or a doctor.) Shop owners, forced to shut down, took the brunt of the economic slide. A few shops remained open for about three hours a day, but many essential provisions and medicines were in short supply. Roadside vendors struggled to make a living. Others, like those involved in construction work, were left high and dry, as were school and college going students. The online classes were of little or no value to 90 per cent of rural children, especially those from the impoverished, low-income households who had no smart phones. Educating children through the digital medium proved to be an illusion and only a small number of those with means managed to get some benefit from online classes. The government has admitted that the reported 4 lakh deaths in India is not altogether accurate since deaths among the migrant workers who rushed to their own villages in faraway states is unknown. Rural India faced devastation and in urban areas, it was not much better.

It is never too late to revisit our cache of knowledge, to relearn, and to share our learning. An effective network of health care providers in each area, treatment protocols, availability of drugs and the quick establishment of oxygen beds would have helped far more than untimely lockdowns, poor public sanitation, and a paucity of oxygen

Chapter 11 The Pandemic and the Rural Doctor

supply. When the pandemic was no longer a threat, we were left with an economic and nutritional debacle, both of which are still to be properly addressed.

All estimates made in the early months of 2021 when vaccines became available in India confirmed that it would take eight to ten months to vaccinate an adequate number of people in our country. During that time, those who were unprotected while waiting for the vaccine would be vulnerable to infection. That was precisely what happened. As lockdowns were relaxed, the virus began to mutate and spread rapidly. There was this other simple protective and preventive measure that we could use to halt the virus.

However, there is one dilemma: Major pharmaceutical companies around the world have invested trillions of dollars in the manufacture of vaccines. One can understand their need to recover costs and make profits by selling vaccines to every country. But it should not mean that we sacrifice millions of lives in order to make it okay for the companies. Sadly, this is happening. Drug control authorities round the world and (ironically) WHO itself chose to dismiss or stay indifferent to the sustained efficacy of Ivermectin. Medical professionals who work in super-specialty hospitals are none too happy about a drug that will drastically reduce hospital dependency.

The saddest part of the story is that the media has apparently chosen to look only at one side of the coin. What other explanation is there for the shrill publicity given to expensive drugs like Remdesivir and several newer drugs while the success, safety, and ease of use of Ivermectin is treated with deafening silence? If patients can recover quickly with a tablet that can be taken at home, we can undo lockdowns, open up business and tourism, and run colleges and schools without waiting until the whole world is vaccinated. None of this is to say that vaccinations are not necessary. What we are trying to reinforce is that we should use the simpler, safer, quicker method of mass prophylaxis with Ivermectin as soon as possible. If properly planned it can be done in a matter of days.

To put it simply, it made very good sense to Ivermectinise the world while going ahead with vaccinations at the same time. Given the crumbling economy of many poor countries, universal vaccination was a long way off. Every single COVID patient was a risk to herself and the rest of the world. And sadly, now we know that vaccine related complications (neuropathy, myocarditis, coagulopathies, myalgia) and deaths have reached alarming proportions.

In conclusion, I quote Michael Capuzzo a six-time Pulitzer shortlisted writer from his article on Ivermectin titled, *"The Drug that Cracked COVID"* He writes: *"I do not know of a bigger story in the world than this."*

Kavery Nambisan, MBBS, FRCS (London)

Dr. Kavery Nambisan is from the southern state of Karnataka, India. She graduated from St John's Medical College in Bangalore, trained in surgery in the UK and obtained the Fellowship of the Royal College of Surgeons from London. She has spent most of her surgical career in different parts of rural India including Bihar, UP, Tamil Nadu and Karnataka. She has been a governing council member of the Association of Rural Surgeons of India and is an honorary faculty at the department of humanities in St John's Medical College, Bangalore. She is also a writer and novelist, and was married to the poet and journalist late Vijay Nambisan. Her most recent work is a medical memoir titled A Luxury Called Health which was published in 2021.

Europe

Chapter

12

Netherlands

Dr. Rob Elens

My Experience with Ivermectin

The first time I heard of Ivermectin was during tropical medicine training. In 1995 I trained in tropical medicine at the Royal Tropical Institute in Amsterdam. There, I first came into contact with all kinds of infections and their treatment. While there, I heard of the drug Ivermectin, which helps in the treatment of river blindness.

From 1996 to 1999, I worked in a mission hospital in Malawi, Africa. For 3 years, I treated an awful lot of infectious diseases there. Most of them were malaria, tuberculosis, worm, and bacterial infections.

I was responsible for the purchase of the medicines which we did through a non-profit organization in Amsterdam (International Dispensary Association Foundation, IDA Foundation). Of course, quite a bit of the work consisted of treating malaria with drugs such as Fansidar, chloroquine, hydroxychloroquine, and paludrine. Because we could buy all kinds of medicines cheaply, we were never without medicines.

During that time, I learned a lot about what parasites and worms can do to the human body.

Malawi has a large lake where a parasite that causes snail fever, or bilharziasis, is found. The treatment of snail fever is praziquantel, a drug I had never heard of before.

Unfortunately, I could not buy Ivermectin at IDA, and had to treat scabies with Benzyl benzoate.

After these 3 years working in Malawi, I moved to England with the family to train as a family doctor. There, Ivermectin was available for the treatment of scabies. Ivermectin is a popular drug for deworming horses. In all these years, there have never been any problems with the availability of this drug, especially if a doctor had written a prescription. In the southeast of England, where I trained, there were many people who owned horses.

Chapter 12   My Experience with Ivermectin

BEFORE COVID-19

After working for 8 years in Malawi and England, I moved back to the Netherlands, where I worked as an acting general practitioner for several years before starting my own practice in Meijel, a village in North Limburg.

In April 2020, we were dealing with a huge increase in sick people who all appeared to have COVID-19. There were days when I had to do 10 visits to people who were sick in the home situations and also 10 consultations at the practice. All were COVID-related cases. In 3 weeks, I submitted 26 people to the hospital, of which 13 died one to two days after admission. They were all older people, but otherwise not seriously ill.

When the hospital announced a freeze in admissions, I worried about how to proceed with the increasing number of my patients. Surely there must be a solution that we, medical frontliners, could adopt? Until then, the advice was to take paracetamol and wait for things to get better or worse. Sadly, the turn of events was for the worse. Eventually, a friend told me to watch a video of Dr. Zelenko, who had developed a treatment protocol for COVID-19 consisting of azithromycin, hydroxychloroquine, and zinc.

I watched that video and researched that the combination of these drugs was biochemically sound, I asked my pharmacist if she had this medication.

These medications were available in the pharmacy, and together in an afternoon we established a local protocol where we would start treating people with high-risk COVID-19 with a combination cocktail of hydroxychloroquine, azithromycin, and zinc orotate.

My first patient was a man of 86 years old who did not want to go to the hospital because, by now, it was known in the village that one out of two COVID-19 patients sent to the hospital would die. He emphatically said he did not want to go to the hospital and he agreed to my protocol. I visited him every day, and he got a little better and better. On the fourth day of treatment, he sat at the breakfast table and was completely healed. I was very impressed with the speed of the effect of the treatment on this very sick, old man.

This is how I treated 9 other people with all the same results. I thought to myself, this can no longer be a coincidence and this should be known throughout the Netherlands because this is a possible treatment for this severe COVID-19 infection.

I was interviewed by a local media company about my COVID-19 treatment experience. After the video was posted on the Internet, within a few days it had 500,000 views. In my naivete, I thought I would get a call from the minister of health to make a plan together to make Holland recover from this COVID-19 pandemic.

To my surprise, I instead got a call from a health inspector asking if I had taken informed consent from my patients, and if I was aware that this protocol is an off-label treatment and that it could have possible dangers.

I was not aware of any harm except that there was a theoretical chance that QT prolongation of the heart muscle could occur with the combination of azithromycin and HCQ. However, I had performed an ECG and assessed renal function for all of my patients, so I knew exactly what I was doing.

His tone was very invasive, and he implored me to stop prescribing hydroxychloroquine.

Because of this admonition, I discontinued the protocol with my next patient, although I believed this case was an excellent opportunity for this type of treatment. Against my better judgment, I did not do it. After a few days, his condition deteriorated and he was admitted to the hospital, where he died after two days.

Chapter 12   My Experience with Ivermectin

This bothered me a lot for several days because my aspiration as a physician is, of course, to make people better with the right cocktail of drugs, medication, supplements and other advice. This completely contradicted my belief, as a physician, in adhering to the Hippocratic Oath.

Finally, I looked in the mirror in the bathroom and said to myself that I will decide which medicines to use to fight a disease, and not the inspector.

I made every effort to make it possible to prescribe these drugs. I wrote to professional groups, asked the ministry to do research, but no one wanted to cooperate in a study of this therapy for COVID-19.

I did have contact with some people who had seen my video, and together we then created a website: www.zelfzorgcovid19.nl containing advice on supplements that can be taken to strengthen the immune system and fight COVID-19.

ALLEGEDLY IN VIOLATION OF THE PHARMACEUTICAL AFFAIRS LAW

Soon, Ivermectin was getting coverage in the news as an effective remedy for COVID-19. Some doctors called me to ask how and why the protocol works. We made it possible for people to request a prescription through the website.

But most of general practitioners (GPs) did not want to prescribe these drugs, and so they stuck to the damning guidelines of instructing patients to use paracetamol, wait at home, and to only call an ambulance if their conditions worsened.

We started using Ivermectin in the dosage advised by the Front Line COVID-19 Critical Care (FLCCC) Alliance, with very good results.

About a year after communicating with the health inspectorate,

309

they came by again for an interview and asked if I had made another prescription with hydroxychloroquine since they had prohibited me from doing so. I said that I just continued prescribing these drugs when I thought it was necessary, and made some people better with hydroxychloroquine and Ivermectin who were suffering from a persistent COVID-19 infection.

This did not please the inspector, who requested information on my patients. The inspector decided that I had violated the medicine law and fined me 3,000 euros.

I was fined €3,000 for a prescription of hydroxychloroquine (HCQ) and €3,000 for a prescription of Ivermectin.

This fine was paid by a donor, but I made an appeal, which at the time of writing is still pending.

The law states that I can only prescribe off-label drugs if it is also in a standard or protocol. At that time, there was no standard or protocol, just advice and guidance. The standards and protocols were evolving, and the drug law says that if so, off-label medications can be prescribed in consultation with the patient and pharmacy.

I always consulted with the pharmacy and the patient when prescribing these drugs, and I made sure I always had an ECG to check for QT issues.

I was very impressed with the effect of the drugs because almost everyone with a severe COVID infection healed within 4 to 7 days. People who had mild disease usually got better with a combination of supplements consisting of zinc, quercetin, vitamin D, C, and NAC in appropriate doses.

VIDEO ATTENTION AND TV APPEARANCES

Meanwhile, I had been on national television because of my video. This appearance on national television gave me a kind of national fame. On one hand, I was extolled as a healer with a potential therapy, but on the other hand, was dismissed as a quack. The issue of these remedies was discussed in Parliament, but the minister concerned dismissed them as quackery and no motion was passed.

When the inspectorate came to the practice for the third time to discuss a few things, I told him that we had started a survey with doctors and a data system to collect information on COVID treatment from medical frontliners.

I told that to the inspector and two weeks later the inspector published a warning that any doctor who prescribed Ivermectin or HCQ could be fined €150,000!

In addition, each pharmacist was asked to pass on the names of doctors who were giving out prescriptions with Ivermectin or HCQ.

I had never seen this happen in the Netherlands before regarding a treatment protocol for an infection.

Off-label use of drugs is very extensive in the Netherlands, and I think every doctor in the Netherlands does that at least once or twice a day. There are about 50,000 doctors in the Netherlands, so that covers nearly 100,000 prescriptions a day. There had never been a fine issued for off-label drug use, and I had the first fine ever issued in the Netherlands.

A local pharmacist from Venlo Arjen Ypma contacted me.

He was wondering why this warning from the inspectorate was being communicated throughout the Netherlands. He shared that at first, he had ignored this warning but after a week, he thought: "This (warning) is really weird. Do I really have to activate some kind of click function to report doctors ?!"

After finding out that there is a staggering amount of evidence that this combination of drugs was effective in treating COVID-19, he again got in touch with me.

In a year, our group had 19 doctors of various specializations: geriatrics, occupational medicine, complementary medicine, and family medicine. Without realizing it, we became a cohort of doctors who were answering requests for help from people all over the country.

More doctors got involved as people were appealing for prescriptions of Ivermectin and Hydroxychloroquine(HCQ), because their own family doctors refused for fear of being fined.

The time came when my own pharmacy did not feel like dealing with the inspectorate anymore and refused to give further prescriptions. So, I sent all my prescriptions to Arjen's pharmacy. A few more pharmacies joined us who were able to deliver medication to those who needed them.

There were many people who were not getting better, and they asked for help through the website. So, we created an online system that allows us to send information securely to the pharmacies. In all, we answered 4,000 requests, 3,000 of which were for prescriptions of Ivermectin and HCQ, which were all sent by the pharmacy.

This system of dispensing medicines "out of the radar" never happened before. Later on, it became clear to us that this had to do with the temporary approval of the newly developed experimental gene therapy, also known as the vaccine, that was believed to make the COVID-19 infection disappear from the face of the Earth.

Unfortunately for us, another pharmacy informed the inspectorate because it saw a prescription coming through from Arjen's pharmacy. The inspectorate decided to raid Arjen's pharmacy. He was compelled to surrender all the prescriptions he had made that contained Ivermectin and hydroxychloroquine.

CHALLENGING THE INSPECTORATE

By that time, there were 19 doctors, all of whom used Arjen's pharmacy to deliver medicines to their patients. Eventually, the inspector fined each doctor according to the number of prescriptions. The names of all the doctors who issued the prescriptions were known, and the fines ranged from €3,000 to €12,500.

My 104 prescriptions containing Ivermectin and HCQ were naturally among those found in Arjen's pharmacy. In a very comprehensive 445-page report, I was again told I had breached the Medicines Act, and my fine was doubled. I was not satisfied that I was being fined simply for treating people and began to challenge the fine. As this fine is an administrative fine, I had to go through a number of committees to challenge it.

Together with my lawyer, Sobar Kouja, we went into the fight, believing that this fine was unjustly imposed.

Three years later, after several appeals to the Commission, we finally arrived before an administrative judge in Lomond.

The case was filed in February 2023, and we found the judge's ruling in his July 2023 decision disappointing in that he found that I had breached the Medicines Act. However, after considering all the information, the Disciplinary Committee ruled that there were no Level 1 evidence-based guidelines and standards in light of the circumstances at the time I prescribed Ivermectin and HCQ to my patients. In other words, the Disciplinary Committee found that I had not contravened the Medicines Act, while the Administrative Law Judge found that I had contravened the Medicines Act. Despite these conflicting decisions, what is important to me is that no one has died as a result of prescribing these drugs, and no serious side effects have occurred.

I will appeal against this fine and will continue to fight the case in the Court of the Council of State in The Hague in 2024.

IVERMECTIN CREAM

All COVID-19 patients I have treated have been cured within four to seven days by prescribing Ivermectin, HCQ, and azithromycin. Our group of doctors has faced a huge wall to get the drug prescribed.

Hospital doctors and general practitioners did not cooperate, and customs confiscated shipments from India and China if they thought they contained HCQ or Ivermectin.

However, for HCQ, it was possible to obtain it from medicine vending machines in the evenings and on weekends.

As for Ivermectin, there was also a case of a patient on a ventilator in the ICU who could not take oral medication, so he got better after applying Ivermectin cream, which had just been launched at the time. We therefore advised the patient to massage his feet, legs, and back with Ivermectin cream every day so that Ivermectin could enter the patient's body through the skin. This was continued for several days, and the patient recovered very well.

CREATE PROTOCOL

We set up a professional group of doctors, the Dutch Tele doctor Association (www.NTG.nu), to develop software for the study of pulmonary COVID and the treatment of vaccine injury. This is a kind of online center where people can enter complaints.

Although there are now few requests for help for acute COVID, a great many people suffer from long-term symptoms of post-vaccination and Long-COVID-19, such as significant fatigue.

We have now also developed a protocol for this based on documents from Switzerland and the USA (from the FLCCC). We intend to use this protocol in the future. It's a kind of first-line second opinion center, where we're going to digitally input patients' symptoms and treat them with a combination of supplements and drug therapies.

Ivermectin will play a major role there as well.

Under the Pharmaceutical Affairs Act, it is up to the expert groups to decide which standards and treatments are approved. Our protocols are based on that.

We assume personalized medicine. It means that the patient decides whether the treatment employed was ultimately effective. The knowledge gained there is then used again for the next patient.

We now offer personalized medicine over the phone to many doctors who have their own practices.

If the initial approach does not work, the patient can always go to the practice of the partner doctor for follow-up tests and consultations.

I am very pleased to have 19 colleagues who believe that prescribing effective medicines can help people.

Together we have taken the Hippocratic Oath. The Hippocratic Oath means that we do no harm to patients and advise the best possible treatment.

Ivermectin has been used in the treatment of Long COVID with very good results.

Overall, all colleagues are determined to prescribe Ivermectin if they think it is necessary.

We have now launched a crowdfunding campaign, and the Dutch public has donated about €100,000 towards the fines and legal fees.

The fight is not over yet, but we will fight to the end until all fines are waived.

Rob Elens, MD

Born in Rotterdam on 27th of June 1962. Started my study with Physiotherapy from 1980 till 1984 in Rotterdam. Then I started to study Medicine at the Erasmus University from 1984 till 1991. I also worked in Several hospital in the department's surgery, Obstetrics Gyn, Anesthesia, Accident and Emergency and then worked for 3 three years as a medical officer in Charge at the Phalombe District hospital in Phalombe Malawi as a tropical doctor. Trained as a GP in United Kingdom in Barnstaple from 2000 till 2005. Then I moved back to the Netherlands where I worked in 35 practices before obtaining my own practice in Meijel from 2010. I have been working there ever since. Studied in Orthomolecular medicine to find out what the origins of diseases and integrate that knowledge into my practice. Married three children living in Venray.

Africa

Chapter

13

Nigeria

Dr. Philip Chidi Njemanze

A Tale of Ivermectin, Prayer, and Resilience in a Monastery During the COVID-19 Pandemic

In the tranquil setting of half-century-old monastery nestled on the outskirts of bustling City of Owerri, Imo State, Nigeria, a peculiar tension began to envelop the lives of twenty nuns as the shadow of an invisible enemy approached. It was the spring of 2022, and the COVID-19 pandemic had laid siege to the world. In the quiet halls of the monastery, where prayer and devotion were the cornerstones of life, a new prayer emerged: one for protection against an insidious virus.

Sister Mary Agnes, an 88-year-old nun, had been a pillar of strength and solace for her fellow sisters for decades. Her unwavering faith had been a source of inspiration to all, but it could not shield her from the relentless virus. Sister Mary Agnes had contracted COVID-19, and her condition was rapidly deteriorating. She had pre-existing conditions of hypertension and chronic obstructive pulmonary disease (COPD). She was hospitalized, leaving the monastery in a state of unease.

Dr. Ihenacho, a compassionate physician with a heart as vast as his medical knowledge, found himself at the intersection of science and faith. He was called upon to care for Sister Mary Agnes and had the formidable task of preventing an outbreak within the tight-knit community of nuns. His face shielded behind layers of protective gear; Dr. Ihenacho felt the gravity of the situation. "We cannot let this virus breach these sacred walls," he whispered to himself.

The initial presentation of Sister Mary Agnes was concerning, to say the least. An 88-year-old Nigerian female patient presented with severe general weakness, anorexia, shortness of breath, cough with productive sputum, loss of concentration, loss of memory, prosopagnosia, and pedal edema. The present illness started two days before admission with weakness, dyspnea, and disorientation. She had a history of long-standing isolated systolic hypertension and COPD.

The blood pressure was 170/88 mmHg, and the heart rate was 90 bpm. The oxygen saturation was 69%. The body mass index was 30. The initial blood sample analysis revealed hematocrit (HCT) of 23.1%, hemoglobin (Hb) of 7.7 g/dL, white blood cell count (WBC) of 12,500/mm^3, erythrocyte sedimentation rate (ESR) of 50 mm/h, clotting time (CT) of 5 min, platelet count of 225,000/mm^3, and prothrombin time (PTT) of 17s. Malaria parasites were seen in the blood. There was electrolyte imbalance showing hyponatremia (sodium 120 mEq/L), hypokalemia (potassium 2.7 mEq/L), hypercalcemia (calcium 12.2 mg/dL), and hypochloremia (chloride 74 mEq/L). The magnesium level (1.9 mEq/L) was normal. The D-dimer (4,201 ng/mL) level was raised.

The cardiac troponin I (cTnI = 0.06 ng/mL) was raised, suggestive of myocardial infarction. She was of blood group A, Rhesus positive. Serology tests including hepatitis B antigen, hepatitis C antigen, and HIV test were negative.

The liver function enzymes such as aspartate aminotransferase (AST, 47 IU/L) were raised but alanine aminotransferase (ALT, 8 IU/L) was within the normal range. The total bilirubin (0.89 mg/dL) was normal, but conjugated bilirubin (0.83 mg/dL) was raised, suggestive of hepatobiliary involvement.

Fasting blood sugar (FBS, 114 mg/dL) was slightly elevated. Lipid profile: total cholesterol (TCHOL 185 mg/dL), low-density lipoprotein (LDL 101 mg/dL), high-density lipoprotein (HDL 50 mg/dL), triglyceride (TG 170 mg/dL), and very low-density lipoprotein (VLDL 34 mg/dL) showed hypertriglyceridemia. Urinalysis was normal.

The initial ECG revealed ventricular arrhythmia with a heart rate varying (VR 60 to 115 bpm) and atrial rate (AR 75 to 375 bpm), suggestive of paroxysmal atrial fibrillation. There was a deep Q-wave suggestive of myocardial infarction and low amplitude R waves due to coronary ischemia.

Two-dimensional echocardiography examination revealed end-diastolic volume 35.5 mL, and the posterior wall thickness was 1.71 cm; the systolic volume was 19.7 mL, and the posterior wall thickness was 2.01 cm. There were intracardiac clots extending from the mid-septal to the apical septal walls. The cross-sectional area of the clot measured 2.91 x 2.24 cm. In the long-axis view, the clot size measured 3.53 x 1.89 cm. There was dyskinetic wall motion abnormality of the apical septal wall. There was mitral regurgitation. The ejection fraction was reduced to 44.5%.

A repeat blood sample analysis done 10 days later showed HCT of 45.6%, Hb of 15.2 g/dL, WBC of 7,900/mm3, ESR of 40 mm/h, CT of 8 min, platelet count of 280,000/mm^3, and PTT of 27 s. The electrolytes were within the normal range. The oxygen saturation rose to 93-94% range while off the oxygen administration. The patient's clinical condition significantly improved.

The control ECG revealed a normal ventricular rate (75 bpm) and atrial rate (AR 75 bpm), suggestive of normal sinus rhythm. There was a deep Q-wave suggestive of a prior myocardial infarction and low amplitude R waves due to coronary ischemia. The control 2D-echocardiography conducted 20 days later revealed end-diastolic volume 31.8 mL, and the posterior wall thickness was 1.3 cm; the systolic volume was 10.6 mL, and the posterior wall thickness was 1.47 cm. There were no intracardiac clots. There was normal wall motion. The ejection fraction was reduced to 66.7%.

The patient tested positive for COVID-19 with a COVID-19 Ag test kit (SD Biosensor) and SARS-CoV-2 RT-PCR assay.

The patient was managed for acute respiratory distress syndrome, myocardial infarction, severe anemia, hypertension, and septic shock. The patient received anticoagulation treatment at prophylactic doses (LMWH – enoxaparin 40 mg s.c. once daily).

As Dr. Ihenacho tended to Sister Mary Agnes in the sterile confines of the hospital, he couldn't help but ponder an unconventional idea. Ivermectin, a humble anti-parasitic drug, had shown promise as a potential treatment for COVID-19. Could it also serve as a shield, a guardian angel, for the nuns who were in such close proximity to Sister Mary Agnes?

The decision weighed heavily on his shoulders, as the use of Ivermectin for COVID-19 prophylaxis was not yet sanctioned by health authorities. Dr. Ihenacho consulted his medical colleagues and prayed for guidance. The risks and benefits danced in his mind like warring angels.

He had prior experience with Ivermectin for River Blindness prophylaxis. He prescribed the drug in the hinterlands where many patients with Onchocerciasis presented with blindness.

However, this was the first use of Ivermectin for COVID-19 treatment and prophylaxis in a closed community. There was apprehension on safety issues and possible drug reactions without significant benefits. Dr. Ihenacho also prescribed the use of steam inhalation twice daily for the nuns.

Dr. Ihenacho made his choice. He decided to provide Ivermectin prophylaxis to all the nuns in the monastery, a decision fraught with uncertainty and the potential for controversy. It was a delicate dance between faith and science, with the lives of the nuns hanging in the balance.

As the days turned into weeks, the monastery became a place of heightened tension. The sisters questioned their faith, the science, and the wisdom of their decision. But Dr. Ihenacho's steady hand and compassionate heart reassured them that they were making the right choice. In the daily morning Mass, the nuns gazed at the firm face of Dr. Ihenacho who attended Mass to get reassured that their colleague was doing well.

And then, as if guided by a divine hand, a miraculous turn of events unfolded. Sister Mary Agnes, against all odds, began to recover. Her vital signs became normal and remained stable, with rising oxygen saturation levels from the low 70s to low 90s. Dr. Ihenacho a few days later broke the news that she was now off the oxygen support. The virus, which had threatened to claim her life, was vanquished. Her story became a beacon of hope and a testament to the power of faith and science working hand in hand.

The weeks passed, and no other nun within the monastery fell victim to the virus. The tension that had gripped the community slowly dissipated, replaced by a profound sense of gratitude and relief. The nuns came to understand that their faith had not wavered; it had, in fact, been fortified by the alliance between science and the divine. There was an unusual strength, confidence, and renewed devotion to Our Blessed Virgin Mary, whose intercession was credited with the victorious turn of events.

As Dr. Ihenacho briefed the nuns in the monastery on the precautionary measures to be taken, he knew that he had been a humble instrument in a remarkable chapter of resilience and triumph. In the hushed corridors of the monastery, where the whispered prayers of nuns had once filled the air, a new prayer emerged—a prayer of gratitude for the science that had saved them and the faith that had sustained them.

And so, in the midst of a pandemic that had tested the world's resolve, a group of nuns and a compassionate doctor had woven a tale of resilience, courage, and the unwavering belief that even in the darkest of times, the human spirit, fortified by faith and guided by science, could emerge stronger than ever before.

Philip Chidi Njemanze, MD

Academician (Prof.) Prince Dr. Philip Njemanze, MD (Hons), was born on 15 March 1962 at Owerri, Imo State, Nigeria, in the royal family of the Njemanze. He is the Chairman of the International Institutes of Advanced Research and Training, Chidicon Medical Centre, Owerri, Imo State, Nigeria. He is an Academician of the International Academy of Astronautics (IAA), the highest UNESCO body for Space Research. He was a former Principal Investigator of the National Aeronautics and Space Administration (NASA) of the study of the Brain in Space. He is also a Distinguished Medical Practitioner (DMP) of the Federal Republic of Nigeria. He went to school at St Paul's Catholic Primary School, Owerri. His secondary education was at Government Secondary School, Owerri. In 1986, he completed his medical education at Rostov State Medical Institute, Order of Friendship, Rostov-on-Don, Russia (former USSR). He undertook postgraduate training and fellowships in Neurosurgery, Neurology, and Angiology at Klinikum Grosshadern, University of Munich, Germany, GUY's Hospital London, and Bowman Gray School of Medicine, Winston Salem, North Carolina, USA. He has over 200 published works including two dozen US and UK patents. He is married to Mrs. Felicia Njemanze, and they have three children. See citations at www.chidicon.com

Chapter
14

Zimbabwe & South Africa
Dr. Jackie Stone and
Professor Colleen Aldous

An Ethical, Clinical, and Regulatory Analysis
Ivermectin in COVID-19 Treatment in Zimbabwe

We present the implementation of an empirically developed, Ivermectin-based, sequenced multidrug regimen in Zimbabwe, for the treatment of COVID-19, that have been used since 2020. This chapter examines the historical context, ethical considerations, regulatory responses, and the clinical experiences of healthcare professionals during the pandemic. The narrative is constructed around a series of snapshots, providing insights into the decision-making processes and the grassroots level response to the healthcare crisis.

INTRODUCTION

The COVID-19 pandemic, emerging in 2019, presented significant challenges to healthcare systems worldwide. Initially, there were no specific antiviral treatments or vaccines, leading to an urgent search for therapeutic options.

In Zimbabwe, a country with constrained healthcare resources, the situation was especially critical. The capital had only 17 understaffed ICU beds and lacked accessible internal medicine physicians. However, several primary care doctors with extensive experience in infectious disease and combination therapies played a crucial role. These doctors, skilled and ethical, were proactive in their approach to patient care, often collaborating on potential treatments, contributing to saving many lives in Zimbabwe.

Zimbabwe's low COVID-19 mortality rate has been partially attributed to its young population, with half of its citizens under age 25. However, this does not fully explain the disparity with South Africa, which experienced significantly higher mortality despite having a similar demographic profile. For instance, South Africa recorded 102,595 deaths out of 60 million people. Zimbabwe was predicted to have over 25,000 deaths and yet we reported only 5,725 deaths out of our population of 15 million, indicating that other factors contributed to saving approximately 20,000 lives.

Moreover, Zimbabwe experienced only three waves of COVID-19 deaths, with the last occurring during the Delta variant in 2021, whereas South Africa had five waves.

A major difference between the two countries was Zimbabwe's early and widespread adoption of Ivermectin in January 2021. Recognized for its effectiveness in early treatment protocols and prevention, Ivermectin became a key component of Zimbabwe's approach, particularly when vaccination alone was not fully preventing hospitalizations and deaths. Its use during the Delta and subsequent Omicron waves may have contributed to Zimbabwe achieving herd immunity with fewer casualties.

This chapter delves into the decision-making process and events leading to the implementation of Ivermectin in Zimbabwe's COVID-19 treatment regimen. It explores the challenges faced by healthcare professionals, including the limitations of standard care and an overburdened healthcare system. Zimbabwean doctors, combining first-world training with third-world experience, brought a unique perspective, often at odds with western experts, to the treatment of infectious diseases.

Ivermectin, a WHO-listed essential drug, was known for its antiparasitic properties and had anecdotal antiviral uses.

Its introduction into Zimbabwe's COVID-19 treatment was a complex decision involving clinical observations, historical precedents, and the urgent need to address a health crisis.

This chapter will provide a comprehensive analysis of the factors influencing Zimbabwe's response to the pandemic. It aims to explore the balance between immediate life-saving measures, scientific rigor, and ethical responsibilities in healthcare. It is a story of resilience and innovation under dire conditions. The chapter is divided into two parts, with the first covering events prior to January 26, 2021, and the second detailing subsequent developments.

PART 1
Historical Context and Precedents
Early Observations (1995–2016)

The history of alternative treatments in Zimbabwe, especially the utilization of silver, has roots extending back to the mid-1990s. This period marked the beginning of a trend towards innovative, non-conventional therapies in response to severe medical conditions. Notable examples include the treatment of HIV patients in London and the use of nebulized silver for managing cystic fibrosis.

This historical narrative follows a timeline that starts with these initial applications and leads to the introduction of silver generators in Zimbabwe in 2016. The story underscores a traditional and community-centric approach to healthcare, illustrating how local practices have adapted and incorporated alternative methods in response to health challenges. This evolution reflects a broader narrative of adaptability and resourcefulness in the face of medical adversity.

The SARS Experience and Silver (2003)

The 2003 SARS epidemic marks an important historical reference for the use of silver in treating viral infections. Research papers demonstrating the effectiveness of silver against coronavirus strains in laboratory settings laid out the scientific foundation for consideration of its use during the COVID-19 pandemic. However, the natural resolution of the SARS outbreak meant that these findings saw limited practical application during that period.

The Onset of COVID-19 and Response in Zimbabwe
Initial Clinical Experiences and Challenges (Early 2020)

As 2020 began, the world, including Zimbabwe, was confronted with a rapidly escalating pandemic. The novel coronavirus introduced a health crisis that precipitated socio-economic challenges, straining Zimbabwe's medical and economic infrastructure. Healthcare workers in Zimbabwe faced a significant learning curve as the virus manifested unpredictably and severely.

The initial COVID-19 cases in Zimbabwe reflected global trends of uncertainty and high infectivity. Primary care physicians, often the first responders, witnessed a surge in patients with varying symptom severities. The virus impacted all segments of society, from the impoverished to the affluent. Zimbabwe's healthcare system, already under strain, struggled with the increasing caseload.

Frontline workers, predominantly general practitioners and medical officers, were thrust into a critical situation. For over ten months, beginning in March 2020, they treated a wide spectrum of COVID-19 cases. This included the majority with mild to moderate symptoms and those who, due to limited resources, could not access intensive or high dependency care. Patients were managed in various settings, including outpatient rooms, local clinics, homes, and even in parked vehicles outside overwhelmed hospitals.

Healthcare workers also played a key role in community education about the virus and preventive measures, facing the emotional impact of dealing with death and its effect on families. Their dedication was evident in their long working hours, including weekends and holidays. Their experiences provided invaluable insights into the disease's progression and treatment effectiveness.

Despite these challenges, their commitment to evidence-based medicine persisted. They adhered to national guidelines, using supportive treatments, steroids, and anticoagulants, as needed. However, the persistently high mortality rates highlighted the inadequacy of these measures. This harsh reality, mirrored in even more resourced nations, underscored the urgent need for effective treatments.

This pursuit was driven by clinical necessity and ethical responsibility. Healthcare workers' experiences symbolized a frontline battle with limited resources against a formidable, poorly understood adversary. Their observations and clinical decisions paved the way for considering alternative treatments like Ivermectin and nanosilver, offering hope in an environment dominated by uncertainty and loss.

Regulatory and Ethical Considerations

During the early stages of the COVID-19 pandemic, Zimbabwe's regulatory bodies and healthcare professionals faced a complex ethical and regulatory environment. The urgent need for effective treatments contrasted with the limitations of a healthcare system constrained by resources and a regulatory framework tailored for conventional medical challenges.

The ethical and regulatory considerations of using complementary medicines and WHO essential drugs, not yet registered in Zimbabwe, presented a challenging intersection of urgent medical need, ethical responsibility, and regulatory adaptability. Authorities grappled with providing optimal care while maintaining medical ethics and regulatory prudence.

Ethically, the situation was complex. On the one hand, there was a moral imperative to act quickly against a novel, deadly virus. On the other, the obligation to ensure treatments were safe, effective, and scientifically sound. The use of Ivermectin, known for its safety but unproven efficacy against COVID-19 in vivo, sparked intense debate.

At the heart of this ethical discussion was the principle of beneficence – the commitment to do good and prevent harm, balanced with the need for scientific rigor. This was challenged by the urgency of the pandemic and the slower pace of traditional clinical trials, complicated by the need to respect patient autonomy in treatment decisions during a health emergency.

Zimbabwe has regulatory bodies, the Medicines Control Authority of Zimbabwe (MCAZ) and the Medical and Dental Practitioners Council of Zimbabwe (MDPCZ), which are both tasked with public protection. The MDPCZ had limited public guidance and engagement, while the MCAZ played a more active role.

The Medicines and Allied Substances Control Act governed the MCAZ's operations, overseeing medical treatment authorization and public safety. Normally, the approval process is thorough, but the pandemic required a more responsive approach.

In response, the MCAZ considered compassionate use – allowing access to unapproved drugs for life-threatening conditions when no alternatives existed. This required balancing potential risks and benefits and making decisions with incomplete information.

Initially, MCAZ demanded extensive data for medications not yet registered in Zimbabwe, but the first wave and lockdown made communication difficult. Consequently, discussions between doctors and MCAZ officials led to the importation of SAHPRA-approved nanosilver from South Africa under an institutional Section 75, facilitated by Dr. Ingrid Landman and me (Jackie Stone) with the Ministry of Health and MCAZ. SAHPRA is the South African Health Products Regulatory Authority.

An institutional Section 75 was issued in August 2020 for nanosilver importation. The MCAZ, within its regulatory constraints, strived to facilitate the use of products to alleviate COVID-19 symptoms.

Clinical Experiences and Challenges (August 2020 to January 2021)

By August 2020, frontline healthcare workers in Zimbabwe were recognizing the effectiveness of a specific treatment protocol for early-stage COVID-19. This protocol included nanosilver, zinc and its ionophores (like doxycycline), and vitamins D and C. Later stages of the illness required steroids and anticoagulants, based on blood testing.

However, as more severe cases emerged and resources like oxygen and adequate staffing dwindled, it became evident that this protocol was insufficient for patients presenting in advanced stages of the disease. Insights from Australia, South Africa, and the US suggested Ivermectin as a potential treatment, with reports of significant improvements in critically ill patients.

Three years on, the understanding of Ivermectin's role has evolved. Beyond its antimicrobial and anti-inflammatory properties, it was found to prevent thrombosis and support cardiac function under hypoxia, addressing issues seen earlier in the pandemic.

I (Dr. Jackie Stone), unfamiliar with Ivermectin's veterinary use, knew it as a safe, WHO-essential drug used in humans, particularly for treating Norwegian Scabies in Australia. Its portrayal as a "horse dewormer" was perplexing to me. In Zimbabwe, Ivermectin was registered for animal use and widely available in farming supply stores. Some pharmacies and patients had independently sourced Ivermectin tablets from Asia.

On 7 August 2021, the situation became critical. My clinic struggled with oxygen supply. With hospitals overwhelmed, waiting patients deteriorated in parked cars. Discussions with South African colleague Dr. Martin Gill, who observed improvements in patients self-administering Ivermectin, led to a combined treatment protocol incorporating Ivermectin and silver. The results were remarkable.

Patients had been informed about Ivermectin through social

media, especially from Professor Thomas Borody's viral posts in mid-2020. A primary care practitioner in Zimbabwe successfully established a dosing protocol for Ivermectin, Doxycycline, and Zinc. From 8 August 2020, patients self-administering Ivermectin as part of the treatment protocol showed notable survival rates. Once silver, Ivermectin, and Doxycycline were combined with Zinc, Vitamin D, and Vitamin C, survival rates improved significantly, and all treated contacts also survived. This approach was also effective in protecting healthcare workers.

On 19 September 2020, these treatment protocols were presented in a CME session, leading to widespread adoption by doctors and patients. As the second wave loomed, information about the protocols spread, preparing the population for the virus's arrival.

During the second wave in December 2020, the disease spread rapidly. Despite lockdowns, cases and deaths surged. Hospitals adhered to conventional protocols, excluding Ivermectin and Silver, and saw high mortality rates. Patients, aware of alternative treatments, often refused hospitalization, opting for home-based care using the established protocol.

In the capital city of Harare, as resources became scarce, home-based care using the protocol became more common. Nurses assisted patients remotely, using WhatsApp for communication and monitoring, with home visits for assessment and necessary interventions. This approach allowed for effective triaging and treatment, demonstrating adaptability and resourcefulness in a crisis.

An ABCDEF approach

In response to the COVID-19 pandemic, healthcare professionals in Zimbabwe adopted an ABCDEF approach for patient management:

A. **Assessment:** Comorbidities and medical history were evaluated in order to record initial observations.

B. **Breathing:** Breathing was assessed to determine if the patient required oxygen and/or needed to start nebulization.

C. **Cannulation:** Blood collection for laboratory analysis was performed. Key tests included a full blood count (to assess prognosis and secondary bacterial infections), LDH (as a marker of lung necrosis), LDH/Lymphocyte ratio (predicting disease severity), CRP (to determine the need for steroids), and D Dimer (to assess the need for anticoagulation).

D. **Diabetes, Doctor, Drugs:** Blood sugar levels were checked, and medication needs assessed. At this point, a doctor was usually consulted. Hypoxic patients (experiencing very low oxygen levels in the tissues), often received IV Dexamethasone while awaiting CRP results. High-risk patients received Low Molecular Weight Heparin.

E. **Exit:** Before the nurse left, the need for home nursing was evaluated and arranged if necessary.

F. **Family:** Close contacts were advised to undergo a 5-day prophylaxis course. Family members were trained to monitor and manage the patient's condition, often using WhatsApp for communication.

However, by early January 2021, this system became overwhelmed. The medical team utilized a central location, the Highlands Presbyterian Church's Gazebo, for training groups of family members in patient care. This site was chosen for its ventilation and central location, previously used in disaster responses.

My testimony reveals challenges faced during this period. On 15 January 2021, a video of mine teaching a patient COVID-19 care went viral without my patient's consent. Subsequently, Professor Rashida Ferrand filed a complaint against me, leading to an inspection by an illegally assembled team from the Medical Council and police intervention. I faced accusations and legal challenges, resulting in my temporary house arrest and a recommendation to go into hiding.

Despite these challenges, the spread of information on social media led to significant sales of Ivermectin. However, on 23 January 2021, Professor Ferrand and Public Health Physicians recommended against Ivermectin use, citing "Insufficient Evidence."

This narrative highlights the complexities and difficulties faced by healthcare workers in Zimbabwe during the pandemic, balancing patient care, regulatory compliance, and personal safety.

Following a change in Dr. Andrew Hill's recommendation in his review, Zimbabwe faced a critical period marked by the loss of prominent figures. Three Cabinet ministers, Professors James Hakim and David Katzenstein, both renowned in medical research, and three influential businessmen passed away. The country experienced a peak in COVID-19 deaths, reaching 70 fatalities per day.

In response to this crisis, primary care physicians convened over a weekend and composed a letter, dated Sunday 24 January 2021. This letter, included in the appendix, was hand-delivered to the Permanent Secretary of Health on the morning of 25 January 2021, coinciding with the peak of daily deaths. By the evening of 26 January 2021, the Ministry of Health requested the Medicines Control Authority of Zimbabwe (MCAZ) to approve the importation of Ivermectin under a bulk section 75. This approval made Ivermectin widely accessible throughout Zimbabwe, which subsequently became the world's largest importer of the drug. It was believed that much of this supply also reached neighboring countries, especially South Africa, due to widespread awareness spread via WhatsApp messages.

The emergency authorization for the importation and use of Ivermectin was a significant move by the Ministry of Health and

MCAZ, illustrating their adaptability in the face of the pandemic. This decision marked a departure from conventional treatment protocols and acknowledged the exceptional challenges posed by the pandemic. It demonstrated an effort to balance the urgent need for effective treatments with patient safety considerations.

Additionally, this decision highlighted the importance of international collaboration and information exchange in shaping local health policies and regulatory responses. Reports of Ivermectin's efficacy in other countries and collaboration with respected frontline clinicians globally played a crucial role in its inclusion in Zimbabwe's treatment protocols.

Division between the Regulators

The division regarding the use of allopathic and unregistered complementary medicines during the COVID-19 pandemic extended beyond the medical community to regulatory bodies in Zimbabwe.

The main contention arose not with the Medicines Control Authority of Zimbabwe (MCAZ), but with the Medical and Dental Practitioners Council of Zimbabwe (MDPCZ). Some members of the Public Health Physicians Council reportedly utilized the MDPCZ to hinder the use of certain repurposed therapies that were considered safe. There were notable conflicts of interest among members of the Medical Council, including its chairperson. These conflicts, combined with their lack of frontline experience and reliance on epidemiological data from outside Africa, raised concerns about their decisions and actions.

Unfortunately, the Medical Act in Zimbabwe limits the Ministry of Health's ability to intervene in disciplinary matters, rendering the Medical Council seemingly beyond reproach. This situation highlighted the challenges in the healthcare regulatory framework, particularly in the context of an unprecedented global health crisis.

Division between the doctors

Ivermectin's introduction in Zimbabwe created a significant divide among the medical community, unparalleled by any other drug. The College of Primary Care Physicians of Zimbabwe (CPCPZ) frontline doctors largely supported its use, citing positive outcomes. In contrast, other primary care physicians were strongly against it. Many specialists privately used Ivermectin but publicly questioned its efficacy, aligning with mainstream narratives. Interestingly, these physicians prescribed Remdesivir, despite its debatable impact on hospital death rates. The media further fueled this debate.

Internationally, many frontline doctors humorously labeled Public Health Physicians with "Ivory Tower Encephalopathy", suggesting a disconnect from practical realities. This criticism extended to epidemiologists, questioning whether their rise to regulatory power during the HIV pandemic was due to compliance, a quest for recognition, and a statistical rather than empathetic focus. Concerns were raised about their reliance on WHO guidelines, perceived as uncritical acceptance of information from an unelected body, significantly privately funded.

The situation in Zimbabwe was positively influenced by doctors in the Ministry of Health who maintained a balanced perspective and were open to hearing both sides of the debate. This approach was partly attributed to connections between military doctors and the collaborative nature of the relatively small medical community. The Permanent Secretary of Health, with his pragmatic Air Force background and familiarity with Crew Resource Management in Aviation, played a crucial role. His approach potentially prevented the loss of many lives, including key family members and breadwinners.

Dr. David Scheim, a former professor of MIT in the USA likened the collaboration between frontline doctors and the Ministry of Health to "raising Lazarus from the dead", highlighting the remarkable and rapid coordination that occurred over three days, which had a significant impact on the pandemic's trajectory in Zimbabwe.

PART 2
Implementation of Ivermectin: Clinical Observations and Public Health Implications
Observations on the Ground during the second wave

As the COVID-19 pandemic progressed in Zimbabwe, healthcare professionals' observations became vital for real-time data collection. Once Ivermectin was officially approved, doctors freely prescribed it, meticulously documenting their findings. Their experiences provided crucial insights into the disease's progression and the immediate impact of various treatment strategies in a rapidly evolving and challenging context.

Notably, specialist physicians, public health physicians, and public and private hospitals did not incorporate Ivermectin into their treatment regimes. This led to patients refusing hospitalization, aware that their Ivermectin treatment would be discontinued. Primary care physicians were thus compelled to manage critically ill patients who were staying within their homes, even those with oxygen saturation as low as 55%, with oxygen and nursing support. The strong doctor-patient relationship in Zimbabwe, fostered by a tight-knit community culture, played a significant role in this scenario. Primary care physicians, deeply invested in their patients' wellbeing, often managed very ill patients at home rather than referring them to hospitals where outcomes were perceived to be worse.

General practitioners (GPs) described the experience as challenging

Chapter 14   An Ethical, Clinical, and Regulatory Analysis

yet rewarding, likening it to a pilot "flying by the seat of their pants." The pulse oximeter became an essential tool, and businesses related to home oxygen, nebulizers, and home nursing services saw significant growth. Specialists criticized primary care physicians for handling cases they believed should be referred to hospitals, leading to tense exchanges highlighting the differences in patient outcomes between home-based and hospital care.

The focus on prophylaxis for contacts of COVID-19 patients was intense, with patients and their families educating others on preventive measures. This proactive approach, similar to data from regions like Uttar Pradesh and Peru, showed an immediate effect with a sharp downturn in deaths. By 26 February 2021, the official death rate in Zimbabwe dropped to zero per day, with a rolling average of 3 deaths per day.

During this period, the Zimbabwean COVID Frontline Clinicians Society was formed, comprising doctors who signed the letter to the Permanent Secretary. They engaged in daily discussions on patient care. I was advised by the Medical Council to cease practice, played a role in coordinating home care and prophylaxis.

My observations led me to explore COVID-19 as a vascular occlusive disease rather than a respiratory illness, aligning with findings from Dr. David Scheim's research. This realization sparked collaboration with U.S. and South African clinicians, leading to data collection and analysis. Despite some doctors' reluctance to participate due to regulatory concerns, the group analyzed 104 patients treated with their protocol, demonstrating a mortality rate of less than 1% compared to 35.4% in similar patients receiving standard care in state hospitals. This collaboration and research marked a significant step in understanding and responding to COVID-19 in Zimbabwe.

343

Observations on the ground after the second wave

By late February 2021, Zimbabwe had successfully controlled the second wave of COVID-19. However, during this time, I faced significant challenges. I had received a notice of disciplinary action from the Medical and Dental Practitioners Council of Zimbabwe (MDPCZ) and criminal charges filed by the Registrar of the Medical Council. The specifics of these proceedings are beyond the scope of this discussion, but it is important to note that the disciplinary hearing on 26 March 2021 was criticized for procedural irregularities and was perceived as a biased trial. This action was seen as a deterrent to doctors using Ivermectin.

Following the letter to the Ministry of Health, all doctors who had signed it received threatening letters from the Council. This coincided with the rollout of the Sinovac and Sinopharm vaccines in Zimbabwe. While vaccination was not mandatory, it was strongly encouraged, and travel was restricted for unvaccinated individuals.

Dr. Agnes Mahomva was vocal in the media, advocating for the safety and efficacy of vaccines in preventing hospitalization and death. Many patients chose vaccination and discontinued Ivermectin prophylaxis. However, during the Delta wave, several fully vaccinated doctors and many others succumbed to the virus, indicating that vaccines did not entirely prevent hospitalization and death. This revelation led to the realization that higher doses of Ivermectin might be necessary, and Primary Care Physicians found themselves managing an increasing number of cases as hospitals continued to avoid prescribing Ivermectin.

To address this, the College of Primary Care Physicians of Zimbabwe organized a series of Zoom lectures to discuss the use of Ivermectin, Silver, Doxycycline, and vitamins D, C, and Zinc. Following the re-adoption of Ivermectin, a significant decrease in

Chapter 14   An Ethical, Clinical, and Regulatory Analysis

deaths was observed.

The Medicines Control Authority of Zimbabwe (MCAZ) authorized the use of Ivermectin in specific pharmacies, allowing doctors to access the medication while reporting any side effects or adverse outcomes. Despite these developments, the Medical Council pursued disciplinary action against me. In August 2021, my license was restricted, and I was not allowed to present a defense due to a backlog of cases. The Council also pursued criminal charges, seeking to use my case as a deterrent for other doctors.

The collection and publication of data on Ivermectin became crucial for its widespread prescription, a move fully supported by the College of Primary Care Physicians. This period highlighted the complex interplay of medical practice, regulatory actions, and the evolving understanding of COVID-19 treatment strategies in Zimbabwe.

The Role of Professional Medical Associations

Within the College of Primary Health Physicians of Zimbabwe, specific professionals played a critical role in gathering and sharing observations from individual practitioners during the COVID-19 pandemic. These efforts provided a vital forum for healthcare workers to exchange experiences, discuss treatment outcomes, and formulate informal treatment guidelines. This collective endeavor was especially important as official guidance continued to evolve.

The College organized two significant Continuing Medical Education (CME) accredited training sessions. The first, held on 19 September 2020, was a comprehensive 5-hour session focusing on the SIDDZ protocol. It featured discussions led by both primary care doctors and specialist physicians, covering the FLCCC protocol, local treatment strategies, and the importance of stringent diabetes control.

The second session, occurring during the Delta wave, consisted of a

345

series of lectures delivered twice daily over two weeks via Zoom. These lectures, coordinated by Dr. Ingrid Landman, who oversees education and heads the Mashonaland section of the College, concentrated on various treatment aspects for managing COVID-19.

Simultaneously, there was a concerted effort to publish the data collected from the second wave as part of a retrospective observational clinical trial. This initiative aimed to formally document and analyze the treatment approaches and outcomes, contributing to a broader understanding of effective COVID-19 management strategies in Zimbabwe.

Initiation of Clinical Trials

The initiation of clinical trials for Ivermectin in Zimbabwe in 2021 was driven by two key factors: the drug's observed potential in treating COVID-19, and the global demand for scientifically validated treatments. Healthcare professionals, recognizing the positive patient outcomes from off-label Ivermectin use, aimed to establish a structured research framework to rigorously assess its efficacy and safety. The objective of these trials was to transcend the limitations of anecdotal evidence, providing robust data necessary for regulatory approval and broader clinical application.

I collaborated with international experts like Dr. David Scheim, Dr. Martin Gill, Professor Colleen Aldous, and Drs. Barry and Jerome Dancis throughout 2021. Within Zimbabwe, I worked with various health professionals, including Professor Ndarukwa, who co-authored the paper that was eventually published. Professor Ndarukwa's involvement was instrumental, particularly in facilitating the ethical approval required for a retrospective analysis.

The consensus was that a retrospective observational study using data from Zimbabwe's first and second COVID-19 waves would be

Chapter 14 An Ethical, Clinical, and Regulatory Analysis

the most effective approach. This study aimed to leverage the wealth of real-world experience and data accumulated during these periods, providing a more comprehensive understanding of Ivermectin's impact in a controlled research setting.

Monitoring Safety and Efficacy

In the context of the COVID-19 pandemic in Zimbabwe, where extensive clinical trials were not feasible, safety and efficacy monitoring became a crucial aspect of the healthcare workers' observational approach. The close monitoring of patients treated with Ivermectin and silver was essential to gather important data on these treatments' safety profiles and potential side effects.

In this scenario, frontline healthcare workers effectively assumed the role of researchers. They meticulously documented their clinical findings and shared these insights with the broader medical community for peer review and evaluation. This practice of systematic observation and data collection was vital, particularly for those doctors who later contributed their meticulously gathered data to the retrospective observational trial.

However, it is important to note that more data could have been available for this study. Unfortunately, many junior doctors were hesitant to submit their findings, fearing potential repercussions. This situation underscores the challenges faced in environments where the collection of comprehensive clinical data is hampered by concerns over regulatory or professional consequences. Despite these challenges, the data collected through these observational methods provided valuable insights into the treatment of COVID-19 with Ivermectin and silver in Zimbabwe.

Ethical Practice and Patient Consent

During the critical period of seeking effective treatments for

347

COVID-19, the ethical principle of patient consent was emphasized by physicians in Zimbabwe. Despite the urgency, healthcare providers ensured that patients were fully informed about the investigational nature of Ivermectin and silver treatments. This process involved obtaining consent in a manner that respected the patients' autonomy and their right to make informed decisions regarding their care. Upholding this ethical practice was not only a professional duty but also a fundamental aspect of maintaining trust between patients and healthcare providers.

The experiences of healthcare professionals in Zimbabwe during the pandemic underscore the dynamic nature of clinical practice, especially in response to a public health emergency. While their observations do not replace the need for randomized controlled trials, they provided critical insights that helped shape the country's treatment strategies during this challenging time. These experiences also highlight the adaptability, resilience, and innovation of medical professionals when confronted with unforeseen and rapidly evolving health crises.

Challenges

The process of obtaining trial approval in Zimbabwe underscored the challenges inherent in conducting research in a resource-limited environment, especially during a health crisis. The extensive paperwork required, the necessity of a Good Manufacturing Practice (GMP) facility for the trial substances, and the multiple rounds of questions from regulatory bodies posed significant obstacles. These hurdles were compounded by the additional burden placed on healthcare workers who were also the primary investigators in these trials, balancing their clinical responsibilities with research demands.

The paper that eventually resulted from this effort has been

Chapter 14   An Ethical, Clinical, and Regulatory Analysis

recognized as a landmark study, mirroring the findings of Dr. Sabine Hazan's research. This achievement stands as a testament to the dedication and tireless efforts of the team involved. The collaboration in this research was not just local; it involved researchers from South Africa and the USA, who played crucial roles in compiling and presenting the data. This international cooperation and the unwavering determination of the research group members underscore the importance and impact of global collaboration in scientific research, particularly in challenging circumstances like those faced during the COVID-19 pandemic.

Description and Findings of the Study on Ivermectin-Based Treatment for COVID-19 in Zimbabwe

The study titled "Changes in SpO2 on Room Air for 34 Severe COVID-19 Patients after Ivermectin-Based Combination Treatment: 62% Normalization within 24 Hours" was conducted in Zimbabwe in response to the COVID-19 crisis, where medical facilities and treatment options were limited. This retrospective research analyzed the effects of Ivermectin (IVM)-based combination treatments on severe hypoxic COVID-19 cases, examining patient data from August 2020 to May 2021.

Key Findings

1. **Treatment Efficacy:** The study reported significant improvements in oxygen saturation (SpO2) levels within 24 hours post-IVM administration in 34 patients. There was an average increase of 55.1% at 12 hours and 62.3% at 24 hours. This outcome is particularly notable compared to standard care outcomes where decreases in SpO2 and pulmonary function were more common.

2. **Treatment Approach:** The decision to include IVM in the treatment

349

protocol was based on its preliminary efficacy, safety profile, and its established use in various diseases. Over 20 randomized clinical trials (RCTs) on IVM treatment regimens have been conducted.

3. **Patient Recovery:** All patients in the study, who were treated with a combination of IVM, doxycycline, and zinc, recovered. This included patients treated in clinics and at home, highlighting the potential effectiveness of the treatment.

4. **Safety Profile:** No serious adverse effects were noted with IVM, though transient effects like blurred vision were observed in some cases, especially at higher doses. The practice of increasing IVM doses for patients not initially responding to treatment proved generally successful.

5. **Study Limitations:** The retrospective nature, lack of control groups, randomization, and follow-up are significant limitations. These factors mean that while all patients in the study survived, definitive conclusions about mortality benefits cannot be drawn.

6. **Comparison with Other Studies:** The findings from Zimbabwe align with studies by Hazan et al. 2022 and Babalola et al. 2021, suggesting enhanced efficacy of the triple therapy of IVM, doxycycline, and zinc compared to IVM with other adjuncts.

7. **Potential Mechanisms of Action:** The study proposes mechanisms for IVM's effectiveness against SARS-CoV-2, including competitive binding with the virus's spike protein, reversing virally induced blood cell clumping, and activating the cholinergic anti-inflammatory pathway.

This study provides significant insights into the potential efficacy of IVM-based combination treatments for severe COVID-19 cases, especially in resource-constrained settings. The rapid improvement in SpO2 and patient recovery are promising, but the study's limitations

Chapter 14   An Ethical, Clinical, and Regulatory Analysis

necessitate a cautious interpretation of the results. These findings highlight the need for more structured research to conclusively determine the efficacy and safety of such treatments.

Conclusion

The exploration of Ivermectin-based treatment for COVID-19 in Zimbabwe, as detailed in the study focusing on changes in SpO_2 on room air, marks a significant contribution to the global response to the pandemic. This chapter highlights the challenges and innovative approaches undertaken in a resource-limited setting to address a public health crisis.

Reflection on Key Findings

The study's findings, demonstrating rapid and notable improvements in oxygen saturation levels among severely hypoxic COVID-19 patients following Ivermectin-based treatment, are encouraging. However, these results must be viewed in light of the study's limitations, including its retrospective nature and the absence of randomized control groups. The noted safety profile of Ivermectin, particularly its tolerability even at higher doses, is key to the feasibility and adaptability of the treatment.

Ethical and Regulatory Implications

The ethical and regulatory challenges discussed in this chapter reflect the complexities inherent in emergency healthcare decision-making. Balancing the urgency of administering potentially life-saving treatments with the commitment to scientific rigor and safety standards is challenging. Zimbabwe's regulatory response, marked by flexibility and collaboration with healthcare professionals, serves as an example for managing similar crises.

Global Context and Implications

This chapter underscores the significance of integrating local healthcare responses into a global framework. The collaborative efforts and insights from international research have profoundly influenced Zimbabwe's approach to COVID-19 management. Conversely, Zimbabwe's experiences contribute essential knowledge to the global understanding of handling infectious diseases in challenging settings.

The Way Forward

Future directions, informed by Zimbabwe's experience with Ivermectin-based COVID-19 treatment, emphasize the need for continued research and collaboration. Structured clinical trials are necessary to definitively assess the efficacy and safety of these treatments. There is a call for the development of healthcare systems that are adaptable and responsive to emerging crises.

The journey of Ivermectin-based treatment in Zimbabwe during the COVID-19 pandemic exemplifies the resilience and ingenuity of healthcare systems in the face of extraordinary challenges. It highlights the importance of clinical experience, evidence-based medicine, patient autonomy, ethical considerations, and regulatory flexibility in managing public health emergencies. Zimbabwe's experiences and lessons learned contribute valuable perspectives to the global conversation on pandemic management and set the stage for future innovations in global health.

Jackie Stone
MBChB, BSc MED Hons, MRCP, FRACGP, D Av Med, and FACAsM

Dr. Jackie Stone, a seasoned primary care physician in Zimbabwe, is renowned for her effective COVID-19 treatments, significantly influencing pandemic management debates. Her medical journey began at the University of Cape Town, focusing on infectious disease management. At St Bartholomew's Hospital in London, she contributed to HIV pandemic strategies, advocating for early triple therapy, and recognizing the limits of single-drug treatments.

Stone's medical philosophy embraces diverse treatments, blending traditional Western and alternative methods. This approach was highlighted during her tenure in Dubai, where she was part of a SARS 1 emergency response team. Working with a diverse patient demographic, she incorporated treatments from Chinese and Ayurvedic medicine. Her interest in integrative medicine grew in Australia, leading to her involvement in using silver as adjuvant therapy for multiple infections, including multi-drug resistant HIV, upon her return to Zimbabwe in 2015.

During Zimbabwe's COVID-19 crisis, Dr. Stone's successful treatment methods, diverging from global protocols, sparked controversy and professional challenges. Yet, her dedication to patient care and relentless pursuit of effective treatments, even amidst adversity, renders her story profoundly inspiring and a testament to her medical commitment.

Professor Colleen Aldous

Professor Colleen Aldous, a healthcare scientist and full professor at the University of KwaZulu-Natal's College of Health Sciences, is known for her diverse work in health sciences, focusing on research and mentorship. Her academic contributions, coupled with her role in public health debates, particularly during the COVID-19 pandemic, highlight her multifaceted expertise.

A central element of her career was advocating for Ivermectin in treating and preventing COVID-19. She has been instrumental in discussions about its efficacy, frequently challenging mainstream medical views. During the pandemic, Aldous emphasized the risks of solely relying on a limited group of experts opposing Ivermectin, highlighting the potential implications for human life.

Her engagement with Ivermectin extended to analyzing clinical trials and promoting its possible benefits. Aldous underscored scientific evidence supporting its use, demonstrating her commitment to examining all effective treatment options and prioritizing patient care.

Professor Aldous's career is distinguished by her steadfast dedication to healthcare research and education. Her approach is marked by rigorous scientific methods and a proactive stance in addressing medical challenges with innovative strategies. Her significant impact on public health and medical practice, particularly evident during critical times like the COVID-19 pandemic, underscores her as an influential figure in the medical field.

Chapter

15

South Africa

Dr. E.V. Rapiti

Ivermectin Saved My Patients with Severe COVID and the Vaccine Injured

I am a frontline General Practitioner (GP) working in the sprawling suburb of Mitchells Plain, Cape Town, which has a population of one and a half million people. In this chapter, I will share my experiences using Ivermectin and other repurposed drugs to successfully treat over 3,000 COVID patients with a 99.98% success rate. My greatest achievement was treating over 1,100 severely ill patients who were infected by the Delta strain with a success rate of 99.95%.

During the early days of treating patients with the highly virulent Delta strain, I developed a set of clinical criteria symptoms and used only two simple bedside tools, peak flow meter and an oximeter, to make an early diagnosis of COVID pneumonia without needing to do costly X- Rays or scans in about five minutes.

Part 1
INTRODUCTION – HOW I GOT INVOLVED TREATING COVID

I first heard about COVID-19 in March 2020, while I was recovering in hospital from a major heart attack. The President of South Africa, Mr. Cyril Ramaphosa, shut down the entire country and declared a state of emergency. Everyone in the hospital was struck by shock and apprehension that we were dealing with an extremely deadly virus that could potentially annihilate the entire human race because there was purportedly no treatment for the infection.

I knew nothing about the disease, and it was the first time in my 45-year career that I heard that the world was being locked down because of a viral epidemic. I am familiar with previous flu epidemics like the Spanish flu and the Asian flu, but this flu came across as far more deadly than anything we had ever encountered in human history.

It was only much later that I discovered in my practice and through my reading that the infection was not as serious as it was made out to be by the various experts, academics, local and world health authorities, other regulatory health authorities and all the media.

I saw this new outbreak as a major healthcare challenge for frontline doctors like me, where a virus was at war with the human race. The soldiers in this war were the frontline doctors and nurses, who had to leave their comfort zones and defeat this virus. I was determined to understand as much as I could about this new "killer" disease to find a solution to destroy it. I was prepared to go out and do battle with this virus against the advice given to healthcare professionals, by our health authorities that they should not see patients in their rooms.

I was not comfortable with the idea of treating patients without seeing and examining them. I wanted to see patients in the way that I had always done and that was to take a proper history, examine them, do tests, make a proper diagnosis and then treat them. To not see and examine patients was certainly not the way I practiced medicine. During the COVID-19 pandemic, most of my colleagues treated patients through their car windows and, without examining them, issued a script. While I was recovering in hospital, I made a concerted decision to find a solution to this so-called deadly virus, and I am pleased to say, as you will read later, that I managed to find a cheap, effective, and safe solution to tame this infection.

Shortly after I was discharged from hospital, I became very curious to learn everything I could about this new virus that was wreaking havoc in the lives of the citizens of the world. I listened to several lectures and the opinions of local and international experts as well as specialists in virology, infectious diseases, pathologists, pulmonologists, immunologists, and epidemiologists.

I closely followed the announcements/advice given by the scientists from the U.S. Centers for Disease Control and Prevention (CDC), the Food and Drug Administration (FDA), and the World Health Organization (WHO).

From my early days in medical school, I had an abiding respect for anyone with the title of Professor and believed everything that they said or uttered, without questioning their credentials. I saw myself as a student, once more entering medical school, trying to grasp as much as I could about this new and baffling disease.

Frontline doctors were strongly advised and informed by local and international experts that there was no treatment for COVID and that frontline doctors were instructed to send patients home to isolate. If patients became breathless, doctors were instructed to immediately refer the patients to hospital without seeing them. In a nutshell, frontline doctors, like me, were told to stand idly and do nothing.

Frontline doctors were told to stay home if they felt it was too risky to be at work. Many doctors closed their rooms and never saw patients for a long time fearing for their own lives. It was a difficult time for patients who desperately needed to see a doctor for help. Patients were left to fend for themselves because the hospitals were too full to see patients.

This advice to turn away patients without seeing them was hard for me to accept. My patients placed so much trust in me in the 40 years that I got to know them that to turn them away would have, rightly, been interpreted as my letting them down in the worst time of their lives. I could not live with such a thought. I was prepared to die in the line of duty helping patients rather than to sit back and do nothing, while my desperate patients suffered alone, in what was dubbed as one of the worst health crises to strike humanity.

I went to my rooms and attended to patients as I always did, against the advice on billboards that adults over 65 years should remain at home. I was 71 and heading for retirement. I decided to banish any idea about retiring and to battle with this virus to save my patients from dying. I saw myself as a medical soldier that was prepared to die in the line of duty, out of an abiding respect to my oath, than to hide in the bunkers of safety, while patients were left to die, abandoned and unattended. I learned quite early in my medical career that not every condition needed medications. Merely being seen and being examined by a caring doctor was most reassuring to patients and enhanced their healing. All patients needed to hear was that they were not seriously ill. People and patients, throughout the world, during COVID-19 were gripped in a trance of unending fear that they were at risk of dying at any time through regular media broadcasts. The captured mainstream and social media played a huge role in instilling fear in the world's citizens by dishing out fake information.

The two deaths in my practice had a major impact on me. It compelled me to find a solution. I accidentally listened to Dr. Pierre Kory speak on YouTube about the effectiveness of Ivermectin, which was banned by our health authority, SAHPRA (South African Health Products Regulatory Authority).

Dr. Kory came across as a very sincere doctor, who made a desperate plea for Ivermectin to be used for the treatment of COVID to save lives. He invoked my irrepressible curiosity about Ivermectin, so I watched every video on YouTube and read every article about the successful use of Ivermectin to cure COVID by doctors from Asia, Africa, and South America.

I listened to a lecture by Dr. Mobeen Syed on the mechanism of action of Ivermectin and several other lectures on the safety, efficacy, and versatility of this very inexpensive drug. I was totally fascinated to learn about the wonders of Ivermectin, which was discovered in 1973 by Dr. Satoshi Omura.

- https://www.nature.com/articles/ja201711

I later read about the amazing success stories of how Uttar Pradesh, a state in India with a population of 240 million, almost the size of the US, managed to bring down the death and hospital rate significantly to as low as 5,000 cases by issuing Ivermectin, Vitamin D and Zinc to all its residents. In the US, on the other hand, where doctors were strongly discouraged from using Ivermectin and Hydroxychloroquine to treat COVID, they had over 1 million deaths. The US with just about 4% of the world's population, accounted for 17% of the world's COVID deaths in spite of spending the most on healthcare compared to any other country in the world.

In June 2021, when the state of Uttar Pradesh in India was hit by the deadly Delta strain, the state introduced the widespread prophylactic use of Ivermectin, which reduced the incidence of new cases by a staggering 97.1%. The WHO praised the state of Uttar Pradesh for its swift handling of the outbreak but refused to acknowledge the role of Ivermectin to wipe out the disease.

- https://weeklyblitz.net/2021/10/08/covid-cases-in-indian-uttar-pradesh-drops-by-97-1-percent-because-of-ivermectin-use/

Dr. Swaminathan, a WHO scientist, warned India in a tweet not to use Ivermectin because of safety issues. This was an absolute lie, because Ivermectin, which was on the WHO's essential drug list, ranks as one of the safest drugs on the WHO's drug safety list.

- https://vigiaccess.org/

She was challenged by the Indian Bar Council for misleading the Indian government. Then Dr. Swaminathan immediately retracted her tweet.

By information outlets like Trial Site News, The Expose. The Epoch times, on Rumble, Bitchute and Telegram channels that several outstanding highly credentialed doctors were de-platformed on Facebook, Twitter, and YouTube for sharing their successes

Chapter 15   Ivermectin Saved My Patients with Severe COVID and the Vaccine Injured

using Ivermectin to treat COVID. These lectures and articles in the alternative media outlets left me unshakably convinced that Ivermectin was highly effective against COVID. It was extremely safe. With the best safety track record of all drugs and it was extremely cheap and easy to produce.

I was left totally dumbstruck to learn that the U.S. FDA and the WHO remained totally opposed to the use of a repurposed safe drug like Ivermectin to treat COVID, even though it was on the WHO's essential drug list and there was a great deal of evidence for its efficacy against COVID.

The WHO had always supported the idea of doctors using repurposed drugs to treat illnesses because it was a far cheaper and a quicker option than to create new drugs. New drugs could take 10 years to produce and cost an arm and a leg. The WHO's opposition to the use of a safe drug like Ivermectin has destroyed much of its credibility amongst members of the health profession and in the world.

It dawned on me, much later, that big pharma and other vested interests played a huge role to influence the negative opinion of the WHO and other public health authorities on the use of Ivermectin to treat COVID.

The scientist, Dr. Satoshi Omura from Japan discovered the drug from actinomycetota on a golf course. He, together with a scientist, Dr. William Campbell, who worked for MSD, discovered the drug. Both these doctors won the Nobel Prize for Physiology or Medicine for discovering Ivermectin in 2015.

Ivermectin was used worldwide against two major tropical diseases, Onchocerciasis (river blindness) and Lymphatic Filariasis. Approximately 3.6 billion doses were safely administered to rid the world of these two tropical diseases.

- https://www.ncbi.nlm.nih.gov/pmc/articles/PMC8383101/#bib4

Around August 2021 Dr. Satoshi Omura, the Nobel co- laureate for the discovery of Ivermectin, and colleagues conducted a comprehensive review of Ivermectin's clinical activity against COVID-19. They concluded that there was a preponderance of the evidence demonstrating major reductions in mortality and morbidity.

- https://www.ncbi.nlm.nih.gov/pmc/articles/PMC8383101/#bib2

A Google Scholar search for a meta-analysis on Ivermectin treatment for COVID revealed that there were seven such studies. Six of the seven meta-analyses concluded that there was considerable evidence for Ivermectin's efficacy to substantially reduce COVID-19 mortality.

- https://www.ncbi.nlm.nih.gov/pmc/articles/PMC8005369/

MAINSTREAM JOURNALS UNWILLING TO PUBLISH POSITIVE RCTS ON IVERMECTIN TO TREAT COVID-19

One of the main objections by most public health authorities to the findings of the many Randomized controlled trials (RCT)s done on the efficacy of Ivermectin to treat COVID-19 effectively was that these studies never appeared in the mainstream scientific journals. The reality at the time was that most mainstream medical journals did not want to publish articles that favored the use of a cheap repurposed drug like Ivermectin. This was most likely due to pressure from big pharma, who were the main sponsors of most mainstream medical journals. Quite a few pharmaceutical companies were busy trying to produce a drug to treat COVID and make a huge profit out of it because it was becoming evident that the vaccines were not achieving what was expected of them.

Fortunately, the publication of five RCTs on the treatment of COVID-19 with Ivermectin, which showed multiple clinical benefits from using Ivermectin over controls, appeared in the journals of major scientific publishers. Almost all of these studies that favored Ivermectin were statistically significant with p-values<0.002.

- https://www.ncbi.nlm.nih.gov/pmc/articles/PMC8383101/#bib24

OVERWHELMING EVIDENCE FROM PERU

There was a 14-fold decrease in all-cause mortality in the ten states in Peru from May 2020 to November 2020, when Ivermectin was widely used to treat COVID. This was followed by a 13-fold increase in all-cause mortality from November 2020 to February 2021, when the use of Ivermectin to treat COVID was prohibited by the new president.

- https://www.semanticscholar.org/paper/Ivermectin-for-COVID-19-in-Peru%3A-14-fold-reduction-Chamie-Quintero-Hibberd/211a1c80097e9a53ef94ea8bf246c90458c82577

This was overwhelming evidence for the efficacy of Ivermectin

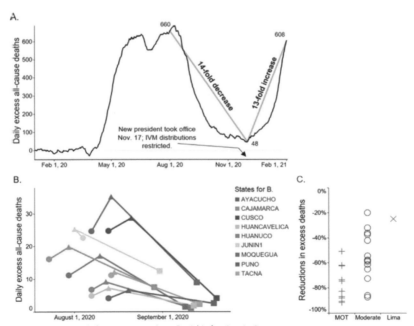

Figure1. Ivermectin's success against Covid infection in Peru

to significantly reduce all-cause mortality during COVID, yet this vital evidence was totally overlooked by all the world's major health authorities, which is nothing short of criminal.

IVERMECTIN IN THE TREATMENT OF MULTIPLE CANCERS

The authors of a research article, written by Dr. Melotti and colleagues, which appeared in PubMed, in October 2014, stated that Ivermectin was safely used on >200 million people to protect them against river blindness. The authors of this study also found that Ivermectin had an additional therapeutic use as a WNT-TCF pathway blocker to treat WNT-TNC dependent diseases, which included a range of cancers. They mentioned that Ivermectin inhibits the proliferation of cancer cells and encourages apoptosis of multiple cells.

- Melotti A, Mas C, Kuciak M, Lorente-Trigos A, Borges I, Ruiz I, Altaba A. The river blindness drug Ivermectin and related macrocyclic lactones inhibit WNT-TCF pathway responses in human cancer. EMBO Mol Med. 2014 Oct; 6(10):1263-78. doi: 10.15252/emmm.201404084. PMID: 25143352; PMCID: PMC4287931.

The role of Ivermectin to successfully treat cancer will be discussed at length later in this chapter.

IVERMECTIN IN SOUTH AFRICA

I learned, only after I had done a great deal of research into Ivermectin, that there was a group of people in Cape Town, who had been using Ivermectin to treat COVID. The liquid form of Ivermectin was widely available to the general public because South Africa was a huge farming country. I am convinced that the work done by these groups of activists all over the country helped to save many people from dying of COVID in South Africa by making the liquid version highly accessible to the public. Many of these activists worked underground, so they managed to escape prosecution from the health authorities.

During my research on Ivermectin, I came across an NGO group, SAHARI, which was founded and headed by Ms. Shabnam Palesa Mohamed, an attorney, journalist, and an activist, who promoted the use of Ivermectin to treat COVID and networked with the public to make the drug available to the public. This group boasted of a membership of over 100,000 on Facebook. They were pulled down from all social media platforms because of their pro–Ivermectin stance. It was too late because the majority of South Africans became familiar with the drug before they were pulled down.

Shabnam was a great asset to me in my fight to help patients with COVID. We teamed up to fight the atrocities in healthcare against society perpetrated by trusted organizations like the WHO, government agencies, academics, and the media. The general public and the non-critical healthcare workers implicitly trusted all these institutions for honest advice. As an alternative media journalist, Shabnam was my gateway to the world to share my success stories on how to treat COVID complications most effectively. Mainstream media shut me off completely, and in the process, denied the public and the medical profession access to my protocols and approach to diagnosing COVID with the least effort and expense, which could have saved millions around the world.

The citizens of South Africa networked into groups and made Ivermectin freely available to anyone afflicted with COVID. A group of females calling themselves the "COVID angels" were tutored by Ms. Terry Herholdt on how to use Ivermectin.

I was introduced to Terry by one of the COVID angels. Terry told me about her experience with Ivermectin for over two decades. She gave me the rundown on how she used Ivermectin to treat a variety of illnesses, long before she started using it to treat patients with COVID. Terry had acquired her experience treating animals on her farm and later, through her research, she discovered its role in treating females with severe menstrual disorders. Her experience with Ivermectin invoked my curiosity about Ivermectin, a drug I did not know much about at the time.

I became extremely curious about Ivermectin after I saw videos and read articles about Ivermectin being successfully used in Africa, Asia, and South America to treat river blindness and COVID. I studied the pharmacology of Ivermectin, its dosages and safety profile because I felt it was a drug I could certainly use in my practice to save the lives of my patients with COVID. Ivermectin seemed to be the answer that I was looking for. You will read later in this chapter; it played a major role in helping me successfully treat patients infected with the Delta strain during the epidemic. I could not have achieved the 99.97% success rate that I did without it being part of my treatment protocol to treat COVID and its complications.

I watched on YouTube and read several articles on the successes that doctors in Asia, the Philippines, South America, and Zimbabwe were having with Ivermectin. I felt a nagging urge to share my new-found information with the citizens of the country and the world.

As a prolific writer to the press for over forty years and a regular guest of several local radio stations on a number of health and socio-political issues, I wrote an article to the media appealing to the South African president, Mr. Cyril Ramaphosa, to make Ivermectin available to the citizens of this country to save lives and our economy, as it was done in Peru, Mexico and the state of Uttar Pradesh.

I was shocked to discover that only one community newspaper, "The Plainsman", published my article. I did not get a single response from any of the other 10 or 20 editors, with whom I had developed a cordial relationship for over 40 years. I realized that the mainstream media and, even, the so-called alternative media in South Africa, like the Daily Maverick and Mail and Guardian, as did the media in many parts of the world, were reliant on the sponsorships of wealthy individuals like Bill Gates and George Soros.

These wealthy individuals were totally opposed to any article that supported the use of Ivermectin or hydroxychloroquine for the treatment of COVID. Bill Gates was heavily invested in vaccines, so any drug that cured COVID was going to scupper his profit agenda from investing in vaccines.

Dr. Tess Lawrie, ranked among the top five researchers in the world and a well-respected researcher for the WHO, published the findings of a huge meta-analysis study of over 27 randomized controlled trials on the success of Ivermectin to treat COVID. She found that Ivermectin reduced COVID fatalities by more than 60% and hospitalizations and complications by more than 90%.

- https://pubmed.ncbi.nlm.nih.gov/34145166/

None of the major medical journals accepted Dr. Lawrie's peer reviewed paper for publication because, even the most prestigious medical journals were following the same narrative, as mainstream media, to discredit the use of Ivermectin to treat COVID regardless of the overwhelming evidence for Ivermectin's efficacy and safety to treat COVID. None of the editors for these prestigious journals provided any valid reasons for not publishing research that showed that Ivermectin was effective.

One of the major reasons why most medical journals were totally opposed to publishing any article that reported favorably on the use of Ivermectin to treat COVID was because it would hurt big pharma, on whom they relied upon for their existence.

Big pharma was busy trying to produce effective antiviral drugs against the Corona virus, so they might view Ivermectin as a huge threat to their profit margins from their patented newly developed antiviral drugs.

The other big reason for pharma's opposition to Ivermectin and other repurposed drugs to cure COVID is that it would have put a complete halt to the use of the experimental COVID vaccine. The vaccine was developed on the false narrative that there was no treatment for COVID. This explains why so many prestigious journals and the media went on a concerted campaign to present a very negative and disparaging view of Ivermectin to the public and to prevent doctors from prescribing it to their patients.

The untested toxic vaccine would never have been given EUA approval if Ivermectin was accepted as an effective drug to treat COVID-19.

DR. HILL AND DR. LAWRIE

Dr. Andrew Hill, a scientist and colleague of Dr. Tess Lawrie in the U.K., conducted a study with a team of doctors, for the WHO to investigate the efficacy of Ivermectin to treat COVID-19 in October 2020 before the roll-out of the vaccine.

Halfway through his study, Dr. Hill posted a tweet stating that countries should stock up on Ivermectin to control the spread of COVID-19. Two days later, Dr. Hill retracted his tweet and refused to explain his decision.

A very shocked Dr. Tess Lawrie contacted Dr. Hill to find out why he retracted his tweet. Dr. Hill's reply to Dr. Lawrie was that if he had to say anything favorable about Ivermectin, it would offend major funders of his university. He made that clear to Dr. Lawrie in her audio recording. He seemed to be unaffected by Dr. Lawrie's concern that by withholding crucial information about a drug that could save lives, Dr. Hill was breaking his Hippocratic Oath, "To do no harm". Dr. Hill shrugged off Dr. Lawrie's comment without any sign of regret or remorse.

- https://worldcouncilforhealth.org/multimedia/tess-lawrie-andrew-hill/

CLINICAL EVIDENCE ON IVERMECTIN AGAINST COVID INFECTION

In the first 19 months of COVID from March 2020 to May 2021, I learned a great deal about Ivermectin, its safety and efficacy to treat COVID-19. I also realized there was a huge effort to demonize Ivermectin by big pharma, public health authorities, medical boards, and a number of academics around the world. Academics, academic institutions, and mainstream media jointly opposed the use of Ivermectin to appease big pharma because they relied very heavily on big Pharma's sponsorship for their survival and existence.

In 2021, Pfizer's revenues had doubled to a record $81 billion from the sales of their vaccines and COVID-19 therapeutic Paxlovid. The group "Justice for Now" revealed that Pfizer's $81 billion revenues was more than the GDP of most countries and accused Pfizer of "ripping off public health systems".

- https://www.theguardian.com/business/2022/feb/08/pfizer-covid-vaccine-pill-profits-sales

But Paxlovid was hardly used in Africa, Asia, India, and South America compared to the US because of the high cost of the drug. These countries relied on Ivermectin and had far better outcomes than the US to combat COVID-19 and reduce mortality from COVID-19.

DR. TIK-TOK AGAINST IVERMECTIN

My views on the safety and efficacy of Ivermectin were well known in Cape Town. I was regarded by the captured or ignorant medical fraternity as the maverick in medicine. A popular Cape Town radio station, Heart 104.9, interviewed a doctor, who went by the name "Dr. Tik-Tok", to share his views on Ivermectin.

This doctor had apparently worked for the WHO, so it did not come as a surprise that he would follow the WHO's narrative, without being critical in his views and opinions especially on Ivermectin. He was vehemently opposed to the use of Ivermectin to treat COVID-19.

Dr. Tik-Tok referred to Ivermectin as "horse medicine", following the example of a scientist from the now disgraced FDA. Dr. Tik-Tok's derogatory views on Ivermectin offended many of the listeners because many members of the public in South Africa, already had first–hand experience of the drug's efficacy to save lives. They also knew about my stance, so they called the station and requested that the announcer to do an interview with me the next day. Dr. Tik-Tok refused an invitation to debate me.

I set the record straight about Ivermectin's safety and efficacy on a radio station interview. I was called by the producer the night before and I agreed to do a ten-minute interview on the early morning drive show with Mr. Aden Thomas, the radio announcer. My interview with the station was widely advertised, so listeners were eager to hear my rebuttal to Dr. Tik-Tok's views on Ivermectin.

The next morning, I was told by the producer that the time slot for my interview was moved to an earlier slot to give me more time. Many of the listeners, who eagerly looked forward to the interview were left highly disappointed when they learned that the interview was over.

The interview went on for over 15 minutes, five minutes more than the allocated time. I managed to set the record straight about Ivermectin, mentioning its history, safety, efficacy, cost, and mechanism of action. In the same interview, I expressed my reservations about the vaccine, which did not go well with the announcer nor with the station manager. The announcer was left gasping for words during the interview because he clearly did not understand the science behind Ivermectin, COVID-19 and the vaccine.

The interview was loaded onto their social media, 12 hours after I was interviewed, and attracted over 30,000 views with the majority of the comments from the public being highly favorable of my views; they saluted me for my outspokenness and bravery. I did not come across to the audience as a hero but as a doctor, who was guided by his conscience and his Hippocratic Oath, "to do no harm", as well as someone, who followed the science and not a paid narrative.

After my stance on Ivermectin was known to the public, I was invited as a guest on a number of alternative media platforms to share my views on Ivermectin and the management of COVID-19. I had the distinct pleasure of being a panelist with great doctors like Dr. Tess Lawrie, Dr. Kory, Prof. McCullough, Dr. Chetty, Dr. Jackie Stone, and Dr. Nathi Mdladla. I am proud to be associated with these ethical doctors of science during the pandemic.

FALSELY CLAIMING THAT IT CAUSES LIVER FAILURE

Dr. Emmanuel Taban, a pulmonologist in Gauteng, South Africa, posted a rather lengthy and damning message on social media claiming that he had been seeing a number of patients in his ward ending up with liver failure as a result of taking Ivermectin. This post went viral and was even reported on by the mainstream media, which helped to perpetuate the false narrative that Ivermectin was a dangerous drug.

I immediately rebutted his post on social media, challenging him on his claim. As far as I was aware, patients were using very low doses of 0.2 mg/kg body weight of Ivermectin. They were using doses that were in the therapeutic range, so there was little chance of patients ending up with liver failure. Ever since Ivermectin was discovered, over 250 million people have been using this drug annually to combat two of the most disfiguring diseases, Onchocerciasis (river blindness) and Lymphatic filariasis.

The safety data on Ivermectin for the past forty years, both on humans and animals, earned it the reputation of being one of the safest drugs on the FDA's drug list and was and remains on the WHO's essential drug list.

I have had the experience of using high doses of between 0.6 mg/kg to 1 mg/kg during the Delta strain and I did not have a single patient with even a mild side effect on this dose, so Dr. Taban's claim that Ivermectin was hepatotoxic was utterly spurious and unfounded.

The most plausible explanation for the liver failure or rise in liver enzymes in patients admitted with severe COVID pneumonia was: patients that were admitted to ICU with respiratory failure probably developed multiple organ failure due to hypoxia of these organs and most certainly not due to Ivermectin toxicity. Hypoxia of the liver results in severe toxicity, which in turn, would adversely affect an individual's breathing, in a bidirectional way. The hypoxia damages the organs and the toxicity from the damaged organs, like the liver, would affect a patient's breathing. Dr. Taban's claim that Ivermectin was responsible for liver toxicity in his patients was plain misinformation, typical of the propaganda dished out by mainstream journalists, as it lacked any scientific justification. He did not refute my rebuttal nor was he willing to debate with me.

It was quite evident that doctors, both in the state sector and in the private sector, were pushing a narrative that favored big pharma by discrediting Ivermectin as an unsafe drug. None of these doctors were interested in listening to the success stories of frontline doctors like me and my other colleagues, who saved thousands of lives from being lost through COVID without any life-support equipment except for a safe, effective, and inexpensive drug like Ivermectin.

Part 2
MY EXPERIENCE WITH COVID-19 TREATMENT

I worked in an extremely poor community, so I diagnosed patients with COVID on clinical grounds as I have done with influenza. I used minimal investigations to reduce my patients' costs without compromising my diagnoses nor my patient's wellbeing. I never ordered the PCR tests to confirm a diagnosis because I learned quite early on that this test was not diagnostic for COVID for a variety of reasons. One of the persons who influenced my decision was Dr. Kary Mullis, the person who discovered the PCR. Dr. Mullis stated in an interview that the PCR test should not be used to diagnose COVID because it was not designed for this purpose.

- https://www.youtube.com/watch?v=-ueVTcOSD1k

Most of my patients recovered on symptomatic treatment. My high recovery rate of 99.88% in patients with the wild type, alpha and beta strains was in line with the Centers for Disease Control and Prevention (CDC)'s view, published in September 2020 that the survival rate for COVID was 99% without much medical intervention.

- https://winknews.com/2020/09/23/cdc-shows-covid-19-has-high-survival-rate-doctor-still-wants-to-see-precautions-taken/

What was puzzling to me were the reasons behind the WHO's decision to declare the COVID outbreak a pandemic when the recovery rate was as high as 99%. According to Prof. Angus Dalgleish, a UK professor of virology, lockdowns are ineffective to stop the spread of respiratory viruses like COVID. In an interview, he mentioned that lockdowns could make the situation worse.

- https://youtu.be/PnJ5T1Enwq4?si=VPsGhh_dqJpu_8W6

South African Health Products Regulatory Authority (SAHPRA) and the U.S. Food and Drug Administration (FDA)'s refusal to approve

Ivermectin on safety grounds is shocking. I failed to understand why SAHPRA, and the FDA could state so boldly that they were not aware of the safety of Ivermectin, after it was widely known that about 3.7 billion doses of Ivermectin were safely prescribed in its 40-year history, and when it was well known that Ivermectin has been and still is listed on the WHO's list of drugs as being the safest drug.

The adverse events recorded for Ivermectin on the WHO's site for adverse events for drugs reveal that Ivermectin is the safest of all drugs compared to Paracetamol, Aspirin and remdesivir. In its entire 40-year history and after more than 3.5 billion doses were dispensed, there were only 7,407 adverse reported events for Ivermectin which is far less than for Aspirin – with 210,217 adverse events: Paracetamol – with 204,875 adverse events and remdesivir- with 11,094.

U.S. FDA and other regulatory health bodies for use to treat COVID-19. Remdesivir chalked up far more adverse events than Ivermectin despite the number of doses being far less than the doses of Ivermectin used worldwide.

- https://vigiaccess.org/

I have no doubt that if I had access to Ivermectin, I could have saved the two patients who died because the early strains of COVID-19 responded extremely well to low doses of Ivermectin.

A GROUP OF SOUTH AFRICAN DOCTORS WON THE RIGHT TO PRESCRIBE IVERMECTIN

In March 2021 a group of South African doctors, headed by Dr. Naseeba Kathrada, took SAHPRA, which is the equivalent of the FDA, to court demanding that doctors be given the right to use Ivermectin to treat their patients with COVID-19. The Judge awarded the case in favor of the doctors and ordered SAHPRA to permit doctors to prescribe the repurposed drug, Ivermectin, to treat their patients.

SAHPRA was forced to comply with the judgment. The doctors had to apply to SAHPRA for a certificate to allow them to stock and dispense Ivermectin to treat their patients.

This was an enormous victory for frontline doctors like me. But it was bewildering to learn that doctors had to apply for permission to prescribe or dispense a repurposed drug that has an excellent safety profile.

Doctors have the right to use repurposed drugs if they have a good safety profile without requiring permission from any regulatory authority. Furthermore, SAHPRA, like the FDA, had no right to advise doctors on how and when to use repurposed drugs. It seems both the FDA and SAHPRA had overstepped their boundaries of power when they discouraged doctors from using Ivermectin.

I received my first stock of Ivermectin in early July 2021, which was the perfect time because we were just getting into the thick of the deadly Delta strain after coming out of the mild Beta strain. Delta was the deadliest strain of all the COVID-19 strains including Omicron.

MANAGING DELTA WAS A GAME CHANGER FOR ME

When the Delta strain hit Cape Town in July 2021, I felt equipped to deal with the condition and to treat it with confidence because I had free access to Ivermectin, and I had gained a great deal of knowledge about the pathogenesis and clinical manifestations of COVID-19.

Prior to the emergence of the Delta strain, Dr. Paul Marik, an infectious disease specialist and a co- founder of the FLCCC, informed his audiences that the pneumonia appeared on day 8, so his advice was that steroids should not be commenced before day eight. This advice, based on my experience, was not applicable when it came to the highly virulent Delta strain infection. Patients infected with the Delta strain presented by day 2-3 with a COVID pneumonia.

During the early days of Delta, I found that patients were

presenting with shortness of breath, fatigue, and cough within two to three days of infection. The Delta strain multiplied 70 times more than the Alpha and Beta strains. It was far more infectious and many times more virulent than the previous strains.

- https://www.nationalgeographic.com/science/article/why-is-delta-more-infectious-and-deadly-new-research-holds-answers

The shortness of breath and cough within two days of illness suggested that the virus multiplied so rapidly that it reached the lungs within two days to cause the cough and shortness of breath.

The early presentation of cough and shortness of breath in patients infected with the Delta strain led me to conclude that the pneumonia of Delta appeared by day two and not day eight. This meant that high doses of steroids had to be introduced early to prevent pneumonia from the Delta strain from progressing into a severe and fatal hypoxia.

In view of the high multiplication rate, I decided to use very high doses of Ivermectin to stop the virus from multiplying. Instead of the recommended 0.2 mg/kg, I increased the doses to 0.6 mg/kg to 1 mg/kg depending on the severity of the clinical presentation of the patients. My aim was to prevent the virus from spreading to the lungs by hitting the infection hard and fast. The teaching in medicine has always been when one was dealing with an overwhelming infection, one had to use high doses of antibiotics and different classes of antibiotics, concurrently, to avoid antibiotic resistance to kill the offending pathogen.

EUREKA MOMENT

I felt that if I could arrest the disease in the viraemic phase with high doses of Ivermectin, I could prevent the complication of pneumonia and get my patients well and back to work within about five to six days. Within the first few weeks, I found that my postulate to treat early, in the viraemic phase, with high doses of Ivermectin was correct because

I found that patients, who were treated early in the viraemic phase returned to work within a few days of treatment. They recovered, fully, without progressing to the stage of pneumonia.

COVID-19 patients develop severe hypoxemia because the spike protein of the virus causes the red blood cells to coalesce and form rouleaux. Ivermectin is capable of separating the clumped blood cells and stopping the hypoxemia.

This was the finding of Prof. Robert Clancy, a widely published immunologist from Australia.

- https://www.youtube.com/watch?v=qWlf7sbomMQ.

The success I achieved from treating the highly virulent Delta strain in the viraemic phases with high doses of Ivermectin before it progressed into pneumonia was like a Eureka moment for me. Eureka, it is an exclamation attributed to ancient Greek mathematician and inventor Archimedes.

My videos depicting my high success rate by treating COVID-19 early with Ivermectin and other repurposed drugs did not go well with the authorities. They viewed my successful treatment of COVID as a threat to their agenda to roll out the experimental vaccines. The authorities and the media kept using the purportedly high death rates from COVID-19 as a tool to drive up the vaccine agenda in a population that was reluctant to take the vaccine.

The response by the general public to the videos of my successful management of COVID-19 on my telegram channel went viral, so being de-platformed by the mainstream media did not stop me from getting my message of hope to the general public.

Many of my followers on my Telegram channel thanked me profusely for recommending the use of Ivermectin early and in high doses. They made me out to be the hero that I did not plan to be; I was merely doing what was expected of any responsible doctor and that is to save lives and do no harm.

My videos, I later learned, went viral all over the world. I had total strangers contacting me from other parts of the world to thank me because my advice had saved their lives.

I shared this experience with a panel of doctors and health activists in a World Council for Health's Zoom meeting. Dr. Kory contacted me about my theory and experience with high dose Ivermectin. After hearing about my experience treating the Delta strain with high doses in the early stages, I was pleased to see that the FLCCC increased the recommended dose from 0.2 mg/ kg to 0.6 mg/kg to treat the Delta strain infection, even though it was much lower than the doses I had used.

I was fully aware that the main side effects of high doses of Ivermectin were nausea, vomiting and blurry vision. These side effects were all reversible, when the drug was stopped or reduced, so there was no need for undue concern. The benefit of high doses saved people in the viral stage and prevented them from ending up with fatal complication like pneumonia or death. The reversible side effects from high dose Ivermectin was a small price to pay to save a life.

DISTINCTION BETWEEN THE VIRAEMIC PHASE AND PNEUMONIC PHASE WAS VITAL

I classified people, who presented with upper respiratory symptoms and no cough as being in the viraemic phase. During the viraemic phase, I used high doses of Ivermectin, Clarithromycin, Doxycycline, Vitamin D3 -5,000 units daily, Zinc 20 mg daily, Vitamin C 100 mg twice a day, Chlorpheniramine 4 mg daily and black seeds (Nigella Sativa). In addition, I advised saline nasal washes and mouth gargles, nebulisation with Colloidal silver and 30 minutes of sitting in the sun. The infra-red rays of the sun seem to accelerate the healing of the pneumonia.

With this approach, patients in the viraemic phase recovered within five days and returned to work on the sixth day without any complications. This approach was a major saving to industry, who lost huge amounts of money through workers being off from work for long periods at a time.

In the very early days of the Delta strain epidemic in South Africa in July 2021, patients presented with a cough and felt out of breath by day three. I interpreted this as a sign of the Delta strain reaching the lungs by day two as opposed to day eight with the previous strains.

I interpreted any sign of lung involvement as an early sign of deadly pneumonia setting in.

I coined the description "Early COVID Pneumonia", which referred to signs of a pneumonia setting in without any signs of crepitations in the lungs on auscultation. Crepitations refers to the crackling sound that doctors listen for, over the lungs, to establish if a patient has pneumonia.

I felt that by introducing steroids at the early stages of the lung inflammation, I could arrest the progress of the pneumonia, prevent the oxygen levels from dropping drastically, and avoid life threatening hypoxia to vital organs like the brain, heart, liver, and kidneys, without requiring supplemental oxygen. I was, in short, nipping the disease in the bud, which is how we should be treating all diseases.

I compiled a set of symptoms, signs, and bedside tests that I used to make a diagnosis of early pneumonia. I managed to make a diagnosis of pneumonia in about 3 minutes without requiring costly and time-consuming chest X-rays or scans, which was beyond the reach of my patients.

SMORGASBORD OF TREATMENTS

COVID-19 was a complicated type of illness. It needed a

smorgasbord of treatments to deal with every possible complication fast and with the appropriate treatment. Ivermectin was one of the important medications, but it was not enough to deal with pneumonia and clotting.

I treated COVID-19 patients individually, so treatment was tailor-made depending on the severity, stage of the illness, complications, and comorbidities. I have always maintained that each patient should be treated individually and not according to dogmatic protocols because each patient responds differently to medications. With children, I used very few medications and they all recovered. I have always believed in the dictum, "use less to get more".

I did not follow the exhaustive protocol of the U.S.-based Front Line COVID-19 Critical Care (FLCCC) Alliance, because I tried to achieve maximum benefit by using the least drugs and least investigations. I did this to avoid the side effects of polypharmacy and to keep patient costs down to a minimum. I was working with an extremely poor community. This approach worked extremely well because I achieved a very high success rate compared to the results in our costly tertiary and secondary hospitals.

IMPORTANCE OF A PEAK FLOW METER READING

I routinely measured the peak expiratory flow (PEF), person's maximum speed of expiration, reading on every patient with symptoms of COVID-19. I found that people who presented with early symptoms of shortness of breath had peak flow readings that were as low as 25% to 50% below the predicted value for people with no history of asthma. This finding was common in patients, who had normal oxygen levels of 96% and above. I found that a low peak flow meter was a major asset in my toolbox for confirming the diagnosis of pneumonia. It was far more helpful than the oximeter reading.

Chapter 15   Ivermectin Saved My Patients with Severe COVID and the Vaccine Injured

I made a diagnosis of early COVID pneumonia with the symptoms such as shortness of breath with or without exertion, shortness of breath on speaking and a low peak flow reading, without crepitations and a normal oxygen reading.

A low peak flow reading supported my diagnosis because a low peak flow was the result of the alveoli becoming damaged. It signified the early stages of the pneumonia setting in.

Early COVID pneumonia was treated aggressively, as I would have treated a pneumonia, with very high doses of steroids of 1 to 2 mg/ kg for five days; Colchicine 0.5 mg twice a day for five days; Ivermectin 0.6 mg to 1 mg/kg for five days, Clarithromycin, Doxycycline, Chlorpheniramine, Aspirin, Vitamin D3, Vitamin C, Zinc, Black seeds, nasal washes with saline water and soda bicarbonate. None of these patients required supplemental oxygen if they could breathe without difficulty, even if their oxygen levels were in the low 90s.

With this approach, every patient that I diagnosed with early COVID-19 pneumonia and who was put on my aggressive treatment for pneumonia, showed signs of recovery by day three and returned to work by day six. This was a great relief to patients; it was a boost to employers because it was a huge cost saver. Patients felt extremely relieved that they did not end up with a dreaded severe pneumonia or land in hospital.

None of the patients wanted to go to the hospital. The hospitals were acquiring the reputation for being places where people seldom returned to their families alive. Patients would plead with me not to send them to any of our hospitals. This placed a huge burden of responsibility on my shoulders because I realized that I was a huge target for the media and medical establishment.

Patients, who had signs of pneumonia on auscultation with normal oxygen levels, were treated the same way as patients with early COVID pneumonia, without oxygen. These patients took about ten days to make a full recovery. During the Delta strain, pneumonia usually set in by day four, one day after early COVID pneumonia. Without timely treatment, healing is delayed by five days, hence I advised the public to seek treatment on the first day of symptoms.

Normal and slightly below normal oxygen levels in the early stages of the infection were extremely deceptive for measuring the severity of disease. I have come across several patients, who presented with severe pneumonia but normal oxygen levels. I treated the pneumonia aggressively, regardless of the normal oxygen levels. The normal oxygen levels meant that the unaffected lung tissue was compensating for the damaged tissue to maintain the oxygen levels.

Many patients delayed seeking early treatment because their oxygen levels were normal, quite unaware of the fact that they were quite ill. Some took as long as three weeks to seek treatment. This delay prolonged their recovery by six weeks. My approach has ways to treat patients according to their clinical presentation and not rely entirely on laboratory results.

Patients and doctors made the mistake of relying too heavily on oxygen levels to determine severity.

Several of my patients delayed seeking treatment during the Delta phase, even though they were breathless because they relied on their oxygen levels to decide on the severity of their illness. Normal oxygen levels were not a good indicator of the severity of the illness.

A delay of one week resulted in so much lung damage that the oxygen levels plummeted suddenly to as low as 80% from a normal of 96%; a one-week delay in seeking treatment, during the delta phase, often resulted in a drop to 60%.

I have had patients who presented with oxygen levels as low as 35% two to three weeks after becoming ill. Patients varied in the way their illness progressed so there was no way of predicting how each patient was going to progress once they contracted COVID-19.

Many patients who were breathless with oxygen levels of 92% were turned away by emergency doctors because our hospitals were too full, and our ER doctors were unaware that a drop in oxygen levels to 92% was a sign of severe lung pathology setting in. Ideally, these patients should have been treated urgently and aggressively for their pneumonia to avoid admission into the ICU.

Many patients with severe pneumonia but near normal oxygen levels were, erroneously, sent home to isolate, by our ER doctors. These patients returned a few days or a week later, terribly ill, needing ICU admission, which could have been avoided if they were treated correctly in the early phase of the disease. I tried hard to share my knowledge and new experience with our specialists, but they shut their doors to frontline doctors like me. One of the great tragedies during the COVID-19 pandemic was that doctors were ignorant about the importance of treating COVID-19 early.

I used home supplemental oxygen liberally on elderly patients with oxygen levels of less than 92%. My rationale was to prevent brain hypoxia and avoid a future neurodegenerative disorder like dementia, memory loss, or decline in normal body functions. Oxygen levels of 92% and less were regarded as a sign that the entire lungs were affected, warranting supplemental oxygen if patients could not breathe on their own.

The elderly were put on strict bed rest because any slight effort, like walking, could drop their oxygen levels significantly, and cause brain hypoxia. The hypoxia of the brain could result in them falling and ending up with a severe head injury. Most of these patients were on anticoagulants, so I had to ensure that they didn't fall due to hypoxia and end up with severe bleeding injuries.

Patients remained on oxygen till they could learn to breathe on their own to achieve oxygen levels above 94%. The average duration for supplemental oxygen was about two weeks. Patients with oxygen levels of 35% to 60% required supplemental oxygen for about six weeks.

There were two main reasons for very low oxygen levels: severe and extensive pneumonia and severe clotting. Patients with high d-dimers were put on a variety of anticoagulants. The choice of anticoagulants depended on the level of d-dimer. Aspirin, Clopidogrel, NOAKS and Heparin were used, depending on the d-dimer level and the way patients responded to treatment.

Low doses of a number of anti-inflammatory drugs were used as maintenance therapy. After two weeks of treatment, Ivermectin was used in lower doses on a twice weekly basis for its anti-inflammatory properties and anticoagulant properties. High doses of Ivermectin were only used during the viraemic phase to kill the virus and prevent its rapid multiplication.

The dose of steroid was reduced to 1 mg/kg till the oxygen levels returned to normal. Budesonide was used for its safety and efficacy especially when used on a long-term basis.

Colchicine was used for its anti-inflammatory properties to act as an adjunct to steroids. An SSRI like Fluoxetine was used for its anti-inflammatory properties as well as to help patients that were anxious. The SSRI was also used to treat any inflammation in the brain and prevent brain fog.

A number of anti-inflammatory drugs were used in low doses to avoid long-term side effects of high doses of a single drug like prednisone. These drugs were used to act synergistically with each other.

Many severely ill patients had to remain on maintenance treatment for up to two to four months.

OXYGEN READINGS EXTREMELY UNRELIABLE DURING THE OMICRON STRAIN

From November 2021 to February 2022, when Omicron 1, 2 was the prevalent strain, and from March 2022 to November 2022, when Omicron 4, 5 was the prevalent strain, I found that patients presented three weeks after being infected with COVID-19. They had extensive widespread pneumonias, and their main symptom was an intractable cough but minimal shortness of breath.

In spite of the extent of their pneumonias and duration of their illness, their oxygen levels remained within the normal range of 96% to 98%, which explains their delay in seeking early treatment. The number of patients who presented during the Omicron phase was considerably much less than the deluge of patients I saw during the Delta phase of the pandemic. This was probably because many citizens had already acquired natural immunity after being widely exposed to the previous strains in the 18 months before the Delta strain became the predominant strain.

92-year female – 3 weeks of pneumonia during the Omicron strain in November 2022

One of my long-standing patients presented to me worried about her blood pressure because she felt dizzy. She casually mentioned that she had a cough for three weeks that wouldn't stop. She did not mention feeling tired. Her oxygen levels were 94%.

On examination, I found that she had extensive crepitations of her entire lungs. I put her on my regimen for the elderly and advised strict bed rest. I prescribed supplemental oxygen, but she did not use it.

Within two weeks, she made a complete recovery dismissing the narrative that the elderly were at risk of dying from the disease. I have seen her recently 12 months after her infection, looking hale and hearty, about to celebrate her 93rd birthday.

I treated several elderly patients with comorbidities like diabetes, COPD, hypertension, and heart failure, and they all recovered fully on my regimen without any complications. I have seen these patients 2 years later with absolutely no trace of their infection or long COVID.

CHILDREN WITH PNEUMONIA

During the Omicron phase, the two-year-old patient that I treated had crepitations. She responded within five days on steroids, low dose Ivermectin, and clarithromycin.

The six-year-old patient had been ill for a week and he could barely stand.

A 9-year-old boy, treated during the Omicron 5 stage, had an oxygen level of 50%. He was put on steroids, a small dose of Ivermectin, and clarithromycin. He made a dramatic improvement within a week. His oxygen levels returned to normal, and he was able to walk with ease, proving that children recovered much faster than adults. I saw him about 18 months later for a minor flu and he showed absolutely no trace of his COVID infection.

A 9-year-old girl's dad did not want her to take Ivermectin. Hospital also feared the outcome and asked me to treat her on an out-patient basis. These types of requests added to my pressure. I had to keep in constant contact with my patients to ensure that they were improving. I was extremely wary of the health authorities coming after me if there was a mishap.

She could barely stand. I put her on my regimen. She made a full recovery within three weeks. She was put on supplemental oxygen. The other two children recovered without needing supplemental oxygen. When the damaged lungs were treated aggressively, the oxygen levels started returning to normal quite rapidly. Children recovered far quicker than adults based on my experience. I feel that the Ivermectin played an important role in helping these children to recover.

From 15 July 2021 to about 15 October 2021, I treated more than 1,100 patients with COVID pneumonia with oxygen levels ranging from 35% to 96%. During that time, I applied my theory of treating hard and early and with this approach, I achieved a success rate of 99.97%. Only three patients died because they presented very late and had severe comorbidities.

Within the first two weeks of treating COVID pneumonias with my regimen, the majority of my patients made dramatic recoveries by the first week and made complete recoveries by the second week. Most of these patients returned to work by the second week. Most of them saw me only twice for their illness. This led me to conclude that COVID, no matter how serious could have been treated on an outpatient basis and could have saved the world tons of money.

The high success rate of my approach to COVID filled me with elation and confidence. I started making videos of my success stories to break the prevailing narrative that the Delta strain is a deadly strain. I wanted to fill the world with hope that there was nothing to fear. I was pleased to meet several elderly people at health conferences on COVID-19 in September 2023. They came up to me and thanked me for my advice because it saved so many of their lives and their family's lives. I was glad to hear that even though many patients could not reach me, my advice on how to manage COVID-19 reached thousands of people, who made remarkable recoveries on my protocol. I could have saved millions more if the popular platforms had not banned my videos.

I made about 600 videos as testimony of my successes, that there was nothing to fear about COVID if the disease was treated appropriately with the right combination of drugs. Only one of my patients during the Delta strain landed in hospital because of dehydration from severe diarrhea but he made a complete recovery. I made these videos to record my success because I did not have the resources to capture my stories on paper. The video recordings were proof of my success in case anyone doubted the validity of my claim that COVID was a highly treatable condition, regardless of its severity.

Within a week, I received a warning from YouTube that my videos of hope were against community guidelines, and I was given a strike for a month by Facebook and YouTube. I was eventually de-platformed from Facebook, but that didn't stop me. I posted my success stories on WhatsApp groups, my Telegram channel, Rumble and on BitChute. I belonged to several groups, who shared my videos widely.

My videos were reaching audiences throughout the world, so the de-platforming did not stop me from spreading the videos of my success.

MY ROOMS BECOMES THE HUB FOR COVID TREATMENT IN CAPE TOWN

My stories went viral throughout the country. Our rooms were inundated with requests from desperate patients, who either discharged themselves from hospital or refused to go to hospital, fearing that they were going to die in hospital. The high death rate of patients on ventilators in hospitals went viral that it was dangerous to be admitted to hospital. People were afraid that if they landed in the hospital that they would never return home to see their loved ones. They were apprehensive of dying alone in hospital.

The high success rates I had treating severely ill COVID patients with a combination of drugs and home oxygen left me convinced that there was minimal need for artificial ventilators. My view was supported by an article written by Jon Hamilton for NPR news on

April 2, 2020. He reported that many critical physicians in a New York hospital that the majority of the patients on ventilators for COVID pneumonia did not survives.

- https://www.npr.org/sections/health-shots/2020/04/02/826105278/ventilators-are-no-panacea-for-critically-ill-covid-19-patients

Several other studies showed that 90% of the patients on ventilators to treat COVID pneumonia did not survive.

- https://www.washingtonpost.com/health/2020/04/22/coronavirus-ventilators-survival/

The street to my surgery was filled with cars from one end to the other with desperate patients seeking my help. My appointment system was rendered ineffective because patients rocked up gasping for breath without appointments. We did not turn any patients away.

I ended up seeing 45 patients a day on some occasions with almost 90% of them having pneumonia.

My staff doubled their working time without complaining. We worked from 8 am to 7 pm without a break. My wife, Joan, with a great deal of experience with patients, helped to handle the calls from desperate callers wanting urgent appointments; helped to triage patients and handled queries from members of the public who demanded to speak to me whilst I was busy treating very ill patients.

My receptionist, Natalie, checked in the patients and escorted the very ill to my emergency/oxygen room. She recorded the patient's vitals, and they called me immediately to see the very ill patients.

There were times when I had about six patients needing oxygen at the same time. It was challenging to attend to everyone, with just one tank. My daughter, Tammy, who had no medical experience, was taught to nebulize patients with oxygen and colloidal silver.

The brief nebulization gave these patients enough relief to wait their turn to be seen.

I was unable to access more tanks of oxygen. None of the suppliers were willing to help me. I was terribly disappointed that not one company from the corporate world was prepared to give me any assistance with additional oxygen tanks, not even my own supplier. To make matters worse, they were closed over weekends, so I had to replace my tanks, way before they were empty, to ensure that I had a supply for weekends, when the suppliers were closed. I felt the suppliers of oxygen in Cape Town had severely let down the citizens in their hour of need. My own supplier for over forty years had an emergency number which they never answered.

Ms. Allie of Big Boy Crockery was a life saver that came to my rescue with free home oxygen machines.

Over 60% of my patients with Delta pneumonia required home oxygen. I was fortunate to come across a lady, Ms. Allie, who worked for a crockery outlet that offered free oxygen tanks to the public, as a service to humanity. Ms. Allie was most helpful and accommodating in helping my patients to access mechanized oxygen tanks at absolutely no cost. She offered her services at very odd hours without complaining once. She saw her work as a service to humanity. Oxygen from private suppliers was far beyond the affordability of the majority of my poor patients. Not even the medical aids were willing to help. This was humanity's cry for help. Medical aids were prepared to pay up to 1 million South African Rand or $50,000 for a futile hospital stay but were not prepared to provide rented oxygen to their patients.

The failure by big corporate businesses in South Africa and Oxygen suppliers in the Western Cape, in that dire time of our life, will be remembered as a terrible blight on their corporate image. It is something that I can never forgive them for. Many of these businesses are known to sponsor sports tournaments to the tune of R5 million to R10 million but they were not prepared to buy a thousand machines for R8000 a piece to save desperate and dying patients.

Chapter 15   Ivermectin Saved My Patients with Severe COVID and the Vaccine Injured

The high number of deaths in our private and teaching hospitals compared to my high success rate compelled a number of very ill patients to discharge themselves from hospital or to refuse to go to hospital. Patients who became very ill came to me immediately rather than going to the hospitals.

I had extremely ill patients tell me that they would rather die in my hands at home than to risk dying alone in an uncaring hospital. I could understand this, because I believe that how we die is as important as how we lived. It was vital for people to die with dignity, surrounded by their loved ones. Once in the hospital, patients never saw their families for three weeks and died alone.

I took on this huge challenge and treated these very ill patients to the best of my ability with the least amount of resources.

SOME OF MY BEST SUCCESS STORIES

1. 38-year-old female

The first patient was a 38-year-old female, who was self-discharged from Groote Schuur Hospital by her husband on the first day she was admitted. He heard about me, purchased an oxygen tank and brought her straight to my surgery. She was completely disorientated.

I put her on my regimen and home oxygen. Within two weeks she made a dramatic recovery. Within six weeks she made a full recovery. I met her a year later and she informed me that she was back to her normal self and enjoying her gym classes.

2. 69-year-old female

The second patient was a 69-year-old female with an oxygen level of 35%, who presented three weeks after she had the illness. When I suggested that I might have to refer her to hospital, she

391

immediately told me that she does not want to go to hospital. She placed all her trust in me. She made a full recovery in about two months and was able to perform her household chores without any limitations and regained all her faculties, physically and mentally.

3. 67-year-old female

The third patient was a 67-year-old female with diabetes. She was admitted to Groote Schuur Hospital for a day. Her daughter was adamant that she does not want her mother to go onto a ventilator. The daughter contacted me to treat her mother. I only offered to help her if her mother was at home.

Late that evening at about 8 pm I was contacted by the daughter, who had discharged her mom. I did a telephonic assessment and emailed a script for the family to obtain her medicines from a 24-hour pharmacy.

Within two weeks of treatment, the lady walked into my consulting rooms, smiling, having gotten her life back.

I visited the lady a year later to do a video of her story and her successful recovery. She looked perfectly normal, without any traces of her infection or near-death experience and was extremely grateful to me for saving her life. It is success stories like these that kept my spirits high and enabled me to withstand the backlash from mainstream media and doctors, who were opposed to the use of repurposed drugs like Ivermectin to treat COVID.

4. 63-year-old Tony, discharged with an oxygen tank, with his oxygen level at 60%

One busy morning in August 2021, as I was about to step into my rooms. I was approached by one of my old regular patients, Patricia, who informed me that her husband was bedridden on oxygen, looking very ill from COVID and was on the brink of dying. She asked me if I could please help her dying husband after she heard about my successful treatment for COVID.

He was discharged from a private hospital after being admitted for two months with an oxygen level of 60% because his medical funds had dried up. He was sent home with an oxygen cylinder. Neither did his doctor nor the hospital contact him after forking out huge sums of money.

When a patient's medical funds dry up in South Africa, patients are left to fend on their own. The only people who come to their rescue are frontline GPs and the state hospitals. His hospital bill for the two months was over South African Rand 750,000 or U.S. $40,000, which is an awful lot of money for ordinary citizens in South Africa. One could understand the anger of many families who lost loved ones in hospital during COVID, after forking out huge sums of money. They felt cheated and let down.

I took up the challenge and treated him with Ivermectin weekly, low dose maintenance Prednisone and Colchicine as well as Vitamin D3, Vitamin C, Zinc, and black seed. When his wife approached me, they had very little funds left, but that did not stop me from treating him. My motto was to help as many people as I could, regardless of their financial status. This was a time when to save lives was more important than to make money, because many were desperate and resources were scarce.

I decided to treat even if they had no money. I felt this was humanity's call for help to health professionals in one of the worst times of our lives. We had a duty to serve humanity.

Tony made a slow but great recovery. Within two months he started walking without supplemental oxygen and picked up a huge amount of weight.

He celebrated Christmas that year with hardly a trace of his past illness. I received a picture of him celebrating his 65th birthday, beaming with happiness, back to his old self again. His wife expressed her sincere gratitude for what I had done for her husband and for saving his life.

5. 27-year-old obese female with 45% oxygen – defies myth that the obese are at high risk of death from COVID-19.

One Saturday afternoon, in September 2021, during the Delta strain, a very obese female was rushed into my room. She was, carried on a chair by four burly men, just before I was about to close.

She was looking confused and had an oxygen level of 45%, I suggested that she be referred to the hospital as all patients had the right to decide where they wish to be treated. In her drowsy state, she indicated quite strongly, by shaking her head, that she did not want to go to hospital.

I put her on my regimen and gave her a note to obtain a portable oxygen tank from my contact, Ms. Allie.

I followed her up for the next two weeks. By the second week she made a complete recovery. Her oxygen levels returned to 95%, looking happy that she did not die. People were gripped by the fear of death during the Delta strain. When they made dramatic recoveries, they felt elated that they managed to escape death.

VIRTUAL CONSULTATIONS

I listened to an interview Dr. Mobeen Syed had with Dr. Melvin De Mello, a physician from India, who had great success treating over 6,000 COVID patients, all over the world with his protocol. With my newfound, tried and tried and tested knowledge on COVID pneumonia, I started treating patients from other parts of the country and the rest of the world over the phone.

After an 11-hour stint at my surgery from 8 am to 7 pm, I attended to my patients requiring virtual consultations from 8 pm to 1 am. I was getting by with just four hours of sleep to meet the demand from people all over requesting my services. I did this for a month and was worried how long this strain was going to persist because I had no help to replace me. Fortunately, I managed to see my patients for the entire Delta strain with just one weekend break. I took calls and messages from my patients even while I was on my break because I realized the need for them to reach me in an emergency.

For some of my overseas patients I had to attend to them at 5 am because of the time differences.

I successfully treated over 120 patients nationally and internationally without a single death.

To combat the censorship that I was subjected to by major mainstream social media platforms, I recorded as many of my success stories treating severely ill COVID patients and posted them on Telegram on my own channel and on all the 20 odd groups I belonged to.

My videos played a major role to make a dent on the false COVID narrative that was being dished out regularly via the various media platforms.

OMICRON SAVES THE WORLD

The Omicron 1, 2 strain, with over 30 mutations, was highly infectious but only mildly virulent; it was extremely resistant to the original COVID vaccines, which were made for the old Alpha strain. There were minimal hospitalizations or deaths from the Omicron 1, 2 infections. I fully agreed with the former Chairperson Dr. A. Coetzee of the South African Medical Association that Omicron 1, 2 was a mild strain and should be treated like a mild flu.

The Omicron 1, 2 strain showed that the clinical presentation could not be predicted by the number of mutations, so I found it strange how scientists with no first-hand clinical experience dared to predict the severity of a forthcoming unknown strain.

Sweden did the right thing by lifting all restrictions and allowing the Omicron 1, 2 strain to spread freely to achieve herd immunity. My own feeling was that Omicron 1, 2 was nature's vaccine that was free and had minimal complications compared to the COVID vaccine.

EVEN BILL GATES ADMITS

Even the "vaccine-loving Gates", who profited heavily from his COVID vaccine investments, conceded that the Omicron strain beat the vaccine to end the pandemic in an interview on German television.

- https://www.youtube.com/watch?v=7J2xV5yGOK8

He seemed to be amused that the virus had saved the world from a pandemic. It was a deadly blow to the Achilles heel of his profit-making vaccine agenda.

- https://www.businesstoday.in/coronavirus/story/covid-19-omicron-to-create-lot-of-immunity-says-bill-gates-318748-2022-01-12

Bill Gates made a $200 billion return on a $10 billion investment on vaccines, yet he promoted himself as a philanthropist that cared for the world.

- https://www.financialexpress.com/industry/bill-gates-making-200-billion-from-vaccines-microsoft-co-founder-explains-math-behind-returns/2092891/

Gates ignores Ivermectin while pushing the vaccine agenda to end the pandemic. Gates totally ignored the role of Ivermectin in eradicating the world of the pandemic, presumably because he could not profit from a cheap repurposed drug, but he, unashamedly, admitted that it was Omicron, and not the vaccines, that saved the world from the pandemic. I mention "unashamedly" because many doctors like myself have been clamoring for the recognition of natural immunity, through infections from innocuous strains like Omicron, to obviate the need for the untried, untested Emergency Use Authorization (EUA) vaccines, but our cries were totally ignored by him.

He could not afford to lose out on his investments. But in January 2023, after making a profit of 10 times on his investment, Bill Gates sold his shares in vaccines, and he hypocritically slammed the COVID-19 vaccines as totally ineffective to combat COVID-19. He went on to say that the vaccines were not infection-blocking and were not effective against the variants. Gates referred to Omicron as nature's vaccine. This is something I said in November 2022, when the Omicron 1, 2 strain replaced the Delta strain. The mainstream media (MSM) and the world was not interested in listening to the views of highly qualified experienced frontline doctors, like Dr. Zelensko, Dr. Chetty, Dr. Jackie Stone and myself, who were having great success treating COVID with repurposed drugs, because journalists from the MSM were beholden to bizarre unscientific utterances of the medically untrained Gates, who was their major funder. They published every word that he uttered.

Gates' admission that Omicron saved the world from the pandemic was a resounding testimony that natural immunity is far superior to artificial, toxic mRNA vaccine immunity, with almost zero side effects.

- https://www.biznews.com/premium/health/2023/01/30/bill-gates-mrna

It was obvious that if Ivermectin was allowed to be used liberally, as it was done successfully in Africa, Asia, and South America, it would have destroyed the plan by big pharma and Bill Gates to push the profit generating vaccine agenda.

Gates and big pharma made billions out of the sale of vaccines. Gates and big pharma's huge sponsorships to academics, medical institutions, medical journals, public health authorities and the WHO enabled them to gag these institutions from telling the world the truth about Ivermectin and about the dangers and inefficacy of the mRNA vaccines, which were no more than toxic gene therapy.

The academics, the MSM and medical institutions were used by their sponsors, big pharma, to demonize Ivermectin and promote vaccines as safe and effective with a number of fake studies. Authentic peer reviewed articles, proving the safety and efficacy of Ivermectin and the dangers of the vaccine were totally rejected without any good reason.

This anti-Ivermectin stance by the media persisted for the entire period of the epidemic, despite there being over 15 randomized controlled trials proving that Ivermectin prophylaxis prevented COVID infection by 88%.

- https://www.researchgate.net/publication/348297284_Ivermectin_reduces_the_risk_of_death_from_ COVID-19_-a_rapid_review_and_meta-analysis_in_support_of_the_recommendation_of_the_ Front_Line_COVID-19_Critical_Care_Alliance_Latest_version_v12_-_6_Jan_2021

Omicron 1,2 ended after being around for about two months.

From March 2022 to about September 2022 I only saw about 241 patients with the Omicron 4, 5 infections in my clinic. This strain was highly infectious, far more virulent than the Omicron 1, 2 but not as virulent as the Delta strain.

About 60% of the patients with the Omicron 4, 5 ended up with pneumonia. They took about two to three weeks to present to me for treatment, unlike during the Delta strain when patients presented in the first two days. Some presented after 3 weeks to seek help, by which time they had presented with an extensive pneumonia but, surprisingly, had minimal shortness of breath.

Unlike the Delta strain, the main presenting symptoms of patients with a 3-week history of an infection from the Omicron 4, 5 strain was an unremitting cough. Very few mentioned that they were short of breath like patients infected with the Delta strain did. As I mentioned earlier, patients with the Delta infection experienced shortness of breath by day two.

Major difference between the Delta strain and the Omicron strains, 1& 2; 4& 5 with the Delta strain, patients became short of breath within about 3 days because the pneumonia set in quite rapidly. The oxygen levels dropped to about 92% quite rapidly within a few days of the pneumonia setting in. A week's delay in treatment, during the Delta strain often resulted in oxygen levels plummeting to about 80% and in some cases to as low as 70% and 60%. Some patients dropped to 45% within about two weeks of being infected with the Delta strain and others to 35% after three weeks of infection.

With the Omicron 4, 5 strain on the other hand, patients with three weeks of pneumonia maintained their Oxygen levels at normal levels of 96% which was quite an anomaly compared to infection with the Delta strain. Their main symptom was an incessant cough. The main reason for patients to present to me, during the Omicron strain infection, was mainly for a persistent cough that did not respond to a variety of over-the-counter cough syrups. These patients were totally unaware of the fact that they had serious lung damage.

It was only after I examined these patients with the Omicron strain, I discovered that most of these patients had extensive pneumonias. The only explanation for this is that they still had good healthy lung tissue, which was unaffected by the virus, to compensate for the damaged lung tissue, to maintain the oxygen at normal levels.

Dispelling the notion of elderly patients with co-morbidities are at high risk I have treated people as old as 90, people in their 70's and several obese patients, elderly with multiple comorbidities, many who presented with very low oxygen levels, and I managed to save them with a 99.99% success rate on my regime and without referring them to a hospital.

My success led me to conclude that the advice given by various public health authorities was based on conjecture and speculation. What is tragic is that these authorities did not revise their stance on COVID, as evidence was emerging, thick and fast, that there was good treatment for COVID and its complications. These authorities weren't prepared to learn from frontline doctors who took the lead and managed COVID very successfully, which was lamentable, because millions of lives could have been saved and the pandemic could have been ended very early or completely avoided if everyone from healthcare worked in a collaborative manner to help society from one of the worst health crises to afflict humanity.

I am convinced that if we adopted the approach used by many frontline doctors to treat all patients early and aggressively, regardless of age and health status, there would have been minimal fatalities, minimal hospitalizations and absolutely no need for the strict lockdown measures that crippled the economies of several developing countries in the world.

My high success rate in treating very ill patients of COVID -19 during the Delta strain, while scores of patients were dying in our hospitals, made me a target for the media. The media were heavily spinning the narrative that COVID was a deadly disease to coerce citizens to take the jab through fear. None of the local mainstream media outlets was prepared to interview me on my successes in treating COVID-19, even though I treated some very ill journalists and their families. Some of these journalists admitted to me that they were under pressure from their editors not to interview people like me or to report favorably on Ivermectin.

I sadly remember being interviewed by a young journalist from

Chapter 15   Ivermectin Saved My Patients with Severe COVID and the Vaccine Injured

NPR, an independent media outlet in South Africa, who presented himself as being totally unbiased. He wanted to know about my experience using Ivermectin to treat COVID. I showed him the pages with 600 names of patients infected with Delta strain that treated successfully using Ivermectin and I mentioned how safe the drug was, even at high doses. I was completely shocked after I saw his report of our interview. He shamelessly wrote disparagingly about me and twisted everything I said.

The drive to promote the vaccine to the public was unabated in spite of the evidence that the Delta strains were resistant to the vaccine which was designed for the Alpha strain.

I realized it was important to stay in touch with my patients, especially those who were critical.

I had about 4,000 numbers on my phone. Patients or family members were instructed to give me a report of the vitals of the patients with COVID on a regular basis after I had treated them. My staff handled my messages, while I was busy consulting and treating very ill patients. My staff were instructed on what to look out for. Patients needing my urgent intervention were brought to my attention immediately by my wife and my staff.

Patients kept in touch with me about their oxygen levels, blood sugar levels and clinical progress.

I would immediately send off a script to the patient's pharmacy for the appropriate treatment to treat the clotting based on the results of their D-dimer levels with a range of anticoagulants, depending on the severity of the clotting.

By keeping in touch with me via WhatsApp, I saved my patients time and money and prevented my rooms from becoming overcrowded. I had to reserve space for the desperately ill. I kept in touch with all my patients as part of my routine. My primary goal was to prevent deaths,

401

avoid complications and keep my patients out of hospital by being extremely proactive. I am pleased that my aggressive and hands-on approach paid off extremely well. I only had two referrals to hospital out of about 1,100 patients infected with the Delta strain; of the 1,100 patients between 70% - 80% had severe pneumonias.

I did everything to stay out of the hawkish media that was out to denigrate and pillory anyone who treated COVID with repurposed medications like Ivermectin or Hydroxychloroquine.

The videos of my successes, which I posted on social media and my Telegram channel, contributed to our practice becoming the COVID hub of Cape Town. Patients from all walks of life and from almost every suburb in Cape Town came to see me for treatment in my rooms in Mitchells Plain.

Our rooms and the street were packed with very ill people and their family members. It was a challenge that I was not prepared for nor was I trained for, but I decided to think on my feet and out of the box to come up with a strategy to meet the crisis head on. I am pleased that my strategy worked. My only regret was that a 24-hour day was too little to save the many people I could not reach due to restraints on my time and resources. After the end of the Delta strain, I felt mentally and physically fatigued. The less virulent Omicron strains gave me the respite that my body desperately needed to recover.

WE SHARED A COMMON GOAL OF SAVING LIVES

My wife Joan, who is my practice manager, took appointments, answered queries, and freed me from taking calls from irate callers demanding to speak to me, about rather trivial issues. I could work unhindered, attending to very ill patients. My receptionist Natalie and my daughter Tammy were equally outstanding. They made my work easy. I mention this for one reason and that is: without our auxiliary medical staff, doctors can achieve very little but rarely are these soldiers in the frontline given the credit that they deserve.

Most of the patients were very understanding and patient, which helped me tremendously in going about my relentless task of saving as many lives as I could without much interference.

We had a few patients who were utterly rude, insulting to my wife and slammed the phone down on her when they could not get through to me, while I was busy attending to very ill patients.

One elderly female, clearly from our former colonial/apartheid era, became quite upset with me for not answering her very long text message for a script for Ivermectin to use prophylactically.

I saw her message in the evening. I was quite irate by her outright effrontery to give me advice on how to run my practice, so I called her to explain the challenges that I was facing. She became totally stroppy with me, insulted me and told me that I was tired and that I should go and sleep. When I told her that I had just finished an 11-hour stint in my consulting room and that I still had four hours of virtual calls to do, she slammed the phone down on me.

She rekindled the ugly memories I had about our apartheid past with her belligerent attitude. She only consulted me because her GP refused to give her a script for Ivermectin. Fortunately, the majority of the patients who came to see me were very patient and understanding, which helped us tremendously when a 24-hour day was too little to deal with the number of desperately ill people who needed help.

I realized that I had five patients from the rest of the country, who were patiently waiting on my call. I composed myself and put the ugly experience behind me and went on treating my patients.

I am pleased that my maturity and years of practice have taught me to be clinical and not to allow myself to get bogged down by emotions. I immersed myself in my work and got on with what I learned to do best, and that was to save lives.

My receptionist Natalie played an outstanding role during the Delta strain infection. Her cool composure helped patients to feel reassured that we will help them to get better. Natalie, like my wife, worked a double shift without complaining. We were all committed to helping as many people as possible to prevent a single death. This was war. We were fighting against a deadly virus. We pulled all stops to win the war.

One of my greatest assets was to be organized and to think fast on my feet. I was a great stickler about being organized and about being prepared, even in crisis. When I was faced with a new challenge, I looked for a way to find a solution. I never gave up easily. I could think out of the box, which is something that is not encouraged in medical schools. We were taught to follow protocols and listen to experts and never dare to question them. Our professors instilled in junior doctors and consultants a strong element of fear not to challenge them to avoid any repercussions or be blamed for being insubordinate. The professors and heads of departments behaved like Gods and dictators. During the COVID epidemic I had to find a solution fast to treat the COVID infection and its complications because I suddenly became the last stop for patients in Cape Town. Every one of my patients refused to go to hospital, so I had to take on the responsibility of saving them with very limited resources.

Patients were filled with a fear that if they landed up in hospital, they would not return alive. The mainstream media played a huge role to create and embellish the fear in people by falsely reporting that a number of people were dying in hospital. This news instilled a fear in people not to go to hospitals when they were very ill. Patients preferred to come to me rather than to go to hospital. The huge demand for my services placed a huge burden of responsibility on my shoulders.

I am pleased that, through my perseverance and determination to find a solution by steadfastly refusing to follow a narrative that spelt gloom and doom, my staff and I achieved a success rate of 99.97% during the Delta strain, which was the deadliest strain of all the strains in the 3 years of the pandemic.

Within a few weeks, I managed to set up my practice to cater for COVID patients. By the middle of October 2021, the number of patients infected with the Delta strain decreased suddenly because of widespread herd immunity. While COVID-19 took much of my time, I made time for my non-COVID patients with chronic illnesses; our state hospitals, sadly, shut their doors to patients with non-COVID illnesses. I have no doubt that many patients with non-COVID chronic illnesses like diabetes, hypertension, ischemic disease and cancer died at home because the hospitals placed far too much emphasis on treating COVID patients.

The elderly suffered the most because they were scared to death to venture out of their homes. Many elderly were left alone, without visits from their children because their children were too afraid that they would infect their elderly parents. Many elderly people must have suffered from unattended depression, out of loneliness and a fear that they were going to die without any help from their children.

The experience I gained from treating patients during the deadly Delta strain gave me a great deal of confidence to treat patients with the mild Omicron strains. I failed to understand why the WHO and other public health authorities took so long to remove the lockdowns and emergency regulations of masking and safe distancing during the innocuous Omicron strain.

The Omicron strains, though highly infectious, were not as virulent as the Delta strain, so all my patients with the Omicron infection responded very well to a high dose of Ivermectin (0.6 mg/kg to 1.0 mg/kg), along with Doxycycline 100 mg bd, Clarithromycin 500 mg daily, Vit D3; Vit C 1,000 mg bd, Zinc 20 mg daily, Aspirin 150 mg daily and Chlorpheniramine as an antihistamine if they presented in the early viraemia phase.

Very few patients during the Omicron strain developed pneumonia compared to patients that were infected with the Delta strain. If patients infected with the Omicron strain presented with pneumonia, their oxygen levels did not plummet like it did during the Delta strain, even if they had their infection for a few weeks.

I did not refer a single patient to hospital, nor did I have any fatalities during the Omicron strain. Only two young males needed supplemental oxygen because their levels dropped to 60%, but they both recovered within two weeks of treatment.

MULTIPLE DRUGS FOR INFLAMMATION AND INFECTION

I used many drugs to treat inflammation caused by the COVID-19 infection. I did this for three reasons, firstly to get the synergistic effect of each drug, secondly to minimize the side effects from using high doses of one drug like Prednisone and thirdly, because one drug was just not enough to treat a multifaceted disease like COVID.

This was particularly important when it came to the use of steroids. I used high doses of steroids to deal with the pneumonia that was spreading like wildfire that had to be tamed and contained in the initial stages of the disease. Many of my patients were elderly with diabetes and other comorbidities. I managed to reduce the dose of steroids in the elderly and people with diabetes by combining them with other inflammatory drugs like Colchicine, SSRIs, Ivermectin and Hydroxychloroquine.

The side effects of drugs like steroids were an important issue when had to use them for periods of 6 to 12 weeks. My initial dose was high for the first week. After the first week, I tapered down the dose of the steroids. I lowered the dose of Ivermectin and only used it twice a week because of its long half-life.

The pneumonia affected the air-sacs and not the bronchi, so we were dealing with inflammation over a very huge surface area. The surface area of the air sacs/alveoli was equivalent to the surface area of a tennis court. The doses we used for severe asthma were insufficient. I used 100 mg in 2 divided doses for a week and tapered the dose to 50mg daily the next week. Colchicine was continued if the pneumonia persisted, or the oxygen levels were not optimal. The Ivermectin dose was reduced for its anti-inflammatory and anticoagulant properties during the phase of pneumonia.

I increased diabetes medication doses for patients with diabetes and severe pneumonia needing high-dose steroids. If diabetic patients were on oral agents, I added a short acting insulin to control their blood sugars till their pneumonias resolved and they no longer needed steroids.

LIBERAL USE OF ANTIBIOTICS

Evidence from the Spanish flu revealed that the majority of the deaths in that pandemic were due to bacterial infections for which there were no antibiotics.

- DM Morens et al. Predominant role of bacterial pneumonia as a cause of death in pandemic influenza: Implications for pandemic influenza preparedness. The Journal of Infectious Diseases DOI: 10.1086/591708 (2008).

I used antibiotics prophylactically to prevent secondary infections in patients with COVID pneumonia, even if they presented in the viraemic phase of the disease. My reasoning was, "better safe than sorry". Clarithromycin had antiviral and antibacterial properties, which was a bonus. Doxycycline was used for its antiviral properties and because it was a zinc ionophore, which helped to transfer the zinc into the cell. Zinc prevented the virus from multiplying. My approach was: "Hit fast and hit hard".

I used Ivermectin in all stages of the disease for its antiviral, anti-inflammatory and anticoagulant properties. The costly, experimental, and toxic antiviral drug Remdesivir and Paxlovid could only be used in the viral stages of the COVID-19. This meant that for the Omicron infection, the viral stage only lasted about 2 to 3 days, so to continue giving antivirals by the third day of an Omicron strain was totally useless and putting the patient at risk of experiencing the unwanted toxic or adverse effects of these drugs.

Ivermectin had several mechanisms of action to kill the virus, so it was unlikely that we would encounter the possibility of a resistance to it. Some of the suggested mechanisms of action of Ivermectin are as follows: it blocks the spike from attaching to the cell; it prevents the virus from dividing or multiplying in the cell, which prevents the virus from proliferating. Ivermectin was a bacteriostatic, which makes it less susceptible to resistance by the rapidly mutating strains. This was evident in my practice when it worked effectively against the Delta and the subsequent Omicron strains, because of its unique properties and multifaceted mechanisms of action.

The use of antivirals like Remdesivir and Paxlovid, as already mentioned, beyond the viral phase made no sense because these drugs are antiviral. These drugs are widely used in hospitals on patients, who were admitted with severe pneumonias. These drugs had no effect on pneumonia. The most likely consequence of using these drugs during the phase of pneumonia is that they cause a great deal of harm through their toxic effects on patients with highly compromised organ functions, due to severe hypoxia. Ivermectin on the other hand can safely be used in all phases of the disease process.

I used high doses of Ivermectin to treat patients with the Delta strain because the Delta strain multiplied 70 to 100 times faster than the previous strains, so I felt that the recommended 0.2 mg/kg was suboptimal to kill the rapidly multiplying virus and prevent complications from it.

An article published on 3 August 2021 by Dr. Santin, McCullough and colleagues in PubMed revealed that patients who were on high doses of Ivermectin ranging from 1,5 mg; 1,6 mg and 3,0 mg over five-day periods experienced minimal and reversible side effects. So, the claim by the WHO, FDA, and several other public health authorities that Ivermectin is dangerous was highly unfounded and misleading.

-   https://www.ncbi.nlm.nih.gov/pmc/articles/PMC8383101/

Unlike other doctors who used Ivermectin for one to three days in low doses to conduct their research on the efficacy of Ivermectin to treat COVID, I used Ivermectin on a daily basis at doses of 0.6 mg/kg to 1.0 mg/kg for between 5 to 10 days depending on the severity of the disease.

Ivermectin had a half-life of 20 hours, so a single dose was grossly insufficient to contain a strain like Delta, which replicated itself at a rate of 70 times faster than the previous strains, which explains the development of pneumonia within three days of the infections. The pneumonia appeared after 8 days, so we had time to introduce treatment with high dose steroids by day 8.

-   https://www.ncbi.nlm.nih.gov/pmc/articles/PMC2751445/

I suspect that many of the studies that showed Ivermectin to be ineffective against COVID-19 was because they used a too low dose of 0.2 mg/kg and for very short periods; some used it for just one day. I used doses ranging from 0.6 mg to 1.0 mg/kg for 5 to 10 days.

Ivermectin alone, beyond the third day of the infection with the Delta strain was totally insufficient because by the third day the pneumonia was starting to set in. Most trials merely used Ivermectin alone to test its efficacy, which was incorrect. Clearly the researchers did not understand the pathogenesis of COVID or the limitations of Ivermectin when COVID pneumonia set in. Ivermectin is a potent antiviral, but it is not an effective anti-inflammatory drug like high-dose steroids. Many researchers, who studied the efficacy of Ivermectin to treat complicated COVID failed to take this into account.

There have been a number of studies that have shown that Remdesivir, hydroxychloroquine, lopinavir/ritonavir, interferon, convalescent plasma, and monoclonal antibody therapy did not reduce mortality in hospitalized patients. The only drug to reduce mortality in hospital patients with severe COVID was high-dose steroids.

- https://www.ncbi.nlm.nih.gov/pmc/articles/PMC8088823/#R1

If the oxygen levels due to COVID pneumonia remained at suboptimal levels for longer periods of up to six weeks, I used Ivermectin on a twice-weekly basis, on Sundays, and Thursdays, primarily for its anti-inflammatory and anticoagulant effects. I also treated the clotting aspects very aggressively with potent anticoagulants because clotting played a major role in rendering patients hypoxic.

Meta-analyses based on 18 randomized controlled treatment trials of Ivermectin in COVID-19 have found large, statistically significant reductions in mortality, time to clinical recovery, and time to viral clearance. Furthermore, results from numerous controlled prophylaxis trials report significantly reduced risks of contracting COVID-19 with the regular use of Ivermectin.

- https://www.ncbi.nlm.nih.gov/pmc/articles/PMC8088823/

Ivermectin is a multifaceted drug making it the ideal choice to treat COVID-19 because it has multiple pathologies According to Zhang et al in the journal "Open Heart" published in 2020 in PubMed,

Ivermectin has antiviral, anti-inflammatory and immunomodulatory properties, which make it suitable to treat patients with COVID-19.

- Zhang et al., 2008, Ci et al., 2009, DiNicolantonio et al., 2020

Ivermectin's antithrombotic properties are very useful to treat COVID-19 which has three types of pathology namely: Viraemia, inflammation (an organizing pneumonia –due to the cytokine storm) and a clotting aspect. Clotting was a serious issue in patients during the Delta strain. It had to be treated very aggressively to avoid the complications of thrombotic events to vital organs like the heart and brain or any part of the body like the limbs or eyes.

Ivermectin, unlike Remdesivir, Paxlovid and Molnupiravir, has an extremely safe 40-year track record with over 3.5 billion doses used worldwide so it could be used to help treat the three facets of the disease: viraemia, inflammation, and clotting with minimal side effects in one go.

LOST CREDIBILITY OF FDA

U.S. Food and Drug Administration (FDA) was misleading the public about Ivermectin. The FDA was guilty of gross misinformation after it sent out tweets and warnings to doctors and the public that Ivermectin's safety was not tested. The FDA sent out a tweet urging doctors and the public not to use Ivermectin to treat COVID-19.

They claimed, "You are not a horse. You are not a cow".

They regarded the drug which saved millions of people in the world from Onchocerciasis or Lymphatic filariasis as not for humans but for horses and cows.

Dr. Paul Marik, Dr. Mary Bowden, and Dr. Robert Apter filed a case against the FDA for demonizing Ivermectin as an unsafe drug, not fit for human use. This stance by the FDA, according to these doctors, had caused irreparable harm to their professional image and careers, as well as to the careers of many other doctors, who lost their jobs and licenses because they used Ivermectin to treat and save their patients from dying of COVID-19.

The case was heard by three U.S. Circuit Court Judges: Jennifer Walker Elrod, Edith Brown Clement, and Don Willet.

Ms. Honold, the defense attorney for the FDA, insisted that the FDA did not stop doctors from prescribing Ivermectin and eventually admitted that the FDA had no right or jurisdiction over doctors when it comes to treating patients.

This admission by the FDA, that they did not stop doctors from using Ivermectin to treat patients with COVID-19, was contrary to the stance that the FDA, the WHO, and Dr. Anthony Fauci, the head of American Academy of Allergy, Asthma & Immunology, and several other regulatory authorities had on the use of Ivermectin by doctors to treat COVID-19 during the three years of the pandemic. It was widely known that all these regulatory bodies were totally opposed to the use of Ivermectin by doctors to treat COVID. Dr. Paul Marik was dismissed by his employer for prescribing Ivermectin and subsequently lost his job for promoting the early use of Ivermectin to treat COVID-19.

The FDA's admission in court that they did not stop doctors from prescribing Ivermectin, after the pandemic was over, was too little too late and criminal, because millions of lives could have been saved if the drug had been made freely available.

The FDA's stance on Ivermectin was unambiguously slanted, through their regular tweets, against the use of Ivermectin to treat COVID-19 during the entire pandemic.

- https://www.theepochtimes.com/article/doctors-can-prescribe-ivermectin-for-covid-19-fda-545658

On 1 September 2023, the judges found that the FDA had overstepped its authority by advising doctors and the public against the use of Ivermectin to treat COVID-19. Judge Don Willet, along with presiding judges Jennifer Walker Elrod and Edith Brown Clement, stated that the FDA is not a physician to endorse, denounce, or advise on a treatment.

The decision to use a well-tested drug is and remains the right of physicians.

The FDA's counsel admitted to the courts that doctors have a right to prescribe Ivermectin and that the FDA has no control over doctors on how to treat their patients. This information was too late when the pandemic was over.

- https://apnews.com/article/coronavirus-ivermectin-fda-doctors-lawsuit-bbc8d4fc726c08940ae4b0da d70170e0

The reason the FDA gave for its decision to advise doctors and the general public against the use of Ivermectin was that they received unverified reports from hospitals that the hospitals were treating a number of patients with Ivermectin toxicity. It was utterly shocking to read that the FDA relied on unverified information to advise doctors and the public on the safety of Ivermectin. This raised a huge question mark on the credibility of the FDA.

- https://apnews.com/article/coronavirus-ivermectin-fda-doctors-lawsuit-bbc8d4fc726c08940ae4b0da d70170e0

The FDA was not able to give scientific data to prove that Ivermectin administered in therapeutic doses is harmful because there is no evidence that Ivermectin is dangerous when given even above the therapeutic doses.

The FDA was corrected by a judge, who sternly refuted the FDA's counsel's explanation that the tweet by an FDA official saying, "You are not a horse", referring to Ivermectin, was an innocent quip and not a command. Its utter embarrassment of the FDA's defense counsel. The judge admonished the FDA's defense counsel for being so facetious about such a serious matter.

FDA – DISPLAYS DOUBLE STANDARDS ON REPURPOSED DRUGS

The FDA's primary duty to the public is to approve new drugs for their safety and efficacy. They also have a duty to report on adverse events of all drugs. They have no right to interfere with a doctor's right to prescribe a repurposed drug because repurposed drugs have a well-known track record for their safety. Doctors have an inherent right to use repurposed drugs, like Ivermectin or Hydroxychloroquine for off-label use, at their own discretion, without requiring the permission from any authority.

Repurposed drugs can be tried without testing because their safety data are already established, as in the case of a 40-year-old drug like Ivermectin. Repurposed drugs have the advantage of saving the 3-12-year test period before they are approved.

Ordinarily, the FDA and other health regulatory authorities have had no problem with repurposed drugs like Aspirin, Viagra, Hydroxychloroquine and SGLT2 (Sodium-Glucose Cotransporter 2) inhibitors. SGLT2 inhibitors were originally developed to treat diabetes, now they are being used as an adjunct to treat heart failure. The FDA's and other regulatory authorities' opposition to well-tested drugs like Ivermectin smacks of downright special intentions.

The American Association of Physicians and Surgeons, in its legal brief in court against the FDA for interfering in the use of repurposed drugs, stated:

"Not only is the use of off-label drugs fully proper, legal, and commonplace, but often necessary to give proper and effective care to patients."

This statement was most apt during the COVID pandemic when

all we had were untested, costly EUA drugs to treat COVID-19, which even if effective, were beyond the reach of citizens in poor third world countries.

- https://finance.yahoo.com/news/fda-misled-public-ivermectin-accountable-144900899.html

OFF-LABEL USE DRUGS WAS THE ANSWER FOR COVID BUT IGNORED

Off-label use of Ivermectin and Hydroxychloroquine, Zinc, Vitamin D, and Vitamin C were necessary to treat COVID-19 during the deadly pandemic. The claim by major health authorities and academic institutions that there was no treatment for COVID when there were so many effective, safe, and affordable treatments, is one of the most unforgivable excuses.

Nations were ruined by futile lockdowns; millions of lives were lost because good and effective treatment was denied to desperate citizens by bureaucrats, politicians, big pharma, and academics, and rich individuals, who had a vested interest in making money out of untested and unproven therapies.

Several frontline doctors, like Dr. Marik (U.S.), Dr. Zelenko (U.S.), Dr. Stone (Zimbabwe), Dr. Chetty (South Africa), Dr. Kory (U.S.), Prof. Carvallo (Argentina) and several other doctors from around the world were achieving phenomenal results with their simple treatment for COVID with 99% to 100% success rates. None of our successes were ever reported on by mainstream media nor were they published in scientific mainstream medical journals.

These doctors, who were pilloried by mainstream media, deregistered by their medical boards and even fired after years of outstanding service by their employers, became the darlings and heroes of the citizens of the world.

HALLIGAN REPORT ON 36 MILLION DEATHS CAUSED BY VACCINES

One of the great challenges for scientists, epidemiologists, and statisticians to try and analyze the efficacy and safety profile of the vaccine was the scarcity of data from the major public health authorities all over the world. Some countries had no data at all. Many scientists and actuaries had to rely on special programs and data from insurance claims to make proper analysis of the effect of the vaccine.

Peter Halligan, a retired investment consultant, conducted an in-depth analysis of the figures and published his observations and deductions on the COVID vaccine in his Substack entitled Peter's Newsletter, which was reported on in The Expose' in October 2023.

Halligan used the European Union's drug regulating authorities' Pharmacovigilance, "Eudravigilance" adverse-events data to estimate the deaths caused by the vaccine and extrapolated it globally.

Based on an under-reporting factor of 40 and the exclusion of deaths from China's use of 3.5 billion doses of the vaccine, the following is a summary of his findings:

1. There were 36 million deaths related to the vaccine.
2. Three quarters of these deaths came from India, with the widespread use of the Astra-Zeneca vaccine.
3. 2 billion dollars were spent on the vaccine alone.
4. If Ivermectin and other repurposed drugs were widely used prophylactically on the entire world's population, it would have cost a mere $160 million.

- https://expose-news.com/2023/05/19/governments-paid-2-billion-for-36-million-deaths/

Fiona Mac Donald wrote an article in the journal "Science Alert" on 12 April 2018 stating that many scientists and editors could be

Chapter 15   Ivermectin Saved My Patients with Severe COVID and the Vaccine Injured

and are corrupt. Journals are forced to publish articles favoring their sponsors like big pharma or risk bankruptcy. They were forced to publish fake articles on climate change and sugar, to name a few, or perish. She wrote the followings:

Most shocking: medical journal editors are paid huge sums by pharmaceutical companies each year.
This is something most of us already know - we see the sponsored pens and all the fancy conferences doctors go on thanks to 'big pharma'.
But that's only a small part of it. The industry also just hands them money directly.

A paper published last year in the British Medical Journal examined how much money editors of the world's most influential medical journals were taking from industry sources.

Of the journals that could be assessed, 50.6 percent of editors were receiving money from the pharmaceutical industry - in some cases, hundreds of thousands of dollars.

- https://www.sciencealert.com/how-much-top-journal-editors-get-paid-by-big-pharma-corrupt

WHY LONG COURSES OF REMDESIVIR, PAXLOVID, AND MOLNUPIRAVIR IS INAPPROPIRIATE FOR COVID?

Administering antiviral drugs like Paxlovid and Remdesivir during the inflammatory phase of the disease was unscientific, costly, and placed patients at risk of a plethora of side effects from these experimental drugs. Some of the serious side effects of the EUA (Emergency Use Authorization) drugs, Remdesivir and Paxlovid, included kidney failure and several severe drug interactions. Paxlovid had about 115 drug interactions via the cytochrome-p450 enzyme pathway in the liver, which should have been of serious concern for the elderly, who were on several medications for a variety of

417

chronic illnesses, like diabetes, hypertension, epilepsy, and arthritic conditions. It was utterly reckless for a regulatory health body like the FDA to approve Paxlovid (https://www.verywellhealth.com/how-to-get-paxlovid-without-seeing-a-doctor-5649541) to be issued over the counter without a prescription for mild symptoms during the Omicron strain because one does not use a highly toxic medication for a condition that is mild and self-limiting as the Omicron strain and when Ivermectin was far more effective, cheaper, and safer.

PAXLOVID- WAS GIVEN FDA APPROVAL TO OBTAIN WITHOUT A PRESCRIPTION

Paxlovid was found to interact with over 650 other drugs, which could result in either an increase or decrease of in the other drug's efficiency.

- https://www.drugs.com/drug-interactions/nirmatrelvir-ritonavir,paxlovid.html

This posed a serious issue for patients on chronic medications for a variety of chronic illnesses, like HIV, epilepsy, hypertension, so it was puzzling why the FDA allowed the drug to be obtained from a pharmacy without a prescription. A drug with so many drug interactions, ordinarily, would have required a doctor's script for the patient's safety. During the safe and largely self-limiting Omicron strain, it made absolutely no sense for patients to go through an expensive course of Paxlovid, with all its attendant toxic side effects.

"TOGETHER TRIAL" ON IVERMECTIN EFFICACY - TERRIBLY FLAWED

A study conducted by Riess and colleagues in Brazil from March 2021 to August 2021 was published in the New England Journal of Medicine, where the authors concluded that Ivermectin was not effective in reducing hospitalization, which was the end point. This article received a great deal of attention from doctors who were opposed to the use of Ivermectin but conveniently ignored the many flaws in the entire study.

There were 679 individuals in the Ivermectin group and 679 in the placebo groups. According to the authors there were 100 events in the Ivermectin group and 111 in the placebo group.

Of the 211 primary events, 178 (80%) were admitted to hospital. Patients were chosen if they had 7 days of symptoms. The Ivermectin group were given Ivermectin 400 mcg/kg for three days.

The authors concluded that Ivermectin was not effective in reducing hospital admissions.

- https://www.nejm.org/doi/pdf/10.1056/NEJMoa2115869?articleTools=true

Despite its numerous flaws, the article was widely quoted in all the media to discredit Ivermectin.

Flaws in the study:

1. Many of the of the outcomes specified in the together trial for Ivermectin were missing in the final report.
2. There were several mid-trial changes to the protocol which is not permitted.
3. The all-cause mortality data was removed from the study.
4. The results for fluvoxamine were released in August 2021, but the results for Ivermectin were released six months later in January 2022, which is highly inconsistent.
5. There seemed to be a problem with the Ivermectin data so scientists who were curious (about the data) requested the data on Ivermectin, but the authors failed to provide it, which was unacceptable.
6. The article in the NEJM does not state what drug was used as a placebo.

7. It emerged that Vitamin C was used, and it has been found that there were 42 studies using Vitamin C, which showed that there was improvement using Vitamin C.

8. Blinding was a serious issue. Ivermectin was given for three days, whereas the placebo was given for 1, 3, 10 and 14 days, which would immediately alert the treating doctor as to who was receiving Ivermectin and who was receiving the placebo.

9. Treatment timing – most studies issued the Ivermectin early in the disease, whereas in the TOGETHER Trial Ivermectin was given much later which accounts for the poor results of Ivermectin in the TOGETHER Trial.

10. Treatment Dose: Ivermectin in the TOGETHER Trial was administered on an empty stomach, which reduced its effective dose to 15% to 40% of the clinically reported dose. My own experience during the Delta strain was I used a dose of 600 mcg/kg to 1,000 mcg/kg because the Delta strain multiplied very rapidly, and this worked to reduce the strain from multiplying and causing serious damage to the body.

11. Different strains: from March 2021 to August 2021 there was a transition from the mild strain to the virulent Delta strain in August 2021, so the dosage used and the period of use were totally incorrect based on my own experience. I used high doses of the drug early from day one for between 5 to 10 days, which explains my high success rate.

12. Conflict of interests: some of the researchers involved in the TOGETHER Trial did paid work for Pfizer, MERCK, Regeneron, and Astra-Zeneca, all of whom were involved in the development of COVID therapeutics. This should be a source of huge concern.

13. Even TOGETHER Trial shows Ivermectin benefit: the trial showed Ivermectin group a 12% reduction in deaths; 23% reduction in

mechanical ventilation and 17% reduction in hospitalization, so it was shocking for the authors of this study to conclude that Ivermectin was totally ineffective to treat COVID.

- https://www.cato.org/regulation/summer-2022/ivermectin-together-trial

The above flaws in the TOGETHER Trial should make it abundantly clear that the trial was poorly conducted; the authors failed to understand the nuances in the different strains and did not follow proper protocols when it came to conducting proper double-blind randomized controlled trials.

One key element in the research of the doctors who conducted research on the efficacy of Ivermectin to treat COVID-19 was that they had failed to understand that the disease had to be treated early with high doses of Ivermectin to yield positive outcomes. The other shortcoming in the knowledge of the doctors performing the research on Ivermectin is that they were unaware that to treat a highly virulent strain like Delta, Ivermectin alone was insufficient to save patients if they presented with pneumonia.

Charles L. Hooper and David R. Henderson of the US CATO Institute, who validated the TOGETHER study, write in a nutshell as follows.

A more accurate interpretation of the findings would be to say that the drug showed promise and that a larger trial may yield the desired statistical significance.

Ivermectin certainly worked for the earlier mild strains of COVID, based on the experiences of doctors in other parts of the world as well as the experiences of Dr. Jackie Stone of Zimbabwe who had easy access to Ivermectin. I did not have access to Ivermectin before the

421

Delta strain appeared in South Africa in July 2021, so I had no personal experience with Ivermectin against the wild type, Alpha, and Beta strains to comment on it. I have no doubt that if Ivermectin had been available to me from the initial outbreak of COVID-19, I would not have had one death in my practice based on the success I had with the drug against the Delta strain.

Most trials on Ivermectin for COVID resulted in poor outcomes because researchers failed to realize that they were dealing with a complex disease that needs a multitude of drugs to treat various aspects of the disease.

Ivermectin in my experience is a great drug in the very early phases or viral phase of the disease to achieve a swift recovery. If the disease progressed to the stage of pneumonia, within 3 days as it did in the case of the Delta strain, about 10 other drugs including supplements and about 3 non-medical therapeutic interventions were needed to cure the disease. Ivermectin played a crucial role in the healing, but Ivermectin alone was insufficient to cure a severe COVID pneumonia or severe clotting.

WHO FOCUSES ON UNTESTED MONOCLONAL ANTIBODIES

In spite of the evidence from countries like India, in Africa, and South America, on the safety and efficacy of Ivermectin to prevent complications and to treat COVID-19, the WHO instead recommended costly monoclonal antibodies such as Baricitinib and Sotrovimab for moderate cases.

- https://apps.who.int/iris/bitstream/handle/10665/351006/WHO-2019-nCoV-therapeutics-2022.1-eng.pdf

Apart from the questionable efficacy of monoclonal antibodies, which were not tried against the highly resistant Omicron strains, monoclonal antibodies were way beyond the affordability of all third world countries compared to the cost, safety, and efficacy of Ivermectin. The high recovery rates, low death, and hospitalizations rates in countries in Asia, Africa, and South America after Ivermectin was used, either as prophylaxis or to treat COVID, was convincing evidence that Ivermectin alone was sufficient to cure the mild strains of COVID in the early phases of the disease, obviating the need for monoclonal antibodies and untested drugs like Remdesivir and Paxlovid, which were merely EUA drugs. It was later demonstrated that both Remdesivir and Paxlovid had poor safety profiles, they did not reduce mortality and were extremely expensive.

Part 3
IVERMECTIN AND VACCINE INJURIES

South Africa started rolling out its COVID vaccine program in earnest from August 2021 in the peak of the Delta strain. According to Prof. Geert Vanden Bossche it was and is strongly inadvisable to vaccinate in the midst of a pandemic because it can affect people's innate immunity and place them at high risk of getting easily infected. Further, vaccines take about 2 to 3 weeks to take effect so there was a strong chance that the vaccinated could get infected in spite of receiving the vaccine. It is common knowledge that if a vaccinated person gets infected, it could over stimulate the immune system and lead to a cytokine storm.

Prof. Geert Vanden Bossche's views were supported by Nobel Laureate, Prof. Luc Montagnier, who stated that history will discover that mass vaccination during a pandemic was a big mistake because it will create variants.

-   https://telanganatoday.com/mass-vaccination-during-pandemic-historical-blunder-nobel-laureate

The most likely reason for the high death rate amongst the vaccinated was because the immune system of the vaccinated was severely depleted so they could not fight common pathogens, as Prof. Vanden Bossche mentioned.

Dr. Kobi Haviv from an Israel hospital told channel 13 news that 95% of the very ill were from the vaccinated, and the vaccinated accounted for 85% to 90% of all hospital admissions. He warned that any further boosters would make the situation ten times worse for the vaccinated.

- https://biotechexpressmag.com/unvaccinated-people-are-not-dangerous-vaccinated-people-are-dangerous-for-others-immunization-expert/

In addition to treating patients infected with COVID-19, I started seeing patients presenting with a variety of injuries that were most likely due to vaccine injuries.

I started equipping myself with knowledge of the various modalities to treat vaccine injuries to help victims because the vaccine-injured were totally ignored by the medical establishments and the state health authorities like SAHPRA. No doctor or health institution was prepared to acknowledge that vaccine injuries existed, fearing repercussions from their employers or the medical boards. This rendered the vaccine injured totally helpless.

Perfectly healthy people were ending up with heart attacks, neurological disorders like shooting nerve pains, vascular problems, and turbo cancers a few months after taking their vaccines.

mRNA – COVID VACCINE ENTERS ALL OVER THE BODY TO CAUSE DAMAGE TO ORGANS- DR. SUCHARIT BHAKDI

According to Dr. Sucharit Bhakdi, the COVID vaccine enters the organs of the body, which it shouldn't do. The spike protein of the vaccine enters deep into the cells of our body; once the spike is inside the cells of our bodies, it turns these cells into spike producing factories that will continue to produce spike protein. The body's immune system will regard these spike proteins in the cells as foreign antigens and will attack the cells with the spike in them, to produce an overwhelming autoimmune response. This autoimmune reaction, in turn, destroys the organs of the body, which explains the high incidence of myocarditis. There is no way of knowing how long these spike proteins will remain in the body, which is an issue of major concern for every health practitioner.

The anti-inflammatory effect on the organs due to the vaccine spike protein was demonstrated in the 15 autopsies done by the famous German pathologist, Dr. Arne Burkhardt, who has taught in the University of Hamburg. His findings confirmed that the causes of sudden death were due to myocardial infarction, arrhythmias, and myocarditis as a result of the inflammatory response to the vaccine's spike protein in the heart muscle.

The abnormal histopathological changes were similar in all 15 patients that were autopsied. In 14 out of the 15 autopsies, the heart was implicated. He showed pathological evidence that the spike protein was found in the heart muscle, which caused the inflammation of the heart muscle. These findings by Dr. Burkhardt provided conclusive evidence that the vaccine was the cause of the cardiac deaths in healthy people who died suddenly. Dr. Arne Burkhardt found that there was a huge presence of T-lymphocytes in the heart muscle, which was abnormal, near the vessels of the heart and dead endothelial cells in the vessels of the heart due to endotheliitis.

- https://links.uwaterloo.ca/Repeal_UW_Mandatory_Vaccination_Policy/end-covax_bhakdi_burkhardt_Dec_10_2021.pdf

Before Dr. Arne Burkhardt conducted the autopsies on patients who died suddenly, the medical world had to rely on conjecture that the vaccine was the cause of the number of sudden deaths amongst previously healthy adults and athletes. The study by Dr. Arne Burkhardt and Dr. Bhakdi provided evidence that the vaccines were the cause of sudden unexplained deaths in previously healthy individuals. This finding rejected the claim by public health authorities and the vaccine manufacturers that the vaccines were not the cause of the sudden cardiac death in healthy individuals that were previously vaccinated.

But the medical authorities who promoted the vaccines refused to acknowledge the findings of Dr. Burkhardt, through which he clearly demonstrated the link between the vaccine and sudden cardiac deaths.

SOME CASES OF VACCINE INJURY THAT I TREATED WITH IVERMECTIN

Bell's Palsy: I successfully treated a 35-year female for a COVID pneumonia. She returned to me about six months after her recovery with a severe left Bell's palsy and an intractable headache. These symptoms appeared two weeks after her employer forced her to take the vaccine, even though she mentioned to them that she had already had COVID. In South Africa, even though vaccines were not made mandatory by the government, big businesses made it compulsory for employees to take the vaccine or face dismissal. The majority of the patients took the vaccine even the case against their will to keep their jobs.

Corporations misinterpreted the labor law by requiring their employees to take the vaccine or face dismissal. Employers in South African turned their backs on COVID to coerce their indefensible employees to take the vaccine or face dismissal.

I treated my depressed patient with Ivermectin and Fluoxetine to stop the inflammation in her nerves that was caused by the spike protein. Fluoxetine was used for its anti-inflammatory properties and its ability to cross the blood brain barrier.

It took her six months of treatment to make a 90% recovery. She still had occasional pain, but she regained full function of her facial muscles. She was dismissed for being off work due to her illness, which she did not cause.

Trigeminal neuralgia: A 69-year retired female health worker came to me with a history of excruciating pain on the right side of the face. This occurred 2 weeks after she took the vaccine. She was perfectly healthy with no chronic illnesses and was looking forward to a quiet retirement. She was kept awake at two o'clock in the morning with intractable pain and regretted ever taking the vaccine.

I put her on a course of Ivermectin and Carbamazepine. She made a complete recovery in about three weeks. I saw her a year later and she was perfectly fine.

The mechanism of action of Ivermectin to treat vaccine injuries is that Ivermectin dislodges the spike protein by attaching to the ACE 2 receptors on the cell membrane to which the spike attaches itself. This is the explanation given by Prof. Robert Clancy, a well-known immunologist from Australia.

- https://www.youtube.com/watch?v=qWlf7sbomMQ

STIFF PERSON SYNDROME-STS – SUCCESSFULLY TREATED WITH IVERMECTIN

In August 2023, a 45-year-old single mother of two children was escorted into my rooms, assisted by her two adult sisters because she was unable to walk on her own. She was totally disoriented and drowsy. Her posture was skew, and her head was pulled to one side by the asymmetrical spasms of her neck muscles; the muscle of her entire body had gone into complete painful spasms.

She was unable to stand or walk. She was in hospital for this condition for about two weeks in intensive care. She was put on artificial ventilation for the two weeks because she lost complete consciousness. When she regained her consciousness, she was discharged from hospital without any treatment for her persistent and debilitating spasms. She was discharged with a gobbledygook diagnosis of, "Functional Neurological Disorder".

She experienced her painful spasms shortly after she took her second Pfizer jab. She too, like so many other vaccines injured patients, took the vaccine because she was forced to take it or risk losing her job. She was a single mother and the sole supporter, so she had no choice other than to comply and take the jab.

Due to her prolonged absence from work, she was dismissed by her employer with no apology or compensation. The employers got away with their forced vaccine mandates by saying that they were merely following the best medical advice at the time. None of these employers were prepared to listen to my views about the adverse events of the vaccines, the failure of vaccines to protect individuals, that natural immunity was superior to vaccine immunity and that there was no need for the vaccines in the first place because there was a cheap and effective treatment, like Ivermectin, for COVID.

The poor lady was angry and bitter for being forced to take the jab. She described herself as bubbly and energetic. She could not accept feeling like an invalid, at such a young age, dependent on her sisters to care for her.

She broke down crying because she could no longer restrain her emotions and anger for being let down by her employer and our health authorities.

I listened with empathy to her, repressing my own emotions about the way she has been treated, and informed her that she had Stiff Person Syndrome caused by the vaccine. She was aware of the diagnosis after watching the story of world-famous singer, Celine Dion, who also suffered from the same condition.

I managed to relieve her spasms through a needle-technique and put her on my protocol for vaccine injuries, which included: Ivermectin, hydroxychloroquine, Fluoxetine, Vitamin D, nicotine chewing gum and much later Nattokinase. I gave her intensive psychotherapy and kept in touch with her via WhatsApp to allow her to communicate with me freely.

I received a report from her siblings that for the first time in six months she slept peacefully right through the night. Her condition was having its toll on the family, her children and her relatives because they all felt helpless when she cried out of pain and the relentless spasms.

She returned to my rooms walking completely on her own, with a huge smile on her face feeling most grateful that she got her life back. She did a video of her story recounting what she had gone through and became a role model of hope for others with the problem.

When she returned to hospital for a routine check-up, her doctors were totally shocked by her recovery, which they described as a miracle. She unhesitatingly told her doctors that her recovery was because she had a miracle doctor, referring to me, who diagnosed her and treated her correctly.

She did not mention my name on my request that she must not divulge my name to our state doctors because doctors working for the state refused to acknowledge that the vaccines were the cause of adverse events to protect their jobs. I also did not want to become a target of the state or state academics for helping patients with vaccine injuries. We were and are living in a dystopian world where the truth is frowned upon. Anyone that dares to speak the truth in science is at risk of being punished for propagating disinformation. It's truly a sick time in the history of the world.

She did extremely well for about six months, when she suddenly developed a full right sided stroke. I suspected it was a clot in the vessels of her brain caused by the vaccine because her blood pressure was perfectly normal.

I resumed my protocol for vaccine injuries. She is making a slow recovery and is regaining power in her paralyzed side. I have put her on Ivermectin because I suspect it's the spike that might have caused her stroke.

It is not uncommon for one patient to have more than one side effect from the vaccine. She was one of them. My advice to people with neurological vaccine injuries is to use a mild anticoagulant like aspirin to prevent a stroke. Fortunately, her spasms did not return, and she was making good recovery from her stroke.

Ivermectin, I remain convinced, plays an important role in the management of vaccine injuries based on my own experience.

Part 4
IVERMECTIN AND CANCER

Ivermectin has powerful anti-tumor activity by inhibiting proliferation, metastasis and angiogenic activity of cancer cells. Ivermectin promotes cancer cell death through apoptosis, autophagy and pyroptosis of cancer cells. Ivermectin can inhibit the growth of tumor stems cells and works best when used with chemotherapy; it can reverse multidrug resistant tumors.

- https://www.ncbi.nlm.nih.gov/pmc/articles/PMC7505114/#bib0110

According to Yoshida and colleagues, repositioning old drugs like Ivermectin saves time and cost because the drug has already been studied and approved with an established safety track record. It makes absolute sense to explore the possibility of using a repurposed drug like Ivermectin to treat cancer, while there is ongoing research to find new drugs to treat cancer.

Yoshida G.J. Therapeutic strategies of drug repositioning targeting

Chapter 15   Ivermectin Saved My Patients with Severe COVID and the Vaccine Injured

autophagy to induce cancer cell death: from pathophysiology to treatment.

- *J Hematol Oncol.* 2017; 10(1):67. doi: 10.1186/s13045-017-0436-9.

TREATING DIFFERENT CANCERS WITH IVERMECTIN
Breast-cancer

Breast cancer is a malignant tumor produced by gene mutations caused by a number of carcinogens; it has the highest incidence of cancer in females with a new case being discovered every 18 seconds in the world. The proliferation of multiple breast cancer cell lines including MCF-7, MDA-MB-231 and MCF-10 was significantly reduced after treatment with Ivermectin.

- Dou Q., Chen H.N., Wang K., Yuan K., Lei Y., Li K., Lan J., Chen Y., Huang Z., Xie N., Zhang L., Xiang R., Nice E.C., Wei Y., Huang C. Ivermectin Induces Cytostatic Autophagy by Blocking the PAK1/Akt Axis in Breast Cancer. *Cancer Res.* 2016;76(15):4457–4469.
  doi: 10.1158/0008-5472.CAN-15-2887.
- https://www.ncbi.nlm.nih.gov/pmc/articles/PMC7505114/#bib0160

I treated one patient with stage 2 breast cancer, for which she was being treated with chemotherapy at our state hospital. She presented to me with severe pain in the cancerous breast. I put her on a course of Ivermectin for five days. She reported to me two weeks later informing me that she experienced considerable improvement after the five-day treatment. I prescribed a daily dose of 0.4 mg/kg daily.

Her treating doctors were amazed by her recovery. I requested her not to inform the doctors that she was on Ivermectin fearing any repercussions from our health authorities. I saw her six months later, and she was perfectly well and off chemotherapy.

Another study found that Ivermectin works as an epigenetic modulator for recalcitrant tumors of the breast. After a course of Ivermectin, the tumor cells became responsive to tamoxifen, which makes Ivermectin a good adjunct in the treatment of multiple drug resistant cancers.

- Kwon Y.J., Petrie K., Leibovitch B.A., Zeng L., Mezei M., Howell L., Gil V., Christova R., Bansal N., Yang S., Sharma R., Ariztia E.V., Frankum J., Brough R., Sbirkov Y., Ashworth A., Lord C.J., Zelent A., Farias E., Zhou M.M., Waxman S. Selective Inhibition of SIN3 Corepressor with Avermectins as a Novel Therapeutic Strategy in Triple-Negative Breast Cancer. *Mol Cancer Ther.* 2015;14(8):1824–1836. doi: 10.1158/1535-7163.MCT-14-0980-T.

Recent studies have also found that Ivermectin could promote the death of tumor cells by regulating the tumor microenvironment in breast cancer. This means that Ivermectin is not only cytotoxic to the cancer cells but also acts by regulating the tumor environment, which encourages the death of the cancer cells.

- Draganov D., Gopalakrishna-Pillai S., Chen Y.R., Zuckerman N., Moeller S., Wang C., Ann D., Lee P.P. Modulation of P2X4/P2X7/Pannexin-1 sensitivity to extracellular ATP via Ivermectin induces a non-apoptotic and inflammatory form of cancer cell death. *Sci Rep.* 2015;5:16222. doi: 10.1038/srep16222
- https://www.ncbi.nlm.nih.gov/pmc/articles/PMC7505114/#bib0185

Colorectal-cancer

In a study that screened the Wnt pathway inhibitors, IVM (Ivermectin) inhibited the proliferation of multiple cancers, including the colorectal cancer cell lines CC14, CC36, DLD1 and Ls174 T and promoted apoptosis by blocking the Wnt pathway. After intervention with IVM, the expression of Caspase-3 in DLD1 and Ls174 T cells increased, indicating that Ivermectin has an apoptosis-inducing effect and inhibits the expression of the downstream genes AXIN2, LGR5, and ASCL2 in the Wnt/β-catenin pathway.

- Melotti A., Mas C., Kuciak M., Lorente-Trigos A., Borges I., Ruiz i Altaba A. The river blindness drug Ivermectin and related macrocyclic lactones inhibit WNT-TCF pathway responses in human cancer. *EMBO Mol Med.* 2014;6(10):1263–1278. doi: 10.15252/emmm.201404084.

Case study

A young 35-year-old male, who was diagnosed with advanced colorectal cancer with secondaries to the liver was brought to me for help with his cancer. He was on chemotherapy under the state hospital. He looked moribund and confused. He was told by the hospital that his prognosis was poor and he was given three weeks to live. He was forced by his employers to take 2 Pfizer vaccines. I suspect that he developed turbo-cancer after the vaccine. He was perfectly healthy before he took the vaccine.

I put him on a course of Ivermectin and Chlorine Dioxide. I also put him on a course of Vit D3, K2 and Vit C.

I followed him up two weeks later. His sister, very gratefully, informed me that by day three he was feeling much better; he was eating and coming back to his senses.

I was pleasantly surprised to hear that he returned to work in three weeks. His doctors were amazed by his miraculous recovery. The family did not inform the hospital that I had used Ivermectin to treat him to protect me from being gas-lit by the state health authorities. I was pleased to hear that, after three months of my treatment, the tumor in his liver had shrunk from 13 cm to 1 cm. He felt extremely grateful that he had turned the corner and that he was on the road to recovery.

I saw him a year later, looking completely well without a trace of being ill. I added Chlorine dioxide to his treatment.

Ivermectin was found to be effective in treating gastric cancers, hepatocellular carcinoma, and urinary tract carcinomas.

- https://www.ncbi.nlm.nih.gov/pmc/articles/PMC7505114/#bib0220

The presence of the mitochondrial fuel acetyl-L-carnitine (ALCAR) and the antioxidant N-acetyl-L-cysteine (NAC) could reverse IVM-induced inhibition. Patients with cancer should not take ALCAR or

NAC if Ivermectin is going to be administered to treat the cancer.

Haematological cancer

In an experiment designed to screen potential drugs for the treatment of leukemia, Ivermectin preferentially killed leukemia cells at low concentrations without affecting normal hematopoietic cells.

- https://pubmed.ncbi.nlm.nih.gov/20644115

Cervical Cancer

Cervical cancer is one of the most common gynecologic malignancies, resulting in approximately 530,000 new cases and 270,000 deaths worldwide annually. The majority of cervical cancers are caused by human papillomavirus (HPV) infection.

- https://doi.org/10.1080%2F21691401.2019.1664560

Ivermectin has been proven to significantly inhibit the proliferation and migration of HeLa cells and promote apoptosis. After intervention with Ivermectin, the cell cycle of HeLa cells was blocked at the G1/S phase, and the cells showed typical morphological changes related to apoptosis.

- https://www.ncbi.nlm.nih.gov/pmc/articles/PMC6496724/

Case study

A 50-year-old female came to see me for a knee injury, looking very ill. She informed me that she was diagnosed with stage II cervical cancer. She was very despondent and was due to go for chemotherapy. I put her on a 5-day course of Ivermectin.

I received a report from her relative that she improved significantly. She regained her appetite and was able to perform her household chores without much difficulty. I am awaiting the report from her treating doctors in the hospital.

Ovarian cancer

Ovarian cancer is a highly malignant tumor with hardly any clinical symptoms. It has a 5-year survival rate of 47%.

- https://www.ncbi.nlm.nih.gov/pmc/articles/PMC6334391/

Ivermectin could block the cell cycle and induce cell apoptosis through a KPNB1-dependent mechanism in ovarian cancer.

Interestingly, Ivermectin and Paclitaxel have a synergistic effect on ovarian cancer, and the combined treatment in vivo experiments almost completely inhibited tumor growth.

- https://www.ncbi.nlm.nih.gov/pmc/articles/PMC7505114/#bib0295

Respiratory system

Nasopharyngeal carcinoma is a malignant tumor derived from epithelial cells of the nasopharyngeal mucosa. The incidence is regional and familial, and Epstein-Barr virus (EBV) infection is closely related to the cancer.

- https://pubmed.ncbi.nlm.nih.gov/31178151

In a study that screened drugs for the treatment of nasopharyngeal cancer, Ivermectin significantly inhibited the development of nasopharyngeal carcinoma in mice at doses that were not toxic to normal thymocytes.

- https://pubmed.ncbi.nlm.nih.gov/30233143

Case study

An oncologist from the US heard about me from a US podcaster and wanted to know about using Ivermectin for cancer. I shared my experiences with her, and how I used Ivermectin and the dosage.

She texted me about 6 weeks later to tell me about a 7-year-old boy, who was sent home with terminal nasopharyngeal carcinoma by the hospital with no hope of recovering. She put him on a course of Ivermectin and within a few weeks she found that his cancer had regressed considerably; he could breathe and sleep better. She was confident that he was going to make a full recovery.

LONG COVID

I have treated approximately 3,000 patients with COVID in under three years and I have not had a single case of Long COVID, COVID-19 sequelae. I do not believe Long COVID exists. Thus far there isn't a definite group of symptoms to describe Long COVID.

One of the reasons that I did not see Long COVID in any of my patients, most probably, was because I used high doses of Ivermectin liberally and early. The spike protein of the virus was trapped by Ivermectin before it reached the rest of the body to cause an autoimmune response and the symptoms of Long COVID. Many South Africans recovered from COVID without any medical intervention so frontline doctors did not see many cases of COVID.

PSYCHIATRIC CONDITIONS MISDIAGNOSED

I saw a number of patients who presented to me with panic attacks and depression; they presented with symptoms of tiredness, lethargy and body aches. Their symptoms resolved completely after their mental conditions were appropriately dealt with. Many patients needed reassurance that they no longer had COVID.

Patients felt totally relieved when they were reassured that their tiredness was due to anxiety or depression because many feared ending up with long COVID or dying from COVID.

The reasons for the high incidence of what is regarded as long COVID by some doctors in the US and the UK is most probably because Ivermectin and other repurposed drugs were not widely used in these countries.

Symptoms of Long COVID are most likely caused by the spike from the vaccine, which has a greater chance of dispersing throughout the body after it is injected into the deltoid muscle, than the spike of the Coronavirus, which is trapped by the respiratory mucosa in the lungs before it could get a chance to reach the rest of the body. Furthermore, the artificial molecule, N1-methyl pseudouridine to replace uridine in the spike of the mRNA vaccine, to make the vaccine stable, seems to make the mRNA vaccine almost indestructible to prolong its side effects in the body.

I have treated one patient with severe brain fog and short-term memory loss after she took the jab. I treated her with SSRI's, Ivermectin, Vitamin D3 for about six months and she eventually made a full recovery.

It would seem many people with long term vaccine injury symptoms are being mislabeled as suffering from Long COVID. We must bear in mind that the COVID virus is first arrested in the mucosa of the upper respiratory tract, then at the level of the lungs; they rarely land in other parts of the body.

The mRNA vaccine, on the other hand as mentioned above, can and does reach all parts of the body within six hours because only about 25% of the vaccine remains in the deltoid; the remaining 75% enters the bloodstream with the aid of the lipid Nanoparticle, which is the toxic carrier of the mRNA vaccine.

EXPERT WITNESS FOR INDIVIDUALS REFUSING THE VACCINE

My knowledge and experience with COVID and the vaccine over the first two years saw me ending up in the CCMA (Council for Conciliation, Mediation and Arbitration) to present evidence as an expert witness on behalf of employees, who were being threatened by their employers with dismissal for refusing to take the vaccine. I presented over 50 hours of evidence in three cases for about six people. My main argument, based on my experience, was that if we treated COVID-19 early with Ivermectin and other repurposed drugs, there would have been no need for a vaccine and no need for the pandemic to be declared.

We won one case. The one case that we lost is being contested by our attorney at the labor courts, which is higher than the CCMA. We feel we were unfairly prejudiced by the commissioner because he refused to accept my evidence as relevant. He relied on the evidence of a relationship officer who neither had any medical training nor an understanding of the law with regards to COVID.

SOCIAL MEDIA'S ACTION TO DEPLATFORM ME DID NOT STOP ME FROM GETTING MY MESSAGE ACROSS TO THE WORLD

When I started witnessing the phenomenal success that I was having with my approach to treat patients with severe COVID pneumonia, I wanted to share my successes with the general public and my colleagues. It came as a great disappointment to me to learn that social media platforms like Facebook and YouTube deplatformed me. My successful treatments for COVID were described by social media's medically untrained fact-checkers as being against community guidelines; a view that I vehemently opposed but there was little I could do to be reinstated. I found it extremely bizarre why social media categorized my videos of genuine hope as being against community guidelines.

Several independent media channels and community stations came to my rescue. I was interviewed on several occasions by Ms. Shabnam Palesa Mohamed on her channels with other doctors to share my experiences about my successful treatment of patients with severe COVID.

I later appeared as a guest on several independent Internet media channels, internationally, to share my successes. These included the FLCCC, the World Council for Health, Child Health Defense, and several podcasters from the US and Canada.

Lovinglifetv.com COMES TO MY RESCUE

One of my greatest platforms was lovinglifetv.com. They offered me a forum page on their platform to post all my memes, articles and videos on their channel. I wrote a memo a day to counter the false narrative dished out by the mainstream media. The producer of the show, Mr. Scott Balson and I developed a wonderful and cordial relationship over the next three years. His channel had a following of over 1 million people. Scott was an outstanding journalist who was totally unafraid to tell the truth, something that the mainstream media would not touch. He earned the great respect of his many followers in South Africa and in other parts of the world.

Mr. Scott Balson together with doctors like me and other activists presented the truth to the world on COVID and the vaccine, on his Internet channel for three years, to counter the false narrative that was being dished out on a daily basis by the captured mainstream media.

One Friday afternoon I was invited by Pastor Wendy McDonald of the Good Hope Christian Centre to do a talk on COVID at their church that evening. I was a bit reluctant because I had heard that most of the religious organizations were promoting the vaccine, so I didn't think that they would be happy to hear my controversial views on the subject. To my surprise, they convinced me that they are open to the truth and alternative views.

That evening, after I presented my talk to the packed congregation of 3000 members and 60,000 viewers, I was pleasantly surprised that

I received a standing ovation and a great deal of praise from Pastor Wendy for my work. I was deeply touched when she honored me as one of the heroes of COVID at a ceremony in her church before Christmas, 2022.

For the next two years, I was invited on a regular basis to talk about several other related issues to her members. Through these invitations, our friendship grew steadily. Pastor Wendy stood out as a woman of great courage with an unshakable conviction to pursue the truth, regardless of the costs.

She allowed our health committee to use her church venue to host our first ever health justice conference in Cape Town in September 2023. The conference was a huge success, which went worldwide. She broadcast the conference to all the members of her five churches in South Africa and her sister churches in the UK, EU and US. Nothing was too much for her to help a good cause. I sincerely hope more religious leaders in the world would follow her footsteps and pursue the truth with the tenacity of Pastor Wendy MacDonald.

When the mainstream media and social media shunned me for my views on Ivermectin, I wrote a poem extolling the wonders of Ivermectin entitled, "Incredible IVY" to beat the banning. I managed to upload the poem on my YouTube channel shortly before I was totally deplatformed. In this poem, I cleverly explain how Ivermectin worked and saved lives as a tribute to Scientists, Dr. Omura and Dr. Campbell for their discovery.

CONCLUSION

The COVID epidemic in the past three years has been the most challenging but exciting experience in my entire 45-year career as a medical doctor. I learned a lot about a totally new disease, which afforded me the wonderful opportunity to put my mind to the test and come up with unique solutions by thinking out of the box. I had the courage to challenge narratives that dismally failed humanity and came up with simple, affordable, safe solutions that worked and saved thousands of lives in South Africa and the rest of the world. Ivermectin played a significant role for me to treat COVID successfully.

Working in a poor economic area with a 50% unemployment rate, I was compelled to find the cheapest and safest solutions to save thousands of people from dying through this serious disease. I am pleased that I found a solution when our hospitals with their sophisticated expensive technology were failing dismally to save patients with COVID. I would not have been able to achieve a high success rate of 99.97% during the deadly Delta strain infection if I did not have free access to Ivermectin.

While hospitals were losing patients in droves, I was saving my patients with the least amount of effort and cost. My work which was recognized by a few fellow doctors here and doctors overseas, as well as by people all over the world, my work was unfortunately never mentioned at all in our mainstream media.

I worked long hours, read a lot, listened to numerous lectures, and educated myself to the best of my ability about the new mRNA technology. This enabled me to advise my patients about the COVID vaccines as accurately as possible as the information about the vaccines emerged daily. I was guided by my conscience and my oath, and I was unafraid to speak the truth. I was pleased to share my knowledge and experience of my successful treatments and discoveries with audiences throughout the world. I was extremely delighted by the wonderful support I received from my very few colleagues and members of the public for my work during one of humanity's greatest challenges for its survival. I did not do anything for fame, nor did I see myself as a hero. I would be satisfied to be remembered amongst the small band of ethical doctors from around the world, who served humanity in its darkest hour, guided by our conscience and our Hippocratic Oath to the best of our ability. We did so at a time, when society was so terribly let down by our medical establishments, health authorities and leaders, and at a time when the careers of ethical doctors were being severely threatened for coming to the aid of humanity in its hour of need.

My success would not have been possible if I did not have easy access to an array of inexpensive, effective, and safe repurposed drugs like Ivermectin, Hydroxychloroquine and several other allopathic and complementary medicines to achieve a 99.97% success treating some of the most ill patients with COVID.

It did not bother me that mainstream media completely ignored my experiences nor that I was deplatformed by major social media platforms for speaking the truth. I managed to get my message to hundreds of thousands of people throughout the world through other independent platforms.

I am eternally grateful to the number of great doctors who shared their knowledge so willingly on this complex topic and to the thousands of well-wishers who supported me throughout this pandemic, which enabled me to carry out my work with the least amount of hindrance. I wish to express my sincere gratitude to the many patients, who trusted me implicitly with their life in one of the most challenging times in our history. Their faith in me gave me the will and confidence to conquer this disease. I have had several wonderful patients, who supported me and prayed for my health and safety by always wishing me well in my quest for justice.

I was touched by the overwhelming support I had from the public.

One patient that stands out for me is Benedict Bergman, who has left an indelible mark in my mind. She was the first patient I treated over the phone for COVID. She was an absolutely remarkable person.

Chapter 15   Ivermectin Saved My Patients with Severe COVID and the Vaccine Injured

She became my bedrock of support when things got tough. We still remain in touch with each other. I treasure her friendship and the friendships of hundreds of other patients like her for their support of my work. It was their confidence in me that gave me the strength to go on.

The success that I achieved to tame one of the worst health crises in modern times was only possible because of the unwavering support I had from my wife Joan, who held the fort for me. Her intervention allowed me to help hordes of desperate patients that urgently needed my attention. She kept the demanding difficult people out of my way so that I could treat patients unimpeded.

My receptionist Natalie and my daughter Tammy were equally exceptional in how they molded themselves for this mammoth task and acquitted themselves brilliantly.

I wish to express my sincere gratitude to Dr. Satoshi Omura and Dr. William Campbell for discovering Ivermectin, which I would consider to be one of the greatest discoveries in medicine.

Even though COVID might be over, we have a bigger challenge and that is the expotential rise in turbo cancers especially in the heavily vaccinated west. The successes I have had from treating very advanced cancers with Ivermectin leaves me convinced that the role of Ivermectin to treat cancers affordably and successively will secure the role of this drug in the future, regardless of the opposition to this drug by big pharma, vested interests, and corrupt academics.

I sincerely hope that one day the entire medical profession will acknowledge Ivermectin as one of the greatest drugs to be discovered and give the two doctors, who discovered it, the just recognition that they so rightly deserve.

My final thoughts on the subject are that a pandemic should not have been declared if we adopted the right approach to treat COVID

443

early with Ivermectin. We could have saved so many lives and the economies of so many countries. Something went horribly wrong during this crisis, and it should never ever be repeated.

Chapter 15   Ivermectin Saved My Patients with Severe COVID and the Vaccine Injured

E.V. Rapiti, MBBS; FCFP; DCH; DMH; Naep Asthma (Dip); MBA

Qualified 1977 with an MBBS;

Other qualifications: Family medicine FCFP; Mental health(DMH) Child Health(DCH) NAEP Dip (Asthma); MBA (Health policy).

Currently practicing as a family physician in Mitchells Plain, Cape Town, South Africa for the past 41 years.

Main focus is lifestyle medicine.

Other interests: Addiction counseling, did module on Opioid management.

Treated over 3,000 patients for Covid with a 99.97% success rate using Ivermectin and other repurposed drugs.

Treated a number COVID vaccine injuries and cancer using Ivermectin.

Developed my own clinical symptoms to make a diagnosis of COVID pneumonia in under three minutes, with the use of X-rays or Scans.

Author of the book: "4 Steps 2 Healing" – a simple self-help book to help substance users and their families to cope with addiction..

Wrote over 5,000 motivational sayings.

Wrote over 700 memes on COVID.

Gives talks at churches and schools on addiction and health issues.

Motivational speaker, regular guest on a number of independent channels about my work on COVID.

Loves reading, good theatre, tranquil music.

Is busy writing a book of his experiences during COVID.

Happily married with two children.

Producer's Note

Japan

Kenji TORII

Producer's Note
And Yet it Works

*A small amount of light pushes away
a large amount of darkness.*
— Dr. Zev Zelenko, July 16, 2020

The great discovery came from Japanese soil. In 1974, Satoshi Ōmura, an Emeritus Professor of Kitasato University (head of the antibiotics division at the Kitasato Institute at that time), collected and isolated a new type of actinomycete from the soil near a golf course in Kawana, Ito City, Shizuoka Prefecture, and discovered the compound Streptomyces avermectinius, an Avermectin-producing bacterium. 2024 marks the 50th anniversary of this discovery, leading to the development of Ivermectin.[1]

In 2021, I decided that a book on Ivermectin needed to be published, and together with journalist Eiichiro Ishiyama, I accepted the role of publication producer and outside editor. Thanks to the full cooperation of Kitasato University and Prof. Satoshi Ōmura in this effort, the Japanese book of "IVERMECTIN - Can Ivermectin become the savior of COVID-19 treatment?" was published by Kawade Shobo Shinsha in December 2021.

The book became a bestseller in the medical book category and received high reviews on Amazon. It was also selected as a "book chosen by the School Library Association."

I should have visited Prof. Ōmura to greet him before

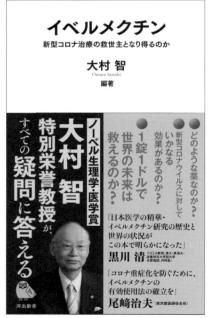

Figure1. "IVERMECTIN - Can Ivermectin become the savior of COVID-19 treatment?"

the book was published, but unfortunately I had to be rude to him due to the COVID-19 pandemic. It was only on April 14, 2023, when I became fortunate enough to meet Prof. Ōmura.

It was a unique opportunity, so I asked doctors from around the world who were saving patients' lives with Ivermectin, "Do you have anything you'd like to say?" I had received a passionate message full of respect and gratitude from the 'Seven Samurai' in the US, Brazil, India, and Africa (the authors of this book, including Dr. Paul Marik, Dr. Flávio Cadegiani, Dr. Jackie Stone, Prof. Colleen Aldous and Dr. E.V. Rapiti).

I translated this and visited the Ōmura Satoshi Memorial Institute at Kitasato University in Tokyo. Although we didn't have much time, I read their messages in front of Prof. Ōmura.He had been listening carefully for a long time, said humbly, "I'm not the only one who helped," and said, "I want to thank everyone." Not too long after that, the Samurai received the following thank-you letters:

Dear friends

Mr. Kenji Torii, the representative of TigerGyroscope, delivered your messages and the latest information.

Your single-minded dedication to medical care in the face of various obstacles deserves praise. Beyond the high mountain, you will find true victory. We are also organizing various pieces of information to provide people with the appropriate information.

I sincerely hope that the day will soon come when all of humankind across the globe will have access to equal and compassionate medical care.

I wish you all good health and great success in your future.

— Satoshi Ōmura, Ph.D.

In the opening conversation found in the quarterly magazine "DOU", published in October 2023, Prof. Ōmura told a very interesting story about his experience with Ivermectin which I would like to share with you here:

> *I got sick with COVID-19 in July, and then recovered in one go once I took Ivermectin. My body temperature was high as my fever climbed, and the antigen test showed that I was fully infected with COVID-19, so I took Ivermectin that night, and I already had a normal temperature by the next morning. It was the first time I took medicine that I made myself. I can now say with confidence that it actually works.*[2]

During the four years of the pandemic, I spent days researching various pieces of information about Ivermectin on social media. There has been a common theory that Ivermectin is ineffective in treating COVID-19, and that it is unsafe and harmful. However, the testimonies of clinicians on the front lines who actually prescribe Ivermectin are quite the opposite of the news in the major media. They all professed, without exception, that Ivermectin was effective against COVID-19.

However, none of the doctors who prescribed Ivermectin to their patients for the treatment of COVID-19 were praised for saving their

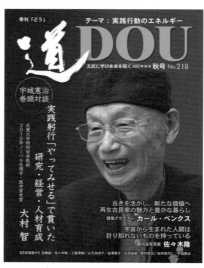

Figure2. the quarterly magazine "DOU"

lives. Rather, there were those who were dismissed from hospitals, deprived of their medical licenses, and sued in court by the Medical Commission were subjected to social sanctions and persecution.

After compiling the testimonies of clinicians from around the world, I was determined in the belief that we must 1) clarify Ivermectin's usefulness and safety, 2) restore the honor of the persecuted doctors, and 3) keep records for future generations. It should not be a world where honesty does not pay.

One of the authors of this book, Dr. E.V. Rapiti, a family doctor from Cape Town, South Africa, gave me the following message while we were planning:

We need to record our successes in a world gone mad. Writing a book of this nature is essential to record our history. There has been a deliberate attempt to discredit the drug. If the public reads it, I have no doubt it will make a difference.

I believe that this book is as important today as when physicist Galileo Galilei published his famous book "Dialogue Concerning the Two Chief World Systems" in which he advocated for the 'heliocentric theory' at a time when the geocentric theory dominated.

If the book is read by future generations 100 years from now, readers will surely understand the foolishness of the human beings who lived 100 years before.

Lastly, articles and research showing that Ivermectin is effective against COVID-19 have already been sent out from the beginning of the pandemic, and the research that has been gaining attention recently will also be kept here as a record.

[CASE 1]

The following is quoted from Chapter 1, "The old and new story of Ivermectin" (written by Satoshi Ōmura) of the book "IVERMECTIN - Can Ivermectin become the savior of COVID-19 treatment?," edited by Satoshi Ōmura:

I received a letter from Dr. Hiroshi Maruta, who is doing research in Australia, saying that Ivermectin could be used as a medicine for COVID-19 and used for treatment. This was around March 2020, when nobody had even talked about the efficacy of Ivermectin on COVID-19.

Dr. Maruta pointed out that Ivermectin inhibits a substance called PAK1 kinase or Diddy's kinase, which transmits signals when viruses bind to receptors and enter cells. Kinase levels increase when the body is infected with bacteria or cancer, and this inhibits immune function. When this happens, antibodies can no longer be produced, leaving the body unable to stop the virus. The proposed mechanism of action was that the body's immunity is restored, leading to production of antibodies, and blocking of the virus when the action of PAK1 kinase is inhibited by administering Ivermectin.[3]

In addition, Hiroshi Maruta, a doctor of pharmaceutical sciences, published the article, entitled "COVID-19: Can be prevented/treated with PAK blockers such as propolis and malaria wonder drugs!," on January 26, 2020 and was one of the first to publish an article.[4]

Prof. Hiroshi Maruta also sent a letter by email to The New York Times urging the WHO, the NIH, and other medical institutions around the world to consider the PAK1 inhibitor Ivermectin, which blocks PAK1, as an effective treatment for COVID-19 infections. Prof. Maruta said he did not receive any reply from the newspaper.[5]

Producer's Note   And Yet it Works

[CASE 2]

On April 24, 2020, the Dominican Republic's "DR1 News" reported on the success of Ivermectin treatment with the headline "Ivermectin is a winner treating COVID-19 patients in DR." [6]

Dr. Johnny Tavarez, a neurologist at the Bournigal Medical Center in Puerto Plata, says that 100% of all the patients treated at the clinic for COVID-19 with Ivermectin have recovered. He says many have made quick recoveries.

Dr. José Natalio Redondo, a cardiologist and founder of the National Network of Medical Services 'RESCUE GROUP' that oversees the medical center, stated on "Dominican Today" (November 30, 2020):

Our results were immediate; the use of Ivermectin, together with Azithromycin and Zinc (plus the usual vitamins that tend to increase the immune response of individuals) produced an impressive variation in the course of the disease; it was demonstrated that 99.3% of the patients recovered quickly when the treatment was started in the first five days of proven symptoms, with an average of 3.5 days, and a fall of more than 50% in the rate and duration of hospitalizations, and reducing from 9 to 1 the mortality rate, when the treatment was started on time.[7]

[CASE 3]

As for Ivermectin in India, Uttar Pradesh (UP state), the most populous state in India with an estimated population of 241 million (as of 2021), the drug was officially approved statewide for the prevention/treatment of COVID-19 in August 2020, starting with the state capital of Agra.[8]

It's undeniable that Ivermectin-based early treatment has made a significant contribution to eradicating COVID-19, such as when 48 districts declared themselves COVID-19-free with a case-positive rate

455

of 0.01% and a recovery rate of 98.7% in UP state.[9]

It's also worth noting that the UP state government's COVID-19 strategy was highly praised and actively supported, including by having WHO field officers accompany the district medical team that visited door-to-door distributing medicine kits (Ivermectin, Doxycycline, Vitamin D, Vitamin C, Vitamin B, Zinc and Paracetamol).[10, 11, 12]

However, the major media outlets were imposing press controls, and as a result had not taken up reporting on any of these successes in India. Even the following official announcement from the Uttar Pradesh state government that the early use of Ivermectin has resulted in low positivity rates and low mortality rates was withheld by the major media:

The Uttar Pradesh government has claimed that it was the first state to have introduced a large-scale "prophylactic and therapeutic" use of Ivermectin and added that the drug helped the state to maintain a lower fatality and positivity rate as compared to other states.[13]

Furthermore, Ivermectin administration to COVID-19 patients had already been tried in Kerala in April 2020, a step earlier than in Uttar Pradesh.

According to the report at the time, a 62-year-old woman from Pathanamthitta, who had been on COVID-19 treatment for 45 days, received Ivermectin every three days starting from April 14, and later tested negative. The Kerala health authority said the 62-year-old woman living in Pathanamthitta had recovered after taking Ivermectin.[14, 15]

In addition, the little-known "White paper on Ivermectin as a potential therapy for COVID-19" was published in India in July 2020 and posted on the official WHO website. The conclusions reached by the Indian doctors were consistent and very clear:

After critical panel discussion, all the attending doctors came to a conclusion that Ivermectin can be a potential molecule for prophylaxis and treatment of people infected with Coronavirus, owing to its anti-viral properties coupled with effective cost, availability and good tolerability and safety.[16, 17]

[CASE 4]

In April 2023, the Kitasato University Medical Center and the Ōmura Satoshi Memorial Institute published a very interesting study in "The Journal of Antibiotics":

The results of the present study demonstrate oral administration of ivermectin prior to SARS-CoV-2 infection in hamsters was associated with decreased weight loss and pulmonary inflammation. In addition, the administration of Ivermectin reduced pulmonary viral titers and mRNA expression level of pro-inflammatory cytokines associated with severe COVID-19 disease. The administration of Ivermectin rapidly induced the production of virus-specific neutralizing antibodies in the late stage of viral infection.[18]

[CASE 5]

In support of this research, on April 18 of the same year, at the 33rd European Congress of Clinical Microbiology and Infectious Diseases (ECCMID) in Copenhagen, the French company MedinCell presented the results of the SAIVE trial (n=399). The results of this 'gold-standard' randomized, double-blind, placebo-controlled trial (RCT) showed a 72% reduction in COVID-19 infections in the Ivermectin group, indicating safety and tolerability.[19, 20]

Prof. Colleen Aldous of KwaZulu-Natal University in South Africa, who is also a co-author of this publication, praised the SAIVE study by saying, "This is the best quality RCT we have yet seen published on Ivermectin." [21]

They also proposed the Totality of Evidence-Based Medicine (T- EBM) Wheel. A T-EBM wheel analysis of peer-reviewed reports on Ivermectin treatment revealed that "on closer examination of each paper, most show signals for efficacy." [22]

[CASE 6]

In January 2024, the peer-reviewed journal "Lung India" published a paper by a research team consisting of members from a university and hospital in the state of Uttar Pradesh and from the All India Institute of Medical Science (AIIMS) in New Delhi.

The paper states that in a retrospective study that included 101 COVID-19 patients with comorbidities who were hospitalized from April 2021 to April 2022, Ivermectin showed promise in terms of increasing survival rates:

COVID-19 patients who were given tocilizumab had a higher risk of death than those who were not given tocilizumab. Nonetheless, Ivermectin (P value = 0.035) and prednisolone (P value = 0.036) exhibited a statistically significant probability of survival in COVID-19 patients.

Thus, it has been suggested that treatment with Ivermectin at an early stage of infection could reduce the viral load, shorten illness, and prevent transmission.[23]

Acknowledgements

I would like to express my sincere gratitude to the clinicians who kindly agreed to contribute to the publication of this book amidst their busy daily practice. This publication would not have been possible without the dedicated support of Dr. Paul Marik, who kindly agreed to edit the book, and the authors of each chapter. I eagerly hope that the knowledge and evidence of doctors backed up by their clinical experience will save as many lives as possible.

Above all, I would like to thank Prof. Satoshi Ōmura, one of the makers of the 'Wonder drug' Ivermectin, from the bottom of my heart and with great respect, for his unshakable strong spirit, courage to face hardship, and untiring devotion full of compassion, which give great encouragement, pride, and hope to humanity.

Furthermore, I would like to thank Mr. Eiichiro Ishiyama of Nantosha Co., Ltd. who has worked with me since the planning stage of this book, for his patience and support. I would also like to take this opportunity to thank all those who have supported the publication of this book.

— I dedicate my heartfelt condolences to all those who were eagerly awaiting treatment with Ivermectin but were denied a prescription and regrettably died. —

References

1. The life and career of Professor Satoshi Ōmura, SATOSHI ŌMURA MUSEUM,
   <https://omura-museum.yamanashi.ac.jp/en/profile/>
2. Opening conversation, Everything is about being useful to others, October 2023, Quarterly Magazine "DOU" (Dou Publishing), No. 218, p8,
   <https://www.dou-shuppan.com/dou218-lp/>
3. Edited by Satoshi Ōmura, IVERMECTIN - Can Ivermectin become the savior of COVID-19 treatment?, December 2021, Kawade Shobo Shinsha, p.50,
   <https://www.kawade.co.jp/np/isbn/9784309631424/>
4. Hiroshi Maruta, COVID-19: Can be prevented/treated with PAK blockers such as propolis and malaria wonder drugs!, 26 January 2020,
   <http://osaka20420.blogspot.com/2020/01/pak.html>
5. Hiroshi Maruta, A Letter to New York Times (2020) : 'PAK1-blockers' against Coronaviral Pandemic, 3 February 2020,

<http://osaka20420.blogspot.com/2020/02/a-letter-to-new-york-times-2020-therapy.html>

6. Dolores Vicioso, Ivermectin is a winner treating Covid-19 patients in DR, 24 April 2020, DR1 News,
<https://dr1.com/news/2020/04/24/ivermectin-is-a-winner-treating-covid-19-patients-in-dr/>

7. Doctor explains 99.3% of COVID-19 patients treated with Ivermectin recovered in five days, 30 November 2020, Dominican Today,
<https://dominicantoday.com/dr/local/2020/11/30/doctor-explains-99-3-of-covid-19-patients-treated-with-ivermectin-recovered-in-five-days/>

8. Deepak Lavania, UP approves use of anti-parasite drug for Covid treatment and prevention, 8 August 2020, The Times of India,
<https://timesofindia.indiatimes.com/city/agra/up-approves-use-of-anti-parasite-drug-for-covid-treatment-prevention/articleshow/77420726.cms>

9. Sharangee Dutta, 48 districts of Uttar Pradesh declared Covid-free; Agra, Ayodhya included, 14 November 2021, Hindustan Times,
<https://www.hindustantimes.com/cities/lucknow-news/48-districts-of-uttar-pradesh-declared-covid-free-agra-ayodhya-included-101636896436280.html>

10. Shailvee Sharda, WHO lauds UP's contact tracing measures for coronavirus control, 14 November 2020, The Times Of India,
<https://timesofindia.indiatimes.com/city/lucknow/who-lauds-ups-contact-tracing-measures-for-coronavirus-control/articleshow/79217186.cms>

11. UTTAR PRADESH Going the last mile to stop COVID-19, 7 May 2021, The World Health Organization,
<https://www.who.int/india/news/feature-stories/detail/uttar-pradesh-going-the-last-mile-to-stop-covid-19>

12. Christine Clark, Home isolation and ivermectin-based treatment kits, 21 May 2021, Medical Update Online,
<https://medicalupdateonline.com/2021/05/home-isolation-and-ivermectin-based-treatment-kits/>

13. Maulshree Seth, Uttar Pradesh government says early use of Ivermectin helped to keep positivity, deaths low, 12 May 2021, The Indian EXPRESS,
<https://indianexpress.com/article/cities/lucknow/uttar-pradesh-government-says-ivermectin-helped-to-keep-deaths-low-7311786/>

14. Pathanamthitta native tests negative for COVID-19 after 45 days, 24 April 2020, Mathrubhumi News,
<https://english.mathrubhumi.com/news/kerala/pathanamthitta-native-tests-negative-for-covid-19-after-45-days-1.4713388>

15. കോവിഡ് പ്രതിരോധത്തിൽ പ്രതീക്ഷയായി Ivermectin; പത്തനംതിട്ടയിലും മരുന്ന് ഉപയോഗിച്ച് ഫലം കണ്ടു, 23 April 2020, News18 Kerala,
<https://www.youtube.com/watch?v=tPMPWChqV-g>

16. Agam Vora, V.K. Arora, D. Behera, Surya Kant Tripathy, White paper on Ivermectin as a potential therapy for COVID-19, July 2020, Indian Journal of Tuberculosis,
<https://www.sciencedirect.com/science/article/pii/S0019570720301025>

17. WHO recognises white paper on ivermectin, 7 October 2020, The Daily Pioneer,
    <https://www.dailypioneer.com/uploads/2020/epaper/october/lucknow-english-edition-2020-10-07.pdf>
18. Takayuki Uematsu, Tomomi Takano, Hidehito Matsui, Noritada Kobayashi, Satoshi Ōmura, Hideaki Hanaki, Prophylactic administration of ivermectin attenuates SARS-CoV-2 induced disease in a Syrian Hamster Model, 25 April 2023, The Journal of Antibiotics (2023) 76:481-488,
    <https://www.nature.com/articles/s41429-023-00623-0.pdf>
19. MedinCell announces positive results for the SAIVE clinical study in prevention of Covid-19 infection in a contact-based population, 5 January 2023, MedinCell
    <https://www.medincell.com/wp-content/uploads/2024/03/20230105_PR-results-TTG-VF-EN.pdf>,
    <https://www.businesswire.com/news/home/20230105005896/en/MedinCell-Announces-Positive-Results-for-the-SAIVE-Clinical-Study-in-Prevention-of-Covid-19-Infection-in-a-Contact-Based-Population>
20. Violaine Desort-Henin, Anna Kostova, Elmozafar Ahmed Babiker, Audrey Caramel, Richard Malamut, The SAIVE Trial, Post-Exposure use of ivermectin in Covid-19 prevention: Efficacy and Safety Results, 18 April 2023, MedinCell
    <https://www.medincell.com/wp-content/uploads/2024/03/Poster-SAIVE-April2023-OK3.pdf>
21. Colleen Aldous, Phillip Oldfield, Large, well-designed randomised control study shows Ivermectin efficacy in preventing and treating COVID-19, 23 January 2023, Biz News,
    <https://www.biznews.com/health/2023/01/23/ivermectin-efficacy>
22. Colleen Aldous, Philip Oldfield, Jerome Dancis, Barry Dancis, The Totality of EBM still points to the efficacy of ivermectin in COVID-19: The Totality of Evidence–Based Medicine Wheel, 27 October 2022, Biz News,
    <https://www.biznews.com/health/2022/10/27/ivermectin-ebm>
23. Azmat Karim, Mohammad Shameem, Anjana Talwar, Deepak Talwar, Impact of comorbidities and inflammatory markers on mortality of COVID-19 patients, 01 January 2024, Lung India, 41(1):p 40-46, Jan–Feb 2024,
    <https://journals.lww.com/lungindia/fulltext/2024/41010/impact_of_comorbidities_and_inflammatory_markers.8.aspx>

Appendix

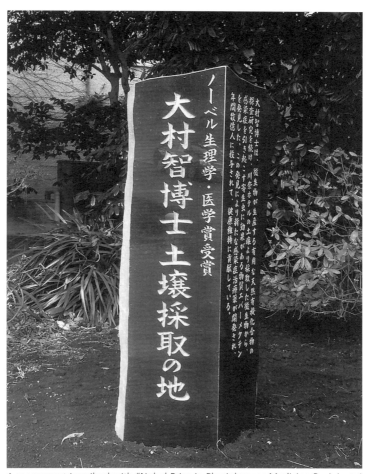

A monument inscribed with "Nobel Prize in Physiology or Medicine Recipient / Dr. Satoshi Ōmura's Soil Sampling Site" on the front. The side of the monument details that from the substance Avermectin, discovered by Dr. Ōmura from soil microorganisms, new treatments for infectious diseases have been developed, contributing to the health maintenance of hundreds of millions of people annually.
©Kawanahotel Golfcourse

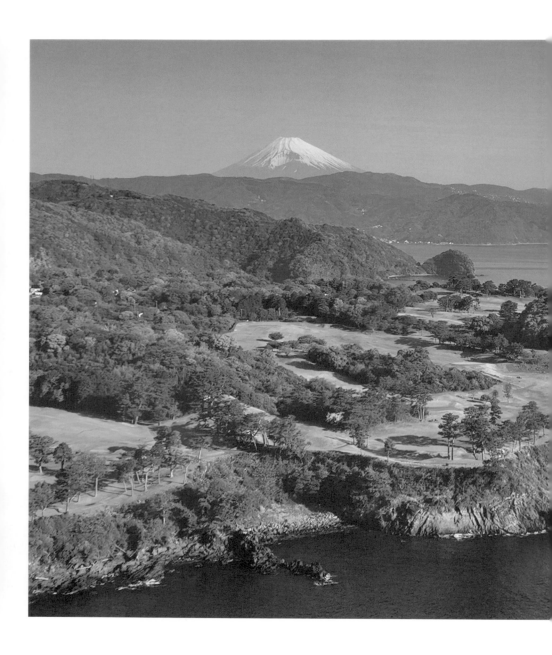

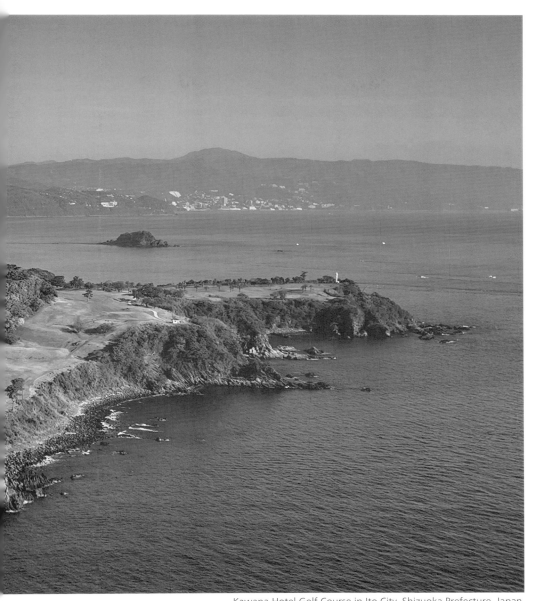

Kawana Hotel Golf Course in Ito City, Shizuoka Prefecture, Japan, where Dr. Satoshi Ōmura discovered Avermectin.
©Kawanahotel Golfcourse

Number of COVID-19 cases per capita by country, number of COVID-19 deaths, vaccination status, etc.

	Tot Cases /1M pop	Deaths /1M pop	Who took one dose vaccine	Median Age	Population /1M
USA	333,985	3,642	*81.39%	38.5	334.8
Canada	128,843	1,538	92%	42.4	38.3
Saint Lucia	163,225	2,215	33%		0.2
Mexico	58,549	2,546	*76.22%	30.6	131.5
Brazil	179,908	3,303	*88.08%	34.7	215.3
Argentina	220,143	2,844	92%	33.0	46.0
Japan	269,169	595	*84.47%	49.5	125.5
Australia	454,687	937	88%	37.9	26.0
China	347	4	*91.89%	39.8	1,448.4
South Korea	673,523	700	87%	45.0	51.3
Philippines	36,800	594	*71.55%	25.4	112.5
Indonesia	24,466	581	*74.00%	32.7	279.1
Thailand	68,069	494	*79.51%	41.0	70.0
Singapore	505,785	341	90%	38.9	5.9
India	32,016	379	*72.50%	29.5	1,406.6
Egypt	4,861	232	55%	24.1	106.1
UK	363,666	3,389	81%	40.6	68.4
Netherlands	501,747	1,336	74%	42.2	17.2
France	612,013	2,556	82%	42.4	65.5
Germany	462,891	2,182	78%	46.7	83.8
Russia	165,454	2,762	61%	41.5	145.8
Zimbabwe	17,373	374	44%	21.0	15.3
Nigeria	1,233	15	42.93%		216.7
South Africa	67,095	1,689	41%	30.1	60.7
World	90,413	899.4			8,117.6

Number of cases and deaths of COVID-19 from Worldometer by February 2024; percentage of people who received at least one dose of vaccine from Our World in Data (unmarked, March 13, 2023; *, December 21, 2023); Median age of population from Our World in Data (2021 to 2023)

編者 ポール・E・マリク（Paul E. Marik）

1958年生まれ。医学博士（MD、FCCP、FCCM）。米国イースタン・バージニア医科大学の医学教授および呼吸器・クリティカルケア医学部長を最近まで務めた。査読付きジャーナル論文を700本以上執筆し、その引用回数は53,000回を超えている。2017年に米国内科学会（ACP）から最も権威ある『全米最優秀教員賞』を授与されるなど、数々の教育賞を受賞している。2020年1月、敗血症に対する安全で効果的な治療プロトコールに基づき、COVID-19病院治療プロトコール（EVMSプロトコール）を確立した。米国に拠点を置くFLCCC（最前線COVID-19クリティカルケア・アライアンス）の共同創設者。近著に『CANCER CARE』がある。

IVERMECTIN
Testimonials by Clinicians Worldwide

2024年11月1日　初版第1刷発行

編者　ポール・E・マリク
発行　株式会社 南東舎
　　　TEL 080-6260-0853
　　　E-mail Ishimic0511@gmail.com
発売　有限会社 柘植書房新社
　　　〒113-0001 東京都文京区白山1-2-10-102
　　　TEL 03-3818-9270
　　　FAX 03-3818-9274

印刷　三永印刷 株式会社
装幀　松田行正

定価は函に表示してあります。乱丁・落丁本は小社にてお取り替えいたします。本書のコピー、スキャン、デジタル化等の無断複製並びに無断複製物の譲渡、及び配信は著作権法上での例外を除き禁じられています。

© Paul E. Marik 2024 Printed in Japan ISBN 978-4-8068-0776-6

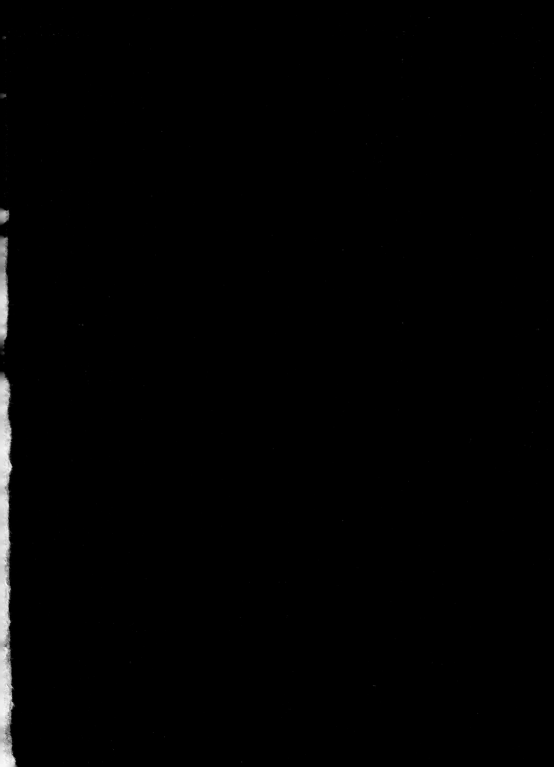